Transformative Learning
in Nursing

Arlene H. Morris, EdD, RN, CNE, is Professor at Auburn University Montgomery School of Nursing, where she received the Distinguished Teaching Award from 2007 to 2010. She is a National League of Nursing Certified Nurse Educator and is President-elect of the Alabama State Nurses Association. She has received several health care/ educator grants and has written chapters for several books, and her numerous articles have been published in peer-reviewed national and international journals. Dr. Morris has presented at local, state, national, and international levels. She has expertise in RN-BSN, BSN, and MSN programs and curriculum revision. She received her EdD in 2007 from Auburn University and worked as a staff nurse in gerontology, medical–surgical, home health, and student health settings. Dr. Morris has taught nursing for 20 years.

Debbie R. Faulk, PhD, RN, CNE, is a Professor at Auburn University Montgomery School of Nursing where she received the Distinguished Teaching Award from 2003 to 2006. Dr. Faulk coordinates the RN-BSN program there. Dr. Faulk received her PhD in 2003 from Auburn University and has over 43 years of experience in a variety of health care settings including critical care, community health, gerontology, management, and education. She is a National League of Nursing Certified Nurse Educator and is the immediate past-President of the Alabama State Nurses Association. She has written chapters in four textbooks and numerous articles in peer-reviewed national and international journals. Dr. Faulk has presented at international, national, state, and local levels.

Transformative Learning in Nursing

A Guide for Nurse Educators

Arlene H. Morris, EdD, RN, CNE
Debbie R. Faulk, PhD, RN, CNE

Editors

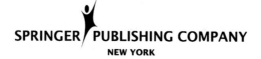

SPRINGER PUBLISHING COMPANY
NEW YORK

Springer Publishing Company, LLC
11 West 42nd Street
New York, NY 10036
www.springerpub.com

Acquisitions Editor: Allan Graubard
Production Editor: Lindsay Claire
Composition: Manila Typesetting Company

ISBN: 978-0-8261-0868-5
E-book ISBN: 978-0-8261-0869-2
12 13 14 15/ 5 4 3 2 1

The author and the publisher of this Work have made every effort to use sources believed to be reliable to provide information that is accurate and compatible with the standards generally accepted at the time of publication. The author and publisher shall not be liable for any special, consequential, or exemplary damages resulting, in whole or in part, from the readers' use of, or reliance on, the information contained in this book. The publisher has no responsibility for the persistence or accuracy of URLs for external or third-party Internet Web sites referred to in this publication and does not guarantee that any content on such Web sites is, or will remain, accurate or appropriate.

Library of Congress Cataloging-in-Publication Data
Transformative learning in nursing : a guide for nurse educators / Arlene H. Morris, Debbie R. Faulk, editors.
    p. ; cm.
  Includes bibliographical references.
  ISBN 978-0-8261-0868-5—ISBN 978-0-8261-0869-2 (e-ISBN)
  I. Morris, Arlene H. II. Faulk, Debbie R.
  [DNLM: 1. Education, Nursing—methods. 2. Attitude of Health Personnel. 3. Students, Nursing—psychology. WY 18]

  610.7307—dc23
                                                                        2012005670

Printed in the United States of America by Gasch Printing

Contents

Foreword

Occasionally, a book comes along as a trailblazer. You are viewing such a book. Drs. Morris and Faulk, through over a decade of exploration, application, and refinement, have created a succinct comprehensive review of transformative learning theory (TLT) that is both contemporary and timeless for nursing education. It is pivotal for the changing times and the future. Situated within adult learning, this work contains ideas and areas for individuals, small groups, and total faculty nurse educators to reflect upon and use to change their educational practices.

The book brings TLT alive for nursing education. It is a thoughtful, unique work that challenges teachers to rethink approaches to courses, content, teaching methodologies, the learning environment, student learning, and expectations of learner achievement. Articulate and clearly written, chapters are laced with practical examples from classroom, clinical, and online areas, as well as nursing practice.

TLT, as presented by the authors, is interwoven with the challenges facing teachers who grapple with issues of learner motivation, authentic teaching and learning, preparation of graduates as lifelong learners, thinking processes and outcomes, and maturing as an educator. From evidence-based findings and personal use, the authors created a transformative thinking model to guide the educator and learner through meaningful interactions.

These authors considered rarely discussed approaches for an educator's use of new material. They believe that learners benefit most from an orientation to TLT and what may be experienced as a participant. In addition, they discuss ethical considerations related to transformative learning. Above all, the rich content is built upon valuing quality nursing practice while committing to valuing others and continually seeking self-improvement as an educator.

I believe that you will find this book a treasure for your library, a gift to yourself and students, and a reference to which you will repeatedly return.

Cathleen M. Shultz
Dean and Professor
Carr College of Nursing
Harding University
Immediate Past President of
the National League for
Nursing (2009–2011)

Contributors

Julie Freeman, MSN, RN
Meren Coordinator-Retention Program
Auburn University Montgomery School of Nursing
Montgomery, Alabama

Cam Hamilton, PhD(c), RN
Assistant Professor of Nursing
Auburn University Montgomery School of Nursing
Montgomery, Alabama

Ginny Langham, MSN, RN
Instructor
Auburn University Montgomery School of Nursing
Montgomery, Alabama

Ramona Browder Lazenby, EdD, RN, FNP-BC, CNE
Associate Dean and Professor of Nursing
Auburn University Montgomery School of Nursing
Montgomery, Alabama

Francine M. Parker, EdD, MSN, CNE
Associate Professor, Nursing
Auburn University
Auburn, Alabama

Marilyn K. Rhodes, EdD, RN, CNM
Associate Professor of Nursing
Auburn University Montgomery School of Nursing
Montgomery, Alabama

Michelle A. Schutt, EdD, RN, CNE
Assistant Professor of Nursing
Auburn University Montgomery School of Nursing
Montgomery, Alabama

Allison J. Terry, PhD, MSN, RN
Assistant Professor of Nursing
Auburn University Montgomery School of Nursing
Montgomery, Alabama

Acknowledgments

We would like to initially acknowledge each of our students throughout our years of teaching. We have learned from the various interactions, and you have helped us to grow individually and to become better educators. We also thank those who have been our teachers; we cannot describe the many ways that your influences have shaped our lives throughout the years. Our colleagues have endured many of our discussions, and provided insights and support that are tremendously appreciated. We particularly want to thank our colleagues who have contributed to this text, as we have witnessed your embracing of transformative learning. We very much appreciate Allan Graubard, executive editor at Springer Publishing, for his vision to support our endeavor and for his guidance and encouragement. Finally, we would like to individually acknowledge and thank our families for their constant love, support, and patience: Kelly, Jared, and Lorie Morris; Gordon Faulk; Cary, Amy, Hana, and Mary Parker Priest; Colbi, Lee, Ford, and Aubrey Carter; and Matthew, Candie, Erin, Lane, and Cameron Faulk.

Preface

BACKGROUND

A number of years ago, during informal discourse, a lifelong collegial relationship began. Through ongoing discussions and a search for approaches to improve our teaching in the discipline of nursing, we discovered transformative learning theory. We began to consider various aspects of this adult learning theory, gradually applying selected premises to individual courses or specific teaching/learning activities. We became very excited as we reviewed, separately and then together, learner responses and outcomes. Our excitement continued to grow when we received comments from other faculty at our school of nursing and from across the country when we presented at nursing education conferences. Our belief in the effectiveness of this pedagogy for education of nurses and belief that it can be used at all levels of educational preparation and professional development created a passion to pursue research and to share our thoughts and findings with other nurse educators.

NEED

We believe this text is important to nurse educators at this particular time for a number of reasons. Demographic and political influences on health care delivery, a focus on quality and safety in light of cost containment and efforts to decrease errors, and an anticipated increased demand for nurses have resulted in a call for nursing education reform. One significant suggestion from this call for reform is to include innovative pedagogies that promote commitment to lifelong learning and ethical comportment.

Another reason this text is critical at this time is that the need for more nurses depends on an increase in nursing faculty. Expert nurse clinicians may enter nursing education with little or no prior background in adult education and find themselves in a sudden disorienting dilemma of being a novice nurse educator. Expert nurse educators can experience disorienting dilemmas in response to the call for radical reform in nursing education. Additionally, there are a limited number of texts with practical teaching strategies that can be used across nursing courses or curricula, and many of these texts are historically overly theoretical or academic and may be overwhelming for the novice nurse educator.

This text is unique in that it provides a foundation for further development of transformative learning as a pedagogy in nursing education with direct application for classroom, online, or hybrid learning environments. Educators who have used transformative principles and approaches share lessons learned, which can be applied in other nursing programs at various levels of education. The text also addresses common learning issues from both learner and teacher perspectives and allows nurse educators to evaluate their own authentic transformation throughout their careers.

In a nutshell, *Transformative Learning in Nursing: A Guide for Nurse Educators* will help readers understand how transformative learning principles and approaches can apply to nursing education and professional staff development, learn effective practices for fostering transformative learning in nursing students and nurses, identify ways to create environments for transformative learning, and determine successful applications of transformative learning across nursing courses.

PURPOSE AND AUDIENCE

Although this text is written primarily for the novice or experienced nurse educator and for graduate students in nursing education programs, it can also be used by professional staff development educators. Transformative learning principles are being used in health care settings to meet adult learning needs for nurses and encouraging positive client behaviors (Phillipi, 2010).

OVERVIEW OF CONTENT

In Part I, Chapters 1 and 2, transformative learning is brought to life as an innovative pedagogy in nursing education. Chapter 1 provides an overview of transformative learning theory and provides an evidence-based background on why this adult learning theory is applicable for nursing education. Chapter 2 presents the transformative learning environment through the lens of the educator and learner and the relationship of transformative learning to educator roles and learner attributes. In Part II, Chapters 3 through 8 provide practical learning strategies using transformative principles and approaches that can be used within various nursing courses and curricula. Suggestions for how these strategies can be used in professional staff development are also offered. Part III, Chapters 9 through 12, situates transformative learning within simulation, service learning, clinical experiences and online learning. Part IV, Chapters 13 through 15, presents transformative learning as it relates to specific educational issues such as student retention, self-regulated learning, and teacher authenticity. Chapter 16 presents a discussion of ethical considerations related to transformative learning, and some concluding thoughts are provided. Finally, in Appendices A, B, and C we provide additional faculty resources. Appendix A includes numerous examples of learning activities for use by our nurse educator colleagues, known and unknown, novice or expert. Appendix B contains examples of case studies that can also be used, revised, or adapted across all levels of nursing education and in staff development to promote critical reflection, self-reflection, and dialogue with the overarching goal of developing a commitment to transformative thinking. Appendix C offers several formatting examples of learning modules for online or face-to-face courses, illustrating use of some of the learning activities and case studies found in Appendices A and B.

REFERENCE

Phillipi, J. (2010). Transformative learning in healthcare. *PAACE Journal of Lifelong Learning, 19*, 39–54.

I

Transformative Learning in Nursing Education

1

Transformative Learning as an Innovative Pedagogy for Nursing Education

Arlene H. Morris and Debbie R. Faulk

Transformative learning focuses on the relationship between personal change and learning.

—Dr. Teal McAteer

We embrace the need for change in nursing education to meet current and future complex challenges, and believe that the transformative learning theory (TLT) offers a practical, innovative approach for nursing education. Each level of preparation in nursing education provides opportunities for learners to develop personal and professional values that are foundational for providing excellence in health care. Benner, Sutphen, Leonard, and Day (2010) express the need for nurse educators to develop and use strategies that promote motivation and lifelong learning—a formation or reformation of ways of teaching and learning instead of using teaching methods that focus mainly on presentation of content. Benner et al. further suggest that teaching strategies must empower nursing students to develop habits of thinking based on evidence for making person-centered clinical judgments. Transformative learning is situated within adult learning and can serve as a guide for developing nursing curricula and learning activities to effectively motivate and empower nursing students to examine and develop new habits of mind, resulting in behaviors congruent with quality person-centered nursing care.

As nurse educators, who were initially nurses and maintain the identity of a nurse, we struggle with how to reach and impact students throughout the nursing curriculum, to set the stage for students to not only gain the unique knowledge of nursing but to become engaged, empowered, and transformed by that knowledge. Use of technical health care–based knowledge is essential to both the roles of nurse and educator and will continue as a basis for knowledge throughout the transition to nurse educator, not only in academic but also in practice settings. Educators in practice and academe must also focus on evidence-based health care knowledge and how nurses use evidence-based educational principles and methods in teaching.

Chapter 1 presents an overview of the TLT including a synopsis of major research in both adult education and nursing disciplines. The chapter concludes with a discussion of transformative learning within the context of nursing education.

TRANSFORMATIVE LEARNING THEORY

A brief overview of the TLT as it applies to the education of adult learners and a short synopsis of research findings from education and nursing begins the discussion for how transformative learning approaches provide an innovative strategy for teaching and learning in nursing education. Mezirow (2000) defines transformative learning as:

> the process by which we transform our taken-for-granted frames of reference (meaning perspectives, habits of mind, mind sets) to make them more inclusive, discriminating, open, emotionally capable of change, and reflective so that they may generate beliefs and opinions that will prove more true or justified to guide action. (pp. 7–8)

Mezirow (2000) suggests that adults develop frames of reference as paradigms for viewing the world through prior learning, life experiences, and instinctual responses. He further suggests that habits of mind form from experiences that are recalled from individual backgrounds or personal history and have an associated emotion. From habits of mind, individuals develop and express points of view. These habits of mind and points of view form an individual's interpretation of the world, thus creating a frame of reference. These familiar and mostly comfortable past frames of reference may transform into new thinking when an adult is exposed to critical reflection such as occurs in educational situations. Mezirow believes that adult learning results from transformation of perspective in response to unexpected events, which he defines as disorienting dilemmas.

Disorienting dilemmas may be sudden or episodic. Reflection regarding disorienting dilemmas can result in sudden or dramatic changes/transformations in points of view or may be latent and occur over time. For example, a nursing student may have developed a habit of mind related to the dying process that was formed from a personal history of a family member's death. From this, the student may have developed a fearful connotation of death, which may lead to fear of caring for a dying person. The student may express the point of view that dying people should be avoided. Using a learning activity that incorporates transformative learning approaches, the student may reconsider previous assumptions leading to a reformation toward a different point of view. The transformation process would involve assimilating new learning from nursing theory and clinical experiences in which caring for a dying person was not actually a fearful experience.

Another example of a disorienting dilemma may be a nursing student whose grandmother was a nurse. This student expresses the point of view during a class discussion that the nurse's role as caregiver is "only to carry out physician orders." A disorienting dilemma occurs when faculty and other students discuss autonomy involved in nursing roles and making clinical judgments. Yet another example is the student who believes he or she is an incompetent learner based on past comments from teachers, classmates, and/

or family members. Experience in nursing school with case studies or with critiquing evidence for nursing interventions could lead to a disorienting dilemma from which the student realizes that critical thinking abilities have actually developed. This realization could change the student's point of view to now consider himself or herself a competent learner, resulting in increased confidence for contributing to class discussions and subsequent nursing care.

Phases of Perspective Transformation

In 1975, Mezirow identified 10 phases in which adult learners achieve new attitudes and worldviews. Mezirow believes that adults develop new points of view from experiencing an initial disorientation (disorienting dilemmas) leading to a final reintegration of a new perspective until the process repeats (see Table 1.1). In 1991, Mezirow added an additional phase of adult perspective transformation, which he called, "renegotiating relationships and negotiating new relationships." In this phase, existing relationships are changed due to an individual's change in perspective and new relationships are developed. An example of this new phase of perspective transformation is the Masters of Science in Nursing (MSN) student who expressed that in a work environment she was not treated as an equal on a health care team until she began to act with more confidence following completion of specific course assignments, which then led to development of different working relationships with physicians and other health care team members.

The example of a nursing student who experienced empowerment and professional transformation during and after a leadership project demonstrates progression through the phases of perspective transformation. Sally, an RN to BSN student, experienced a *disorienting dilemma* when she believed she could learn nothing new about nursing, but needed to complete her baccalaureate degree to progress in her nursing career. In a final class project, which interestingly was not an instructor-developed learning assignment, she assumed the role of leader, which led to comprehensive *self-reflection*. From this reflection, Sally *identified assumptions and habits of mind* that she had previously used in similar situations. When all members of the cohort did not

TABLE 1.1 Phases of the Perspective Transformation Cycle

Phase 1	A disorienting dilemma occurs
Phase 2	Self-examination with feelings of guilt or shame, sometimes turning to religion for support
Phase 3	Critically assessing personal, professional, or cultural assumptions
Phase 4	Recognizing that the process of discontentment and transformation can be shared, acknowledging that others have negotiated similar changes
Phase 5	Searching for and committing to new roles, relationships, and behaviors
Phase 6	Planning a strategy to act on commitment
Phase 7	Acquiring knowledge and skills for implementing strategies for action
Phase 8	Trying and evaluating new roles and behaviors
Phase 9	Developing personal skill and confidence in new roles and relationships
Phase 10	Incorporating behavioral change into one's life based on the new perspectives

Adapted from *Transformative Dimensions of Adult Learning* by J. Mezirow, 1991, pp. 168–169. Copyright 1991 by Jossey-Bass.

follow her lead, or respond to her requests in order to complete the project, Sally *expressed anger* and actually contemplated "just giving up." However, she moved forward by *exploring alternate ways* of getting the followers to take action that would result in a finished project. To her surprise, her *revised actions* worked. Her *self-confidence* as a leader was born. She *developed relationships* with difficult classmates and *strengthened relationships* with peers whom she most trusted. Thus, a disorienting dilemma set in motion a change in perspective related to her leadership role and ultimately led to a change in her career path. The outcome of this transformation process was Sally's belief and confidence that she could become a leader, specifically in the role of nurse educator.

Building upon Mezirow's (1978) work, Cranton (2006) suggests that transformative learning involves a process of exploring and questioning prior perspectives to validate or reform thinking. Cranton further purports that relearning occurs as the learner examines prior or alternative points of view. Like Mezirow, Cranton believes this relearning or transformation may result over time or with a sudden and dramatic change in points of view. In the example of empowerment and professional growth presented earlier in this chapter, Sally's sudden, dramatic change occurred due to a situation that required skill development for a leadership role, but over time, her career choice changed. Cranton's belief that transformation may occur suddenly or over time is mirrored in the work of Horton-Deutsch and Sherwood (2008), who indicate that the learner is continually assessing actions at a deeper level of reflection in order for knowledge to make sense in practice. For example, a deeper level of reflection involving awareness of human dignity can lead to changes in behaviors in clinical settings.

Cranton (2006) proposes that not all learning is transformative or occurs separately from other types of learning. Learning involves multiple processes depending on the motivation and outcomes of what is learned.

Proponents of transformative learning agree that critical discourse is a core approach to determine different perspectives based on others' thinking, valuing, and rationales for behaviors. In this way, personal meaning perspectives can be reconstructed by reviewing one's dominant stories (past experiences) and resultant beliefs and values. This is a reconsideration of an individual's habitual way of thinking that has led to their assumptions and point of view (Brookfield, 1991; Cranton, 2006; Mezirow, 1991). This key transformative approach of critical discourse and other approaches will be discussed in upcoming chapters.

Types of Knowledge Foundational for Transformative Learning

Mezirow (1991) and Cranton (2006) elaborate on Habermas's (1971) three types of knowledge—technical, practical, and emancipatory—that set the foundation for transformative learning:

- Technical (or instrumental) is knowledge that allows manipulation and control of one's environment.
- Practical (or communicative) is knowledge required to understand another person through language.

- Emancipatory knowledge comes from questioning instrumental and communicative knowledge and depends on adult learners' self-knowledge, self-determination, and self-reflective skills.

Nurse educators can use the three types of knowledge in a similar manner as Bloom's (1956) domains of learning (cognitive, psychomotor, and affective), to develop individual learning outcomes and related teaching strategies. A learning activity for the areas of instrumental and communicative knowledge can stimulate learners to question prior habits of mind and points of view, leading to the assumptions that may be driving their view of the self and the world. From questioning and reviewing assumptions, there is a potential for transformative learning to occur that could result in reconsideration of personal assumptions (habits of mind) and the decision to adhere to these.

Technical (instrumental) knowledge is similar to identification of the psychomotor domain in that understanding and actual manipulation of one's self or instruments provide a method to change the environment. For example, a nursing student must have psychomotor skill (technical knowledge) to competently insert a urinary catheter following an accurate assessment of client need. The nursing student must be able to relate the client's complaint of inability to void or complaint of suprapubic pain to a distended bladder and the need for catheter insertion. The client assessment is considered a cognitive domain outcome, which is similar to practical (or communicative) knowledge that necessitates sharing of common meaning through client interaction. Emancipatory knowledge relates to affective learning outcomes in that the learner progresses through responding to reflecting, to valuing, and ultimately to determining if the content will become a part of his or her character (Krathwohl, Bloom, & Masia, 1964). The nursing student must use cognitive and psychomotor skills to insert the urinary catheter. However, the astute valuing of appropriate assessment and early intervention to prevent further complications, together with increased confidence, leads to development of a personal identity of becoming (or being) a nurse.

TRANSFORMATIVE LEARNING RESEARCH IN ADULT EDUCATION

Transformative learning has become the primary paradigm discussed within the adult education discipline (Mezirow, 2009), and as a result, research is prolific in this area. In 2000, Taylor provided an analysis of studies related to the TLT from which he identified eight overriding themes:

- Perspective transformation is unique to adult learners.
- Perspective transformation is a process of change that is not always linear.
- Frame of reference is an elusive concept.
- Triggering events for transformative learning may be sudden, profound, subtle, or trivial events that may arise from an internal or external origin. Uncertainty continues related to why some triggering events result in perspective transformation, and others do not.

- Critical reflection with resultant expression of emotions (affective learning) is at the core of transformative learning.
- The importance of relationships with others involved in rational discourse (based on trust or support) is essential for transformative learning.
- Personal factors provide a context of readiness for change.
- Transformative learning can be promoted in different settings and disciplines.

Snyder (2008) concluded that Mezirow's theory can be operationalized and used as a guiding framework for other research to promote understanding of adult learning in various settings.

TRANSFORMATIVE LEARNING RESEARCH IN NURSING EDUCATION

The use of TLT as a framework for thinking about nursing curricula and development of teaching and learning strategies that foster perspective transformation is underresearched. Research has focused on either the process of perspective transformation or on teaching and learning strategies that promote perspective transformation. A study by McAllister et al. (2006) relates to how TLT was used in the development of a "solution-focused curriculum . . . with the goal of cultivating critical thinkers and knowledge workers . . . nurses who are not only able to work skillfully, strategically, and respectfully with clients, but who also demonstrate discernment, optimism, and vision about nursing and healthcare" (Abstract).

Research in RN to BSN programs describes perspective transformation as effective in the resocialization process (Callin, 1996; Maltby & Andrusyszyn, 1990; Morris & Faulk, 2007; Periard, Bell, Knech, & Woodman, 1991) and learners described experiences parallel to Mezirow's phases of transformation (Lytle, 1989) or involve studies that compare perspective transformations between online and traditional programs (Cragg, Plotnikoff, Hugo, & Casey 2001). Heightened awareness of self-concept and nursing role fulfillment were the most identified changes in perspectives in graduate nursing students, and some participants believed that Mezirow's phases adequately described their experiences in the graduate education process (Cragg & Andrusyszen, 2004, 2005; Faulk, Parker, & Morris, 2010).

Research specifically related to using TLT in development of teaching and learning strategies has mainly come from writers in the field of education. Findings have demonstrated that applying theoretical foundations in planning for teaching and learning strategies can promote cognitive dissonance (conflict in values), critical reflection, and critical dialogue that can then allow individual learners to consider alternative ways of thinking (relearning). Research in nursing related to use of transformative learning strategies primarily focuses on traditional BSN students, returning second-degree students, and returning RN students (for either BSN or MSN programs). Mezirow's Adult Learning Theory (2000) was used as a framework for a study by Morris and Faulk (2007) in which findings demonstrated transformation in perspectives of RN to BSN students based on development of professional nursing values. The changes, which led to increased professional behaviors, can occur through planned learning activities that stimulate identification and analysis of assumptions through reflective dialogue. Ruland and Ahern (2007) found that teaching strategies, such as a reflective writing activity, promoted changes in perspectives in traditional nursing students.

Although research related to transformative learning in nursing is limited, the theory has upheld through critique, evaluation, reevaluation, numerous revisions, and continues to provide an excellent framework to best illustrate how adults relearn. We propose that transformative learning can be used by nursing educators at all levels, and in staff development, while acknowledging that further research would provide supporting evidence for application of the theory in nursing education.

USING TRANSFORMATIVE LEARNING IN NURSING EDUCATION

Nurse educators design curricula and develop learning activities from a perspective that nursing students are adult learners, although some students may continue to transition to adult learner characteristics while in nursing school. The goal of nursing education is to produce graduates who can make sound, rational clinical judgments based on evidence, make strategic decisions, problem solve, and initiate and embrace change. Integrating TLT in nursing curricula can promote nursing students' exposure to the model of respectful discourse, reflection on assumptions, and emancipatory learning to result in choice and conviction for nursing behaviors and professionalism. Nursing and health care organizations, as well as leading health care research entities, have identified the need for an overhaul in nursing education as a result of changes in health care delivery, demographics, and technological and scientific progress (American Association of Colleges of Nursing [AACN], 2007; Carnegie Foundation, 2010; Institute of Medicine, 2011; National League of Nursing [NLN], 2009). These long-unheeded calls for changes to nursing education have culminated in a challenge for nurse educators to consider radical and innovative pedagogies to address the gaps in quality nursing education as more nurses need to prepare to critically plan and provide care for quality person-centered outcomes in ever increasingly complex health care delivery systems (Benner, Sutphen, Leonard, & Day, 2010). "Because practice will only become more complex over time, nurses must leave their formal programs prepared to be lifelong students, with a disposition and skills to be reflective practitioners and expert learners" (p. 4).

Transformative learning provides a model for solving problems, whereby a problem may be defined or redefined, thus allowing reconsideration of previous ways of thinking (Mezirow, 2000), which is applicable to the learning needed in nursing education. Transformative learning approaches can foster a process of formation or reformation of habits of mind in order to evaluate prior perceptions, motivations, and behaviors in both the teacher and learner. Nursing faculty must reconsider content and methods of teaching. Learners must develop astuteness in methods of learning and organizing content that incorporates personal responsibility and accountability to oneself for learning. Transition from a reliance on passive learning methods to active engagement and self-regulated learning must be developed. Nursing graduates can then use a more astute awareness of unique nursing knowledge and skills and exhibit behaviors that reflect personal and professional values within diverse nursing roles, which will continue throughout professional careers and various practice experiences.

Examples of Learner Transformation

The following student comments illustrate empowerment through personal and professional transformation:

During a learning activity where students were asked to identify assumptions related to the value of social justice, John wrote:

> There was a patient that no one wanted to care for because she was over 400 pounds and incontinent. My co-workers would take her lunch tray in late stating, "It won't hurt her to miss a meal or two." This was a type of discrimination to me. As I reflected on why others treated this patient like this, I began to explore my thoughts and assumptions related to people who are overweight. I started asking to take care of this patient every time I worked on the unit. I found that she was one of the nicest ladies I had ever met. I began to see her as a human being, who just happened to be overweight. I put myself in her place and asked how I would feel. As a result, I now treat all patients with dignity. When I hear co-workers making fun or not treating all patients equally, I feel empowered in reminding them that they are there for the patient regardless of condition or whether the patient has insurance or not.

In a clinical journal, Susan expressed her shock and sadness that many of the nurses on her unit often made disparaging remarks about clients from a certain cultural background. Before beginning a nursing program, Susan never thought about saying anything to the staff nurses. She recognized this as a disorienting dilemma because she valued social justice and believed that everyone should be treated equally, but she also wanted to be liked by her coworkers. After a learning activity in which she had to reflect on how she applied the value of social justice in her work setting, she became empowered to speak up against this behavior. She stated, "Had I not had my sense of social justice enriched through the . . . program, I may very well have allowed them to continue to make crude remarks. I actually fear I may have even joined in."

In a capstone project Patsy wrote:

> As a novice nurse I was naïve and at times still feel that way because I do not always have a clear understanding of hospital policies and procedures, especially more so since I am working in a new facility. In the past, I have never liked to complain or fill out hospital surveys that wanted to know their employee's opinion because I felt that in some way administration was trying to figure out who was the potential bad egg that needed to be kicked out of the nest. Also, I felt that I would not have anyone to back me up if I ever spoke up. As ashamed as I am to admit it, as of this past year, I now know who has had my back the entire time, ANA and my state nursing association. This has truly been a transformative experience.

These actual examples illustrate the power of one's point of view in influencing behaviors and reveal how changes in points of view occurred through using the transformative approaches of critical reflection, critical self-reflection, and critical dialogue. From the reconsideration of personal points of view, the learners experienced a change in their perspectives that can lead to lifelong changes in behaviors.

TRANSFORMATIVE THINKING MODEL

In 2007, following completion of a qualitative study using TLT, the editors of this book developed a professional role transformation model to conceptualize how planned transformative learning approaches could be used in nursing curricula to promote learner lifelong transformation for professional role identity. This model evolved through several years' use of TLT to plan learning activities in a baccalaureate nursing program and is informed by ongoing research. The model was revised in 2010 (see Figure 1.1) to include the premise that triggering events for transformative learning may be happenstance and that the process can apply to concepts broader than professional role development. The transformative thinking model (2010) now provides a framework for understanding how transformative learning can be used to plan learning activities and to promote learner reflection on happenstance events.

The transformative thinking model illustrates the process of change involved in transformative learning. Adult learners come to any planned learning experience with prior habits of mind and frames of reference, which have formed their points of view. Learner behaviors and choices are based on current points

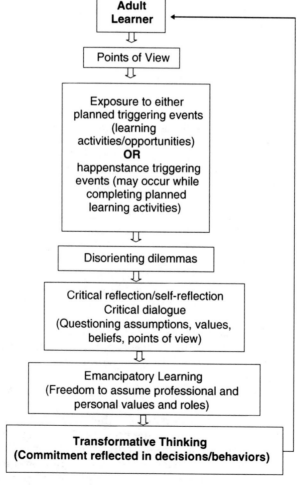

Figure 1.1 Transformative thinking model.

of view. Individuals experience perspective transformation when they critically reflect to identify current assumptions, values, and beliefs (components of their points of view), then critically self-reflect to understand how and why personal points of view may constrain current world views or paradigms or not provide information needed for new situations.

Nurse educators can plan learning activities or seize situations that cause critical reflection and/or dialogue. Learning activities can trigger critical reflection, self-reflection, and/or dialogue to allow examination of thinking, values, beliefs, or behaviors. Further learner reflection, dialogue with self, others, or the educator prompt changes in thinking. Other events can also trigger examination of points of view and habits of mind, possibly impacting changes in behaviors. Openness in thinking allows individuals to make choices to integrate new thoughts or release or revise prior points of view, leading to emancipatory learning, which may result in change(s) in decision making (perhaps not observable) and/or behavior(s). The learner freely chooses new or revised values and roles. From emancipatory learning, commitment to the new ways of thinking is reflected in behaviors. From the commitment and the changed approach to thinking, the cycle continues, and transformative thinking is possible throughout life.

CONCLUSIONS

The TLT can provide a foundation for nurse educators' creation of learning activities that promote lifelong consideration, evaluation, and development of new perspectives throughout the personal and professional life of nurses. Teaching/learning strategies that flow from key transformative learning approaches of critical reflection, critical self-reflection, and critical dialogue can enable learners to become engaged to imagine alternatives to prior held assumptions and their own role in nursing and health care delivery systems during these momentous times. Transformative learning, as an innovative pedagogy in nursing education, can set in motion development of attitudes and behaviors that promote health care system and public awareness of nurses' impact on health care delivery and ultimately in meeting nurses' obligations to society. New perspectives or a renewed commitment can empower nurses, leading to a holistic understanding of the client, the nurse, the profession, and the health care delivery system.

As Kitchenham (2008) so aptly stated "Transformative Learning Theory has changed the way we teach adults . . . and continues to influence adult learning praxis across many disciplines" (pp. 119–120). Transformative learning can promote development of a personal and professional identity and motivation for continual reflection and lifelong learning. Relationship development in educational endeavors can assist learners to consider new ways of thinking and can also support transition to different roles that may result from education. Nursing practice and education are at the precipice for change. No doubt, the call for radical transformation in nursing education will provide the impetus for educators to consider innovative methods of designing and implementing curricula. We believe that transformative principles and approaches can be used at all levels of nursing educational preparation to meet the challenge for nurse educators in the 21st century. The transformative learning environment through the lens of the educator and learner and the relationship of transformative learning to educator roles and learner attributes are examined in Chapter 2.

REFERENCES

American Association of Colleges of Nursing (AACN). (2007). *Joint commission nursing advisory council report on the revision of the essentials of baccalaureate education.* Washington, DC. Retrieved from http://www.aacn.nche.edu/JtComNACReport07.pdf

Benner, P., Sutphen, M., Leonard, B., & Day, L. (2010). *Educating nurses: A call for radical transformation.* San Francisco, CA: Jossey-Bass.

Bloom, B. S. (1956) *Taxonomy of educational objectives, the classification of educational goals—Handbook I: Cognitive domain.* New York, NY: McKay.

Brookfield, S. D. (1991). The development of critical reflection in adulthood. *New Education, 13*(1), 39–48.

Callin, M. (1996). From RN to BSN: Seeing familiar situations in different ways. *The Journal of Nursing Education, 27*(1), 28–33.

Carnegie Foundation for the Advancement of Teaching. (2010). *Study of nursing education.* Retrieved from http://www.carnegiefoundation.org/nursing-education

Cragg, C. E., & Andrusyszyn, M. A. (2004). Outcomes of master's education in nursing. *International Journal of Nursing Education Scholarship, 1*(1), 1–17, article 18.

Cragg, C. E., & Andrusyszyn, M. A. (2005). The process of Master's education in nursing: Evolution or revolution? *International Journal of Nursing Education Scholarship, 2*(1), 1–15, article 21.

Cragg, C. E., Plotnikoff, R. C., Hugo, K., & Casey, A. (2001). Perspective transformation in RN-to-BSN distance education. *Journal of Nursing Education, 40*(7), 317–323.

Cranton, P. (2006). *Understanding and promoting transformative learning. A guide for educators of adults* (2nd ed.). San Francisco, CA: Jossey-Bass.

Faulk, D., Parker, F., & Morris, A. H. (July, 2010). Reforming perspectives: MSN graduates' knowledge, attitudes and awareness of self-transformation (MS #2052) *International Journal of Nursing Education Scholarship, 7*(1), art. 24., doi: 10.2202/1548-923X.2052, Retrieved from http://www.bepress.com/ijnes/vol7/iss1/art24/?sending=11080

Habermas, J. (1971). *Knowledge and human interests.* Boston, MA: Beacon Press.

Horton-Deutsch, S. & Sherwood, G. (2008). Reflection: An educational strategy to develop emotionally-competent nurse leaders. *Journal of Nursing Management, 16,* 946–954.

Kitchenham, A. (2008). The evolution of Jack Mezirow's transformative learning theory. *Journal of Transformative Education, 6*(104), 104–123. doi: 10.1177/1541344608322678

Krathwohl, D. R., Bloom, B. S., & Masia, B. B. (1964). *Taxonomy of educational objectives: The classification of educational goals. Handbook II: Affective domain.* New York, NY: David McKay.

Lytle, J. E. (1989). *The process of perspective transformation experienced by the registered nurse returning for baccalaureate study.* Unpublished doctoral dissertation. DeKalb, IL: Northern Illinois University.

Maltby, R., & Andrusyszyn, M. A. (1990). The case study approach to teaching decision-making to post-diploma nurses. *Nurse Education Today, 10,* 415–419.

McAllister, M., Venturato, L., Johnston, A., Rowe, J., Tower, M., & Moley, W. (2006). Solution focused teaching: A transformative approach to teaching nursing. *International Journal of Nursing Education Scholarship, 3*(1), article 5.

McAteer, T. (2010). Transformative learning in business education. Retrieved from http://www.nationalpost.com/story.html?id=2495255

Mezirow, J. (1975). *Education for perspective transformation: Women's reentry programs in community colleges.* New York, NY: Center for Adult Education, Teacher's College, Columbia University.

Mezirow, J. (1978). Perspective transformation. *Adult Education, 28,* 100–110.

Mezirow, J. (1991). *Transformative dimensions of adult learning.* San Francisco, CA: Jossey-Bass.

Mezirow, J., & Associates. (2000). *Learning as transformation: Critical perspectives on a theory in progress* (pp. 35–69). San Francisco, CA: Jossey-Bass.

Mezirow, J., Taylor, E. W., & Associates. (2009). *Transformative learning in practice: Insights from community, workplace, and higher education.* San Francisco, CA: Jossey-Bass.

Morris, A. H., & Faulk, D. (2007). Perspective transformation: Enhancing the development of professionalism in RN to BSN students. *Journal of Nursing Education, 46*(10), 445–451.

National League for Nursing's Nursing Education Advisory Council's Task Group on Competencies. (2009). *Nursing education competencies.* Special Session NLN Summit 2009. Retrieved from http://www.nln.org/facultydevelopment/pdf/summit_special_session_neac_092609.pdf

Periard, M. E., Bell, E., Knecht, L. & Woodman, E. A. (1991). Measuring effective factors in RN/BSN programs. *Nurse Educator, 16*(6), 14–17.

Ruland, J. & Ahern, N. (2007). Transforming student perspectives through reflective writing. *Nurse Educator, 32*(2), 81–88.

Synder, C. (2008). Grabbing hold of a moving target: Identifying and measuring the transformative learning process. *Journal of Transformative Education, 6*(159). doi: 10.1177/1541344608327813

Taylor, E. W. (2000). Analyzing research on transformative learning theory. In J. Mezirow and Associates (Eds.), *Learning as transformation: Critical perspectives on a theory in progress* (pp. 285–328). San Francisco, CA: Jossey-Bass.

2

Transformative Learning Environments: Teacher and Learner Perspectives

Debbie R. Faulk and Arlene H. Morris

Transformative learning cannot take place simply because either the educator or the learner decides that this is a goal of the learning experience.
—Patricia Cranton

Working from the assumption that transformative learning cannot simply occur because the teacher espouses the theory or because a student values change in perspectives as a learning goal, two questions will be answered in this chapter:

1. How can faculty use transformative learning principles and approaches within transformative educator roles to create an environment in which learning can occur to provide a foundation for nursing practice?
2. How can learners engage in the transformative learning environment, linking unique personal histories (e.g., experiences, learning styles, values, cultures, motivation, competencies) to develop and transform into a competent nurse?

Transformative learning has been described as a process in which the student comes to "own" knowledge rather than memorizing facts (Cranton, 2006). It goes beyond just getting the "right" answer. The goal is to promote reflection, analysis, and synthesis of knowledge that can be applied to a variety of situations. However, the teacher who uses transformative learning principles should be aware that each student brings his or her own history and goal(s) for learning. Often learners' short-term goals are related to assumptions from prior experiences in education, in which the learner believes that the teacher is paid to present facts, which the learner memorizes and repeats back to pass the course. Bean (1996) refers to this as "text parroting," rather than actual learning that results in changes in perspectives and behaviors.

When a nurse becomes an educator, he or she is expected to: fulfill multiple roles, such as a content expert, designer, facilitator, mentor, role model; understand various student learning styles and how these differences impact individual learning; use multiple teaching theories in construction of learning activities; and last but not the least, know how to use evolving adult learning principles. It is no wonder that novice educators are frustrated. Consider the following example:

> Mary considers herself a novice nurse educator although she has been teaching for four years. She is desperately seeking the answer to the question: What does good teaching look like? Although not formally familiar with educational theories, Mary is aware of adult education principles, but is frustrated with students who are not engaged or who do not "own" their learning. She has been reading about transformative learning and has listened as a colleague discussed the merits of using Transformative Learning Theory as a framework for creating learning activities which engage students. She asks the colleague if she can visit her classroom.

TRANSFORMATIVE LEARNING THROUGH THE LENS OF THE TEACHER

The transformative educator fills many of the roles listed above but may take on the additional roles of co-learner, provocateur, and reformist by using transformative learning principles (see Box 2.1) and core approaches (see Box 2.2) to create and plan learning experiences, resulting in significant changes in thinking about teaching approaches. Nurses are accustomed to filling multiple roles concurrently while providing care for clients—often the roles of comforter, advocate, and educator occur simultaneously when performing responsibilities of nursing care. Nurse educators using transformative learning principles can adapt approaches in presenting knowledge by taking on customary roles

---

BOX 2.1 Transformative Learning Principles

1. Learning and relearning occurs throughout life.
2. Learning involves facts, feelings, ethical, intrapersonal, interpersonal, and social issues.
3. Learning can be inward focused or outward focused.
4. Learning is driven by motivation to know, which may include attaining power to navigate through life's situations.
5. Learning is uniquely experienced, based on personal histories and characteristics.
6. Individuals choose to engage in the transformative learning process.
7. Learning can be a shared experience.
8. Learning requires critical or self-reflection to retain, to revise, or to reject prior values, assumptions, habits of mind, and points of view.
9. Learning environments must be open, safe, and respectful of all.
10. Learning approaches and activities promote identification of assumptions and critical reflection of individual meaning perspectives.
11. Learning environments can foster critical or self-reflection.
12. Transformative learning results in changes in perspectives or changes in decisions, which may result in voluntary behavior changes.

BOX 2.2   Core Transformative Learning Approaches

1. Critical reflection: The process an individual uses to learn. Involves pondering new concepts
2. Critical self-reflection: The process of questioning personal values, beliefs, and assumptions
3. Critical dialogue: The process whereby an individual considers new concepts, how this concept fits within the personal point of view, and what revisions to personal assumptions, beliefs, or values may be indicated compared to the other points of view

of content expert and authority, then adding the roles of facilitator, co-learner, encourager, prober, explorer, contemplator, provocateur, or reformist.

Principles of adult education are complex and evolving, no longer simply the transfer of facts in a comfortable environment to meet the needs of adult learners (Cranton, 2006). Novice nurse educators, or nurse clinicians who become educators, cannot be expected to intuitively grasp principles of effectively transferring facts and expect those facts to be used by learners in making clinical judgments. This expectation creates frustration for teachers and learners, which actually hampers learning. It is helpful for nurse educators to consider *how* knowledge is transferred to learners.

Patricia Cranton (2006), a transformative learning educator and author, discussed the various roles of a transformative educator by considering the three types of knowledge (technical, communicative, and emancipatory) that are foundational for transformative learning. Cranton framed her discussion of transformative educator roles within the context of these types of knowledge acquisition. Technical knowledge applies to control of the environment through skill acquisition, communicative knowledge is centered in understanding self and others through language (and is influenced by individual perceptions), and emancipatory knowledge involves development of self-reflection and autonomous choices. These types of knowledge are often used in discussions related to transformative learning. However, to describe the roles of the transformative nurse educator, we use a more familiar framework to nurses by examining educator roles with the context of Carper's (1978) patterns of knowing.

Transformative Educator Roles Within the Context of Patterns of Knowing

Carper's (1978) classic work provided a way to conceptualize complex knowledge that is foundational and essential to nursing. A nurse must use some or all of these patterns of knowing to reflect on knowledge required to provide care. The original four patterns of knowledge included empirical, aesthetic, ethical, and personal knowing. Two additional patterns of knowing, unknowing (Heath, 1998; Munhall, 1993) and sociopolitical (White, 1995), further describe types of knowledge needed by nurses due to changes in current complex health care systems (e.g., unknowing as related to cultural diversity) and development of nurses' roles (e.g., sociopolitical related to health care system planning).

Empirical knowledge includes facts and scientific principles that can be taught and then applied in specific nursing situations. This is somewhat similar to Cranton's (2006) description of technical knowledge. Nurse educators, teaching content that is primarily empirical, may function in the roles of expert, authority, designer, or researcher. In the expert or authority role, the nurse educator provides guidance to learners from a broad and deep knowledge of subject areas and awareness of situations in the "real world." In the designer role, instruction is planned according to learning principles and expected outcomes. In the researcher role, evidence that supports practice is added to the educator's base of information regarding subject content, as well as new knowledge related to methods of instructional design. Furthermore, the nurse educator may design or participate in research studies that add to the body of nursing knowledge itself.

Although empirical knowledge may broaden the knowledge base of nursing students, it is not the most common area in which transformative learning occurs. Cranton (2006) asserts that "though the acquisition of technical knowledge is not necessarily transformative in itself, I see it as having the potential to provide a foundation for transformation" (p. 104). The transformative nurse educator may design case studies that have potential to provide a foundation for transformation. For example, knowledge of specific facts, principles, or theoretical concepts can be applied to the situation within a case study, requiring prioritization or clinical judgment, thereby involving valuing. Additionally, the educator can model, guide, and prompt learners to consider the situation within the case study as it relates to system thinking with various implications or opportunities for team building. Thus, the potential for transformative learning can begin in acquisition of empirical knowledge and continue through application experiences. A case study can be continued through a simulated experience, which provides opportunity for students to progress to other types of knowing.

Aesthetic knowledge includes areas of nursing that are difficult to quantify, including providing care with a valuing of the care recipient or colleague (e.g., therapeutic presence while delivering care). Aesthetic knowledge can be considered as either technical skill acquisition (manner of providing nursing care), communicative knowledge (perceiving self or other as being valued), or emancipatory in that assumptions and values are evaluated and freely chosen. Aesthetic knowledge may or may not build upon empirical knowledge. Clinical, classroom, or online nurse educators may model some of the "art" of nursing, thus filling the important role of the educator as role model. In longer-term relationships with learners, this role may evolve into the role of mentor. The educator's characteristics, including passion for content and for learners, presence, authenticity, and enthusiasm are essential to the role model or mentor role.

In aesthetic learning, the transformative learning educator acts as a facilitator to promote learner-centered and collaborative processes. This necessitates development of a trusting relationship with learners and fostering interpersonal connectivity, which can develop into what Cranton (2006) refers to as communicative knowledge. The transformative educator, as facilitator of aesthetic learning, challenges learners to question assumptions and beliefs while accepting and respecting the learner. Nurses may recognize a similarity of this collaboration to Jean Watson's (2008) human carative factor of valuing and accepting persons for who they are at the moment and for who they may become.

Brookfield and Preskill (1999) suggest strategies to facilitate dialogue that can be used to enhance aesthetic learning:

- exploring and appreciating diversity of perspectives,
- increasing student tolerance of uncertainty or fluctuation of facts or situations,
- verifying students as codevelopers of knowledge,
- respecting students' histories,
- helping students recognize and examine assumptions leading to transformation.

As facilitators of the aesthetic pattern, nurse educators assist learners to access and evaluate resources and experiences needed to become a nurse. Transformative educators design instruction to facilitate aesthetic knowledge by including teaching strategies such as assumption hunting, assumption "busting," and examination of alternative points of view.

Ethical knowing is concerned with determining the most prudent course of action while considering multiple levels of events and potential effects. The transformative educator roles for the ethical pattern of knowing are prober, encourager, dialogue prompter, designer, provocateur, or reformer. Ethical knowing is similar to components of both communicative and emancipatory knowledge, in that students construct knowledge about themselves and others, while identifying sources of personal and social power. When creating learning opportunities for ethical knowing, it is critical that nurse educators realize the importance of being trustworthy, caring, open, authentic, and ready to consider alternatives to personal assumptions or points of view. Kathleen King (2005), an adult educator, eloquently illustrates this point by stating:

> we as educators need to be aware of the consequences of our actions and purposes . . . ethically, adult educators need to respect the rights, beliefs, values, and decisions of our adult learners . . . we need to delicately balance the value we place on transformative learning and the learner's decision to pursue it, or not. We must be careful and mindful to leave room for the learner to say, "I don't want to go there." (p. 17)

Planning for learning experiences that help self and others to evaluate personal resources and values, standards, and expectations for ethical comportment and the context in which nursing decisions are made enhance development of ethical knowing.

Personal knowing involves a deep level of awareness of self and others, discernment of factors that influence human interactions, and potential for self-actualization. As with ethical knowing, personal knowing involves components of both communicative and emancipatory knowledge. Individuals develop personal knowing by becoming more aware of themselves, their values and motivations, and developing astuteness in discriminating underlying elements of interactions with others. Roles of the transformative nurse educator to promote personal knowing include co-learner, explorer, contemplator, reformist, or provocateur. In the role of co-learner, the educator, as a learner along with students, determines how experiences have influenced personal values and behaviors. From interactions through learning experiences that promote consideration of these influences, new knowledge or awareness can collaboratively occur. For example, a nurse educator working with nursing students to determine needs of individuals with lower health literacy shares experience with the students and with the individuals who have health literacy needs. These experiences can stimulate evaluation of assumptions regarding health behaviors and lead to a greater understanding of both the individuals need for health information and a greater shared understanding among the nurse educator and nursing students regarding ways to apply nursing content within this context. Another example may be nurse educators working with graduate students to conduct a root cause analysis for identifying problems within health systems. This shared experience can lead to increased personal knowledge among both educator and students as the process of root cause analysis unfolds.

The transformative nurse educator, as a co-learner, participates in the process of learning, exploring new insights, contemplating assumptions and also consequences, which can result in personal, professional, system, or societal reforms. As the personal knowledge of both nurse educator and learners increases, collaborative interactions invoke critical thinking and development of new understandings. Additionally as provocateur, the transformative nurse educator challenges nursing students to think critically and develop clinical judgment, awareness of themselves, and what they bring as individuals to the nursing profession that stimulates further discourse among learners to evaluate personal beliefs and values—and the cycle continues!

The pattern of *unknowing* is closely related to personal knowing as the awareness of self includes awareness that all is not known regarding the personal self and that everything is not known about others. Opposite to the traditional focus of clustering what is known regarding patients into a diagnostic label or rapidly prescribing interventions, the focus of unknowing is an intentional awareness that the other person (with whom an interaction is occurring) is not yet fully known. This awareness creates openness to the other person, allowing interactions to occur in which underlying needs of the other can be identified. Benner and Wreubel (1989) provide an example in the narrative titled "A Pot of Coffee" in which nursing staff are in conflict with a client over a coffee pot. One nurse's openness to understanding the meaning of the coffee pot to the client resulted in interactions in which the client's actual needs could be identified and eventually met. Roles of the transformative nurse educator in the unknowing pattern are always to be co-learner (being open to what the educator does not know) and role model, to provide a living example of interacting with others in openness, realizing that others' thoughts and experiences are different (i.e., "I didn't know what I didn't know about you, or your needs").

In the *sociopolitical* pattern of knowing, nurse educators must consider influences of variables such as geographic, economic, social, cultural, historical, and political factors related to nursing theory, practice, and research. The sociopolitical pattern of knowing correlates with communicative and emancipatory knowledge in that critical dialogue and reflection are needed for informed critiquing of values such as social justice and identifying whose voices are heard and whose are not heard in dialogues regarding social factors and resultant change. Roles of the transformative educator in this pattern include those in the personal pattern: co-learner, explorer, contemplator, reformist, and provocateur. An additional role is that of informed leader with political acumen. In the roles of co-learner, provocateur, and reformist, learning experiences can be planned to enhance critical reflection and discourse, increase awareness of current policy issues impacting health care and the role of the nurse as policy advocate. During learning opportunities, learners may become aware of the limitations and power of their habits of mind in influencing personal decisions and behaviors, and possible consequences of personal or professional assumptions. A learning outcome may be increased awareness of the inconsistency in expressed values and behaviors.

Overlap and transition between or among transformative educator roles is expected. Transformative learning experiences may be designed with awareness of this overlap or transition among roles within the various patterns of knowing. For example, in the role of co-learner, the educator encourages critical reflection. The educator is aware that insights within the sociopolitical pattern may transfer to the personal knowing pattern, with the learner outcome of behavioral change.

Consideration of Learner Variations

Students in nursing programs are either adults or are in transition from high school into adulthood. In either case, prior life experiences have contributed to assumptions and expectations. As individuals continue to experience life, or through experiences in education, personal assumptions and expectations may be exposed as incomplete or inaccurate. Educators of adults face the challenge of what can seem like a chaotic environment of learner characteristics (i.e., age, personal histories and experiences, culture, current life situations, etc.), learning preferences, and styles. Decisions regarding how to design instruction to meet learner needs are potentially overwhelming as educators must organize content and structure learning activities to encourage learning in a manner that addresses individual attributes.

Individual learner goals are important for engagement and motivation. However, comprehension of facts and self-reflection, which ultimately results in actions based on knowledge and values, is the overarching goal for learners and educators. Principles, approaches, and strategies for transformative learning can be used to enhance student development and attainment of this goal. Educators must be aware that different students may engage in different ways or at different times in the transformative learning process. Cranton (2006) skillfully articulates the relationship of transformative learning and individual learner differences by including a discussion of psychological types and learner preferences and styles in her book, *Understanding and Promoting Transformative Learning*. Rather than reiterate the relationship of learner psychological types to transformative learning, we address transformative learning as a global atmosphere created by using transformative learning principles and approaches to design learning environments where specific learning activities flow from transformative learning approaches. These approaches and learning activities can be adapted for use across all levels of nursing education.

Frameworks for Designing Transformative Learning Experiences

In addition to thinking about the roles of a transformative learning educator within the context of the patterns of knowing, these patterns of knowing can also be used for educators to design transformative opportunities for learners. For example, a nurse educator considers the empirical pattern of knowing when discussing factors involved in handwashing, the aesthetic pattern when encouraging learners to critically reflect about how handwashing is important to prevent suffering, and the sociopolitical pattern when encouraging discussion about changing unit policies to create an environment more conducive to handwashing.

Shulman's (2002) Table of Learning can also be used as a framework for the transformative nurse educator to plan opportunities for learning among the patterns of knowing and as a structure for evaluating outcomes of student knowing. The educator can use this table (see Chapter 8, "Shulman's Table of Learning") to evaluate multiple or sequential outcome behaviors that occur at a specified time for outcome evaluation, or at later times in the curriculum, thereby gauging progression toward becoming a nurse. Nurse educators may also encourage learners to use the Table of Learning as a method for self-reflection to identify personal or professional levels of commitment that occur in actual nursing practice. Shulman asserts that development of commitment and identity occurs as learners:

> internalize values, develop character, and become people who no longer need to be goaded to behave in ethical, moral, or publicly responsible ways. . . . [Commitment] is the highest attainment an educated person can achieve. . . . Commitments always leave open a window for skeptical scrutiny, for imagining how it might be otherwise. (p. 37)

Another framework that can be considered when planning transformative learning opportunities is King's (2005) transformative learning opportunities model. This model can help educators plan learning activities to advance skill development, to provide an image for lifelong learning, and to serve as a guide for students to reflect on personal knowing and knowledge within a content area.

When designing learning experiences, transformative nurse educators must realize that individual learners are at different levels and may progress at various rates through nursing education. Nursing students will not identically retain (i.e., "own" or "know") all knowledge regarding nursing. However, individual learners must have foundational knowledge required to demonstrate behaviors to ensure quality and safe client care. Transformative nurse educators must understand the power of potential further experiences to promote transformative learning that results in continued development and behaviors at higher levels. Thus, instructional design for sequential transformative learning experiences throughout nursing curricula allows multiple opportunities for identifying assumptions, reflecting, committing, and acting/behaving in congruence with new knowledge.

Carper's patterns of knowing provides a framework for viewing educator roles within a transformative learning environment. Shulman's Table of Learning offers another framework for thinking about the development of transformative thinking. In Table 2.1, the relationship of transformative learning approaches

TABLE 2.1 Relationship of Transformative Learning Approaches, Educator Roles, Learner Outcomes

Transformative Learning Approach	Pattern of Knowing According to Carper (1978)	Educator Role(s)	Learning Outcomes (Shulman's Table of Learning, 2002)
Critical dialogue	Empirical	Expert Authority Designer Researcher	Engagement and motivation Knowledge and understanding Performance and action Reflection and critique
Critical dialogue	Aesthetic	Facilitator Role model	Engagement and motivation Understanding Action Reflection Judgment and design Commitment and identity
Critical reflection; critical self-reflection (questioning prior beliefs, values, assumptions)	Ethical	Prober Encourager Dialogue prompter Designer Provocateur Reformer	Engagement and motivation Knowledge and understanding Performance and action Reflection and critique Judgment and design Commitment and identity
Critical self-reflection	Personal	Provocateur Reformist Co-learner Explorer Contemplator	Change in behavior Personal understanding of motivations Engagement and motivation Knowledge and understanding Performance and action Reflection and critique Judgment and design Commitment and identity
Critical self-reflection	Unknowing	Co-learner Role model	Engagement and motivation Knowledge and understanding Performance and action Reflection and critique Judgment and design Commitment and identity
Critical reflection; critical self-reflection; Critical dialogue	Sociopolitical	Co-learner Provocateur Reformist	Engagement Knowledge Action Reflection and critique Judgment and design Commitment and identity

to patterns of knowing, transformative educator roles, and Shulman's (2002) behavioral outcomes are presented. Examination of the transformative learning environment from the student perspective and how learning approaches may impact learners is the focus for the following discussion.

TRANSFORMATIVE LEARNING THROUGH THE LENS OF THE LEARNER

At this time in the discipline of nursing, it is critical to create learning environments in which educators and learners partner to consider and evaluate the power that prior knowledge from media, life experiences, perspectives, and traditional health care has had on individuals' behaviors and to construct new ways of thinking that impact the health care needs of society. Learners may notice that transformative learning principles and approaches to education differ from those used in prior courses and may make choices about when to engage. Cranton (2006) reminds us often that transformative learning is voluntary and if educators try to force learners into the transformative learning process, then, it becomes "brainwashing or indoctrination" (p. 7). As King (2005) so fittingly points out, learners who engage in transformative learning may perceive themselves in a "sea of change." This change allows for openness to others' points of view and perspectives, which may then result in opportunities for growth, but the opportunity for change may seem uncomfortable or even threatening. Changes in thoughts, emotions, decisions, and behaviors may occur intrapersonally, interpersonally, professionally, or socially and may threaten valued relationships. Educators may not be aware of learner transformation as transformation occurs inwardly or gradually, resulting in behaviors that may not occur until after the time of interactions.

Learners in a transformative environment expect educators to set the stage for transformative learning by being authentic, humble, open to learners, and acknowledging their role as co-learner. It is through classrooms (traditional or virtual) that nurse educators build upon life experiences to create transformative learning opportunities (King, 2005). Learners may have no prior experiences in health care delivery, but have prior personal or family experiences, vicarious experiences from exposure to media, and prior educational experiences. These experiences can be used as a foundation for scaffolding new learning or may need reconsideration and reevaluation as learners socialize into the discipline of nursing.

An environment of trust and nonpunitive repercussion or coercion is important for students to be able to dialogue and express values and assumptions as they progress through exchanges with educators and peers. Students must believe that if they choose not to "go there" during critical reflection or dialogue, their grade will not be impacted. In an environment that is open, safe, and respectful, empowerment is the transformative learning outcome. Student empowerment can actually be the starting point for a transformative learning journey (Cranton, 2006). Power sharing, a scary proposition for some nurse educators, allows learners to overcome emotional barriers, which may occur when learners are asked to reflect upon beliefs, values, and assumptions. Transformative educators must be careful to not be perceived as elitist or "holders of all knowledge." An educator's display of humility related to what one knows and does not know is critical to empowering learners. The educator role of co-learner prompts release of "I hold the knowledge" attitude to the mind-set of "Let us find out together." Learners can be empowered by guiding them to access and evaluate various sources of information, thus providing modeling for a lifelong ability to attain and share new knowledge.

A transformative environment from the view of the learner is learner centered to create opportunities for integration of student learning goals, preferences, and characteristics. Student-centered learning is addressed as learners make choices regarding learner and course goals. This allows for a more engaged, rather than passive, learner and can increase self-concept and self-efficacy. Learning preferences are solicited at the onset of courses. Learners can perceive a sense of trust and acceptance of their individualism through submission of specific questions or identification of assumptions before class meetings using email or other social communication tools. In an environment where transformative learning principles and approaches are used to develop learning activities, power is shared, meaningful interactions are encouraged, and diverse points of view are appreciated and respected, learners can believe that they are supported and challenged to change.

As learners experience transformative learning, consequences must be considered. King (2005) notes that transformative learning is often experienced in the affective domain. She states, "[the] intellectual questioning experience can reach into the inner being of the person" (p. 106). Students need to be forewarned that they may have anger, fear, self-doubt, or unhappiness as they experience cognitive dissonance. For example, one student approached a nursing faculty member at the completion of a course, expressing anger that occurred when she reconsidered her prior points of view as revealed by her statement, "I did not expect this course to provoke such strong emotions; I was not prepared for this." Learners should expect that faculty will prepare them for the possibility of experiencing strong emotions during class dialogue or self-reflection and provide a safe environment for follow-up discussion if desired.

Learners will see the transformative learning environment as one of trust and respect, where various points of view can be expressed without fear of coercion or repercussion and where individual learning goals are supported. The transformative learning environment is fostered by an educator who is an authentic, humble co-learner, sharing power with learners, encouraging a spirit of inquiry for new knowledge or reconsideration of prior beliefs and values, and allowing flexible individual progression to commit to new perspectives or behaviors. Learning in this environment promotes attainment of course outcomes and the ability to pursue self-directed lifelong learning. For a listing of characteristics of a transformative learning environment, see Box 2.3.

CONCLUSIONS

Transformative learning principles and approaches can be used to engage learners in the process of learning. In this chapter, transformative learning through the lens of the teacher and learner was addressed by examining the roles of the transformative learning educator within the context of

BOX 2.3 Characteristics of the Transformative Learning Environment

1. Educator is authentic and humble, participating as both expert and co-learner.
2. Learning builds upon prior life experiences.
3. An environment of mutual trust is established.
4. A learner-centered environment is established.
5. An atmosphere of inquiry and respectful dialoguing stimulates expression of points of view without fear of coercion.
6. Power is shared among learners and the educator as co-learner.
7. Lifelong ability to attain and share new knowledge.

Carper's (1978) patterns of knowing and by considering that learners come to every learning situation with various styles and preferences, life histories, and with assumptions and expectations. Characteristics of the transformative environment have been presented to set the stage for a discussion of specific transformative learning strategies and activities within various nursing courses. Chapters 3 through 8 include specific learning activities that flow from the transformative learning approaches of critical reflection, self-reflection, and dialogue, presenting information as to how these activities promote student attainment of course-based learning outcomes.

REFERENCES

Bean, J. (1996). *Engaging ideas: The professor's guide to integrating writing, critical thinking, and active learning in the classroom.* San Francisco, CA: Jossey-Bass.

Benner, P., & Wreubel, J. (1989). *The primacy of caring: Stress and coping in health and illness.* Upper Saddle River, NJ: Prentice Hall.

Brookfield, S., & Preskill, S. (1999). *Discussion as a way of teaching: Tools and techniques for democratic classrooms.* San Francisco, CA: Jossey-Bass.

Carper, B. (1978). Fundamental patterns of knowing in nursing. *Advances in Nursing Science 1*(1), 13–23.

Cranton, P. (2006). *Understanding and promoting transformative learning: A guide for educators of adults* (2nd ed.). San Francisco, CA: Jossey-Bass.

Heath, H. (1998). Reflections and patterns of knowing. *Journal of Advanced Nursing, 27,* 1054–1059.

King, K. (2005). *Bringing transformative learning to life.* Malabar, FL: Krieger.

Munhall, P. L. (1993). Unknowing: Toward another pattern of knowing in nursing. *Nursing Outlook, 41,* 125–128.

Shulman, L. (2002) Making differences: A table of learning. *Change, 34*(6), 37.

Watson, J. (2008). *Nursing: The philosophy and science of caring* (rev. ed.). Boulder, CO: University Press of Colorado.

White, J. (1995). Patterns of knowing: Review, critique, and update. *Advanced Nursing Science, 17,* 73–86.

II

Transformative Learning Approaches and Strategies Within Nursing Courses

3

Transformative Learning in Foundational Nursing Courses

Marilyn K. Rhodes, Arlene H. Morris, and Debbie R. Faulk

> *Transformative learning . . . demands that we be aware of how we come to our knowledge and [be] as aware as we can be about the values that lead us to our perspective.*
>
> —Jack Mezirow

In Part I, Chapters 1 and 2, transformative learning theory (TLT) is suggested as an innovative approach for instructional design at various levels of nursing education and is viewed through the lens of the learner and educator. Part II begins with Chapter 3 in which focus shifts to discussion related to transformative learning within specific nursing courses. Examples of effective transformative learning activities/teaching strategies that have been used in teaching fundamental courses are provided. Fundamental concepts are taught in prelicensure nursing programs at Licensed Vocational Nurse/Licensed Practical Nurse, Associate Degree in Nursing (LVN/LPN, ADN) diploma, and Baccalaureate of Science in Nursing (BSN) levels and in graduate programs that provide entry into nursing practice. Using core transformative learning approaches, the strategies and activities suggested in this chapter can be adapted by educators teaching in these nursing programs and may be considered and/or adapted for use by professional staff development educators.

Using transformative learning strategies in fundamental nursing courses may at first seem unusual as more traditional teaching approaches, such as lecture, are more commonly used in these courses. We believe, however, that critical reflection about content, critical self-reflective activities in which the learner is encouraged to identify previously assimilated assumptions/values/beliefs, and then engagement in dialogue will lead to a greater understanding of foundational concepts of nursing. Additionally, these activities may encourage learners to become more aware of the influence and power that personal points of view have on decision making and behaviors. Educators who use the principles and core approaches of transformative learning acknowledge that all learners begin their nursing careers with assumptions and values assimilated throughout life. Learning the skills of critical reflection, critical self-reflection, and dialogue can lead to a more aware and astute nurse who is committed to value-based person-centered care.

CONCEPTS IN FUNDAMENTAL NURSING COURSES

Nurse educators design curricula to present concepts in a logical manner. Knowledge involved in learning the concepts within fundamental courses includes all patterns of knowing: empirical, aesthetic, ethical, personal knowing, unknowing, and sociopolitical. Giddens (2010) provides an example of different ways to cluster concepts, such as categories of health and illness concepts or professional nursing concepts. Health and illness include concepts such as oxygenation, infection, pain, anxiety, cognition, and sexuality, while examples of professional nursing concepts are communication, advocacy, leadership, ethics, clinical judgment, patient teaching, and safety. Courses considered to be fundamental in nursing curricula include physical assessment/nursing skills, pathophysiology, pharmacology, and introduction to professional nursing concepts. After the complex process of determining *what to teach*, educators must then decide *how to teach* this information. Novice and master educators would agree that the most difficult challenge is to decide which instructional strategy will engage the learner and will be most effective in helping learners meet course and curricular outcomes. Transformative learning can begin in fundamental nursing courses. Critical reflection, self-reflection, and dialogue enable learners to review their thoughts and deliberately reflect on prior life experiences that may result in transformation of perspective, with the ultimate goal of application to fundamental nursing concepts in person-centered situations.

Although nursing fundamental concepts are taught in specific courses or threaded among courses, some content will continue to be foundational. Nurse educators have been challenged to reconsider how these foundational concepts are taught. Benner, Tanner, and Chelsa (2009) recommend that nurse educators focus on formation of nurses by presenting (a) concepts through incorporating nursing theory and knowledge applied in real-life examples from practice, (b) clinical judgment using multiple ways of thinking, and (c) integration of ethical comportment. These authors discourage use of formal lectures about isolated content, favoring a solid integration of theory and application within the context of developing clinical judgment. Additionally, Benner, Sutphen, Leonard, and Day (2010) stress the need for nursing education to integrate knowledge, clinical judgment, and ethical comportment. Transformative learning principles and approaches offer educators who primarily teach in fundamental nursing courses an alternative teaching method that can address the need for changes in nursing education. An example illustrates use of transformative approaches to link theory to application within the context of development of clinical reasoning:

> During the first day of a fundamental nursing course, learners are asked by a faculty member to consider what they have expected from a nurse in actual past experiences when seeking healthcare. This question encourages critical reflection about what roles or tasks are assumed to be involved in nursing. In this manner, learners begin identification of personal points of view about what nurses do, characteristics of nurses, and nurses as a component of the healthcare delivery system. During a subsequent class meeting following presentation of nurse roles, learners are asked to critically self-reflect to identify if the assumptions from the initial activity included any of the actual nurse roles or characteristics and if so,

in what way. Learners are asked to complete a one-minute writing assignment to record their thoughts, then to compare personal responses with those of one or more classmates. From this discourse, learners are then encouraged to compile characteristics and roles of nurses within the healthcare delivery system and prioritize these in application to various scenarios presented by the educator. This exercise can assist beginning nursing students to compare assumptions with what is likely to be encountered in actual clinical experiences.

TRANSFORMATIVE LEARNING APPROACHES

The development of the ability to reflectively think is a substantive goal of all education. Critical self-reflection is a major concept in TLT (Cranton, 2006; King, 2005; Mezirow, 2000). Although various authors use the terms *critical reflection* and *critical self-reflection* differently, we use the term critical reflection to describe a process that an individual can learn, which involves pondering new concepts without critical self-reflection (i.e., deciding "What is in this for me?"). If the individual then decides that he/she desires to further consider the concept, a process of engagement leads to critical self-reflection, which includes bringing into awareness personal background and assumptions and how the new concept relates to past points of view or how personal thinking may need to be revised based on the choice to integrate the new concept into a new personal view (i.e., deciding "Do I want to include this concept in how I look at the world and my place in it?"). There are various thoughts about types of reflection within the context of transformative learning. Cranton (2006) discusses content, process, and premise reflection. These types of reflection for transformative learning are discussed in more detail in Chapter 6.

It is during critical self-reflection that disorienting dilemmas or cognitive dissonance may occur because personal values and beliefs must be reexamined. While critical self-reflecting, an individual may experience anxiety that leads to withdrawal from further reflection about the concept. However, engaging in dialogue with others can help individuals to consider other points of view and to identify personal assumptions that may be foundational to basic values and beliefs. Consider this example of a learner enrolled in an registered nurse (RN) to Baccalaureate of Science in Nursing (BSN) program:

> In a learning activity where a student was asked to critically self-reflect on a "critical incident" that had occurred in a clinical situation, the student chose to write about a difficult preceptorship that she had encountered during her first nursing position shortly after graduation from a two-year nursing program. Instead of focusing on a specific patient situation, the student wrote about the preceptorship and the emotions she experienced when the preceptor made "fun" of her nursing abilities and skills and told her she would never be a competent nurse. The student became so upset while reflecting on her thoughts and actions about the preceptorship, that she told the faculty member she would not be able to continue to think about the situation. Through open and caring dialogue with the faculty, the student concluded that she was ashamed of not standing up for herself and for developing the assumption that all preceptors were uncaring. Although the learning activity lead to extreme anxiety for the student, she was

able to transform a long-held assumption and stated to the faculty member that the activity allowed her to "let go."

Dialogue (or discourse) is also considered essential in fostering transformative learning. According to Mezirow (2000), dialogue involves assessment of personal beliefs, feelings, and values. Dialogue provides a process during which an individual can consider new concepts, how this concept fits within the personal point of view, and what revisions to personal assumptions, beliefs, or values may be indicated compared to the other points of view. The above example regarding the RN to BSN student illustrates this point. Critical reflection, critical self-reflection, and dialogue approaches can be used in specific teaching strategies in foundational nursing courses for traditional classroom or online delivery. The following examples are intended to provide *food for thought* and may be used in other teaching strategies or courses.

Examples of Transformative Teaching Strategies in Pathophysiology and Pharmacology Courses

Content that relates to anatomy, physiology, and the pathologic functions that comprise illnesses or diseases is predominately empirical. Facts also provide the basis for learners to consider desired actions of pharmaceutical interventions to promote healthy body functioning. Owing to the empirical nature of the content in these courses, traditional teaching strategies have included lecture, problem-based learning, or computer-assisted instruction in which facts are presented and learners parrot the information provided.

Use of case studies in pathophysiology and pharmacology courses can provide a shared story experience as a basis for discussing nursing care in either classroom or clinical settings. Information from the case study, such as what would be included in a change-of-shift report, provides a situated experience for learners to relate to a need for understanding the information, determining what other information is needed, and interpreting the information in terms of previous knowledge. Learners who reflect on this information must decide what is pertinent. Further critical reflection helps learners develop clinical reasoning required to determine what nursing care is indicated. The first action that must be taken is for learners to identify how the information relates to their own need to know in their own goal of assuming the role of a nurse.

An unfolding case study might begin with a change of shift report for an individual based on a medical diagnosis, such as "Mrs. X was admitted last night with acute appendicitis," or may begin with the person's experience of distress, such as Mrs. Y has just been admitted stating, "My stomach hurts when I walk." In considering this case study learners can use effect-based reasoning (EBR) to consider either the medical diagnosis or the symptoms as a beginning point for thinking. When combined with a case study teaching strategy, EBR can guide beginning learners in developing clinical reasoning skills.

EBR can promote transformative learning because it requires learner willingness to "open" thinking. EBR exemplifies use of different patterns of thought, forcing learners to consider variables that can produce real or potential outcomes that are intended or unintended. Additionally, the EBR model provides an impetus for thinking that can be examined during teacher/learner and learner/learner dialogue. For example, the faculty can increase the complexity of learner thinking and reflection regarding the case study by adding "what if" questions for learners to identify or anticipate variables. In a learner/learner dialogue, the question "why could this be happening?" can be used to enhance thinking regarding analyses of possible causes or functioning of systems (within the human body or within family or environmental systems).

The use of metaphors as a teaching strategy in empirically based courses can also stimulate transformative learning. For example, in a pathophysiology course for RN to BSN students, a learning activity is used to help learners think about pathologic processes in a different way. Learners are asked to critically reflect on the process involved in a self-selected illness, then to determine a metaphor that would describe the process. Dialogue with other learners is encouraged. In one student example, the metaphor of pressure on a water hose that blocked flow of the water was used to describe the process of hypertension. This metaphor learning activity can also be used in a pharmacology course to describe the intended outcome from pharmaceutical interventions. For example, one student used a metaphor of a dump truck to describe the process of insulin taking sugar into cells.

The metaphor activity fosters transformative learning by encouraging critical reflection about processes involved in empirically based content. From their critical reflection, learners are encouraged to consider other points of view and to consider how they would describe the process to a person for whom they were teaching. Additional anticipated learner outcomes from use of metaphors are increased retention of understanding about the disease process or actions of pharmacologic interventions. Additional learning activities for pathopharamacology-type courses are included in Boxes 3.1 and 3.2.

Examples of Transformative Teaching Strategies in Physical Assessment Courses

Content included in physical assessment courses involves both learning how to relate up close and personally with another previously unknown individual and how to link isolated assessment findings into patterns. In physical assessment courses, learners must integrate technical and communicative knowledge to effectively combine knowledge of facts, how to use the facts, and how to interact with another person. Developing personal skill in the transformative learning approach of self-reflection assists learners to determine any personal assumptions or values that could block interactions. Acquiring the ability to consider points of view of the other person/family/group can lead to development of emancipatory knowledge.

During a class focusing on conducting an interview, learners are asked to contemplate their assumptions by using a case study describing a malodorous, physically dirty, loud client seeking care for abdominal pain in an emergency department. Learners are asked to imagine shaking that person's hand, offering care and compassion, while trying to obtain a health history. Students are then asked to list assumptions about the client's appearance and behavior. Then, more information is made available to the learners: the client works 12-hour days in a coal mine, is hearing impaired, and is seeking care after experiencing food poisoning. Once again, learners are asked to discuss their

BOX 3.1   Health Alteration Reflection Writing Assignment

Outcome(s) of learning activity:

1. Identification of state public health websites for statistical data
2. Increased awareness of prevalent health alterations in home communities
3. Critical self-reflection about why a chosen health alteration is personal
4. Critical reflection regarding pertinent empirical knowledge related to a health alteration
5. Critical dialogue to reveal personal assumptions or points of view compared to those of classmates

Instructions for learners:

1. Access information from a state public health website that identifies recent health statistics for your personal county of residence.
2. From among the top three categories, select one specific health alteration that most surprises you.
3. Write a one- to two-page paper about the selected health alteration that includes the following points:
   - Name, description, and statistical level of occurrence of the health alteration
   - Rationale for your selection of this health alteration
   - Basic pathophysiological processes involved in the health alteration
   - Identification of possible signs and symptoms of the health alteration
   - Holistic implications of the health alteration (physiological, psychosocial, developmental, spiritual)
4. Use the points you have written as a basis for dialogue with a classmate who has identified the same health alteration.
5. Contrast the points of view that are apparent from any variations in the two written assignments.

assumptions and share if and how perspectives changed when more information was provided. When critical self-refection is encouraged in the context of person-centered care, learners explore previously held beliefs to determine if a change is necessary from their previously held points of view to develop respect for individuals who may look or behave differently, thus fostering development of the nursing value of compassion.

In another example of a teaching strategy for a physical assessment course, students are paired to practice assessment skills. Each student has an opportunity to experience the assessment as the nurse and as the client. Pairing begins during the first class meeting at which time an assessment interview is performed. This allows students to practice communication skills as well as evaluate the skills of a classmate and understand how it feels to have someone

BOX 3.2   Health Alteration Virtual Dialogue Assignment

Outcome(s) of learning activity:

1. Critical reflection regarding experiencing one specific health alteration
2. Critical self-reflection to consider nursing care of a person who experienced the health alteration with identification of any areas for improvement
3. Critical self-reflection to consider personal assumptions or points of view compared to paired classmate's point of view

Instructions for learners:

1. Learners will be paired to respond to each other's online postings.
2. Each posting should focus on the holistic aspects of a health alteration, including:
   - A brief overview of a health alteration, addressing issues such as cost, impact on a person's activities of daily living, ability to rest/sleep, ability to seek health care, access to health resources, etc.
   - An example of the health alteration as experienced by a person for whom you have provided nursing care, adhering to confidentiality
   - Critical self-reflection to identify why this health alteration and the issues were selected
3. Read your partner's posting and include the following in your response:
   - Any assumptions that you make about why your classmate may have selected the issue(s) related to the health alteration
   - Any assumptions that you make about the person described by your classmate for whom nursing care was provided
4. Then, reply to your partner's response to verify if his/her assumptions were accurate or not.

ask personal questions. Before beginning, students are asked to introduce themselves and shake hands. Structured questions force the students to reveal something semipersonal, but not health related, to avoid revealing inappropriate or private information to others. For example, questions may include asking about pets. Partners are reassigned each week to help learners practice relating to several different people, for the purpose of increasing awareness of diversity. When evaluating the chest or abdomen, assignments are made for same gender students to decrease potential anxiety among beginning learners. Class discussion includes sharing perspectives, comparing communicating with friends versus strangers, and being in a care-recipient role.

During this peer assessment activity, one student expressed a high level of discomfort in asking personal questions, even though the questions were semipersonal. The student voiced that all of her life she had been taught that personal information was never to be discussed with others; some class members agreed. This disorienting dilemma initiated dialogue about the personal nature of nursing care as well as the professionalism required to provide person-centered care. Dialogue allowed learners to explore realities of nursing as their chosen profession, identify how frames of reference can influence skills, understand the knowledge needed to obtain information, and practice methods for professional interactions.

Before learners become aware of nursing interventions, assessment skills must be learned. This process requires learners to recall previous knowledge to identify potential physiology creating the assessment finding and then to unravel possible conditions to determine the most likely contributing factors. For example, when a student auscultates high-pitched bowel sounds, he or she must identify the finding. Then, the learner must determine what organs and what process is known that could cause that sound (i.e., obstruction or gastric secretions). The student is then encouraged to think further about known facts, to question what the exact process is that would most likely be causing the finding in the particular situation. A format for this thinking is for learners to ask:

- What? (What is the sound I hear? What organ(s) may be involved? What process would cause or contribute to this finding?)
- Why?
- What else?
- What if?
- What then?

Effect-based reasoning (EBR) can also be used as a teaching strategy in a physical assessment course to help learners cluster assessment findings and begin to consider possible plans for client outcomes. In EBR, a direct effect (also known as a first-order effect) is the immediate, direct result of a trigger action without an intervention. A first-order effect will introduce variables that change results, thus creating a second-order effect. Anticipating possible outcomes from second-order effects leads to identification of potential third-order effects. For example, a student gives a newborn a bath (the trigger action) with the intended outcome of taking a clean baby to its mother. The first-order effect is that the infant received a bath. Variables could include low ambient temperature, at which time the newborn became chilled, increasing oxygen need (second-order effect). The baby compensated by increasing heart and respiratory rates (physiologic variable), which created the third-order effect of depletion of blood glucose level exhibited by a lethargic baby (see Box 3.3).

Novice nursing students can begin formulating templates for development of thinking needed for clinical reasoning by using such EBR questions as:

1. If I find _____ during my assessment, I want to also check for _____.
2. If I find a pattern of _____ throughout the assessment, I need to ask further questions about _____.
3. If I do _____, I believe _____will occur in this situation because _____.
4. Then, I will do _____.
5. Depending on the effect of that action, I will consider either _____ or _____.

BOX 3.3   Effect-Based Reasoning

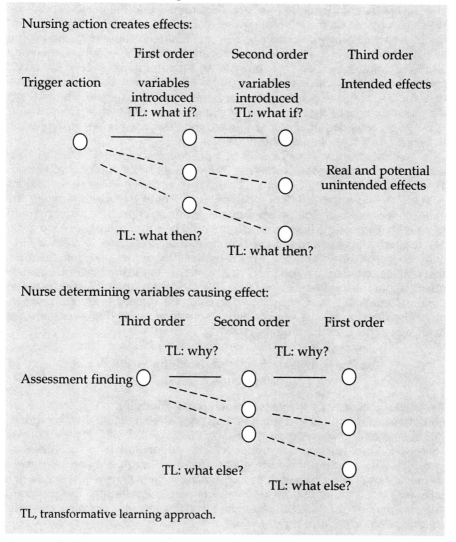

Nursing action creates effects:

Nurse determining variables causing effect:

TL, transformative learning approach.

By using these questions, learners work through first-order effects and identify real or potential outcomes for second-order effects. EBR can expand learner frames of reference when learners must consider other perspectives by using critical reflection and critical self-reflection. These questions can be used in a traditional or online classroom, simulated or clinical settings, and effectively used to recap learning during post-clinical conferences.

For example, learners in a post-clinical conference dialogue assess a person who experienced a cerebrovascular accident. Using the EBR questions, learners discussed that if right-side weakness is found, further assessment is needed to determine if any other symptoms are present. Assessment for fields of vision in both eyes is indicated, along with questions about the person being able to complete activities of daily living. Further post-conference discussion may reveal that students had, in fact, determined that the person could not see objects placed on the left side of a table. From identification of assessment findings that indicate hemianopsia, learners dialogue about how food could be placed on a plate to promote the self-care function of feeding. Depending on the outcome of the person's ability to eat a greater percentage of food with revised food placement, learners discuss possible alternative or additional actions for assessing and planning appropriate care for this patient. The students then identify actions that are within nursing's scope of practice, use previous knowledge, consider other comorbidities, and assess responses of the person in the current situation to provide care.

In another example of using EBR in a post-clinical conference, a client admitted for exacerbation of congestive heart failure has symptoms of nausea. The nausea is the third-order effect. Learners would need to assess for various possible second-order effects. One possibility would be an apical heart rate of 54, concurrent with long-term digitalis administration. The learner would identify that a possible first-order effect would be a toxic digitalis blood level. The triggering event would be medication administration for decreased force of heart contractility. Variables include the severity of the condition, the function of liver and kidneys, and individual response to the medication. Learners must gain empirical knowledge to be able to identify the variables, real and potential outcomes, and accurately interpret assessment findings. Learners must also develop ethical and aesthetic knowledge to develop a commitment to engage in the EBR thinking process.

Examples of Transformative Teaching Strategies in Nursing Concept Courses

Although concepts vary across levels of nursing education, some concepts are ubiquitous to the nursing discipline. For example, safety, quality, communication, and ethical comportment are taught across all levels. Within nursing concept courses, learners are presented with opportunities to consider relationships with another person in a way that may not have been considered before. For example, discussion of transferring a client from a wheelchair to a toilet in a safe manner that includes maintaining client dignity and promotes self-care may be the first time nursing students consider toileting and self-concept needs synonymously.

One of the most fun and challenging responsibilities of faculty teaching in concept courses is helping students to *think like nurses*. In most nursing concept courses, learners are exposed to tools frequently used to guide thinking, such as: assess/diagnose/plan/implement/evaluate (ADPIE), subjective data/objective data/assessment/plan/implement/evaluate (SOAPIE), or a communication guide such as situation/background/assessment/recommendation (SBAR), and so on. These tools help learners to develop patterns to structure thinking. A number of learning activities that have been successful in helping nursing students think like a nurse are offered. In an example of one such learning activity that can be adapted for various levels of nursing education, learners are encouraged to dialogue to promote use of nursing terminology with one another and the faculty member within a safe environment. This learning activity can be expanded by the educator asking learners to explore various nursing roles through discussing rationales for nursing attire, rationales for interprofessional communication techniques, or rationales for nursing interventions to meet a patient's possible physiological, psychosocial, developmental, or spiritual needs. When nursing students first consider rationales for behaviors required for communicating, assessing, or performing basic nursing skills, personal assumptions may be brought to light. During small-group discussion, learners can encounter various points of view in response to the learning activity, stimulating further critical reflection and critical self-reflection for assumption hunting. The assumption hunting may be anxiety provoking for some learners if a conflict in values is discovered.

A second learning activity that can be used in nursing concept courses is for nursing students to write a personal philosophy of nursing. As learners are exposed to the different roles of nurses within the health care delivery system, nursing school experiences can place them in situations that challenge their beliefs and perceptions of self-efficacy to meet the demands of the roles. Learners link past knowledge or renegotiate knowledge to work toward a personal definition and philosophy of nursing. In this activity, learners can compare themselves to a perceived silhouette of a nurse. Learners must first identify how they describe the silhouette of a nurse that requires critical reflection. During critical self-reflection, learners are encouraged to hunt for any assumptions, including answering questions such as "What exactly do nurses do? Which of my needs will be met by becoming a nurse? Am I seeking to meet my own ego need or the needs of another person? How do my personal beliefs and values fit with the *Code of Ethics for Nursing* (American Nurses Association, 2009) or the values identified by the nursing profession?" The learning activity of creating a philosophy of nursing can be expanded to include critical self-reflection regarding motivation for becoming a nurse. In studying motivation for entering the nursing profession, Rhodes, Morris, and Lazenby (2011) found altruism to be the most frequently identified motivator. This nursing philosophy activity encourages learners to identify other personal values and evaluate how important those values are as they begin a nursing career and assume various roles of the nurse. This activity can be revisited in a capstone course by asking learners to critically self-reflect and journal about development of nursing values, assuming the role of a nurse, and the personal transformation involved throughout the nursing curriculum. The two nursing concept learning examples presented above relate to helping learners develop a personal identity as a nurse or to see the need for thinking like a nurse, which is foundational for clinical reasoning in various situations.

In nursing concept courses, learners begin to consider values and ethics of nursing. The *Code of Ethics for Nursing* provides a foundation for development of ethical comportment. Teaching strategies to develop ethical comportment must incorporate awareness that learners of all ages and backgrounds bring personal value systems. Activities that help learners to identify personal values, such as value clarification exercises, can assist learners to develop nursing values. Some students may never have given conscious thought to their values, and some may identify values that contrast with those of nursing, thus creating cognitive dissonance and potential disorienting dilemmas. After critical self-reflection involved in a value clarification exercise, learners can dialogue in self-selected pairs or small groups to discuss personal values that either complement or contrast with the values in the *Code of Ethics for Nursing* or other professional nursing organizations.

Acting like a nurse builds on the ability to think like a nurse, including development of an awareness of others and their needs. A learning activity to introduce ethical comportment includes the concepts of civility and respect for others. The intended outcome is for learners to realize personal responsibility to others in a learning group and other situations in which their behavior influences others. Learners may need to explore personal assumptions of those in the learning group who differ in appearance, speech, mannerisms, interactions, or expression and consider how they will provide nursing care for individuals who differ from themselves.

In this activity related to ethical comportment, learners are asked to complete a 1-minute writing assignment to self-reflect regarding desired behaviors for classmates by answering the question "What would be the perfect classmate?" Building on this assignment, learners then self-identify personal characteristics and areas in which they can improve to facilitate self-learning and awareness of others' needs. For example, after critically reflecting and critically self-reflecting, one learner identified a personal difficulty in interacting with others who do not speak English and voiced that they did not want to be placed in a learning group with these individuals. This led to dialogue with peers and faculty about how she would respond when providing nursing care to those with English as a second language. Although the learner did not respond at the initial discussion, subsequent dialogue with the teacher revealed that further reflection led to transformative thinking.

Other activities that foster awareness of civility, with respect for self and others, are those that promote team building. Often students bemoan group work due to previous experiences when one person produced the work and the group received the grade. A basis for working with members of the health care team can be provided by learning teamwork skills. Teamwork emphasizes the value of every member of the team, the importance of differing perspectives, respect, and communication (Cronenwett et al., 2007). By establishing teamwork as an expectation in a fun, interactive, learner-centered activity, students can internalize the values of working with others in a civil manner (Rhodes, 2010).

Within a learning activity called Teamwork Challenge, learners are asked to participate in various tasks that require exploration of thoughts from all team members and to create a plan to solve a problem. Critical self-reflection questions, such as those listed in Box 3.4, help learners identify personal

BOX 3.4   Teamwork Challenge Reflection Questions

After completing the Teamwork Challenge:

1. What did you realize about yourself that will help you become a better team player?
2. What did you realize about yourself that will help you become a better leader?
3. What attributes did you encounter that create a positive work environment?
4. Think of a previous clinical or class experience. Explain how a better team experience may have created a better outcome.

perspectives that may be challenged. Critical self-reflection may also cause learners to think about their points of view related to working in a team and to determine how they can combine points of view from others to achieve completion of a task. To create an equal opportunity for learners with no health care background, non-nursing problems are presented. After completion of team-building activities, learners are asked to identify five words that describe the learning activity and to answer four critical self-reflection questions. Learner comments have revealed an increased awareness of essential elements of effective teamwork and leadership as indicated in Quality and Safety Education for Nurses (QSEN) guidelines: communication, mutual respect, and shared decision making (Cronenwett et al., 2007; Scheckel, 2009).

Although the learning activities that have been presented for use in fundamental nursing courses are certainly not all inclusive, and may not be unique to nursing education, these activities promote learner critical reflection to consider other points of view, critical self-reflection, and dialogue to enable learners to carefully consider their choice for points of view and resultant behaviors. Additional learning activities and how they can be adapted for use in various nursing education settings can be found in the appendices.

CONCLUSIONS

Nursing continues to be ranked as one of the most trusted professions in the United States. Nurses provide competent, ethical care for people during vulnerable situations. Including transformative learning approaches in instructional design and development of learning activities is especially useful for students learning foundational nursing concepts. These approaches encourage learners to examine personal points of view, previous knowledge, and to consider how current thinking is affected. Students can evaluate personal development of nursing practice by considering *why* they do *what* they do as clinical reasoning and ethical comportment is developed. Dialogue in a safe learning environment gives voice to assumptions, values, and beliefs that when reflectively considered may lead to revision or change in thoughts and behaviors.

REFERENCES

American Nurses Association. (2009). *Code of ethics with interpretive statements.* Retrieved from http://www.nursingworld.org/MainMenuCategories/EthicsStandards/CodeofEthicsforNurses/Code-of-Ethics.aspx

Benner, P., Sutphen, M., Leonard, V., & Day, L. (2010). *Educating nurses: A call for radical transformation.* Stanford, CA: Jossey-Bass.

Benner, P., Tanner, C., & Chelsa, C. (2009). *Expertise in nursing practice: Caring, clinical judgment and ethics* (2nd ed.). New York, NY: Springer.

Cranton, P. (2006). *Understanding and promoting transformative learning: A guide for educators of adults* (2nd ed.). San Francisco, CA: Jossey-Bass.

Cronenwett, L., Sherwood, G., Barnsteiner, J., Disch, J., Johnson, J., Mitchell, P., & Warren, J. (2007). Quality and safety education for nurses. *Nursing Outlook, 55,* 122–131. doi: 10.1016/j.outlook.2007.02.006

Giddens, J. (2010). The immunity game: Conceptual learning through learner engagement. *Journal of Nursing Education 49*(7), 422–3.

King, K. (2005). *Bringing transformative learning to life*. Malabar, FL: Krieger.

Mezirow, J., & Associates. (2000). *Learning as transformation: Critical perspectives on a theory in progress* (pp. 35–69). San Francisco, CA: Jossey-Bass.

Rhodes, M., Morris, A., & Lazenby, R. (2011). Nursing at its best: Competent and caring. *OJIN: Online Journal of Issues in Nursing, 16*, 2. doi: 10.3912/OJIN.Vol16No02PPT01

Rhodes, M. K. (June, 2010). *Teamwork and leadership challenge: A strategy for achieving effective affective learning*. Poster session presented at the Drexel Nursing Education Institute, Myrtle Beach, SC.

Scheckel, M. (2009). Selecting learning experiences to achieve curriculum outcomes. In D. M. Billings & J. A. Halstead (Eds.), *Teaching in nursing: A guide for faculty* (3rd ed., pp. 154–172). St. Louis, MO: Saunders Elsevier.

4

Teaching Acute and Chronic Care Across the Life Span Using Transformative Approaches

Cam Hamilton and Arlene H. Morris

To be authentically present to a patient [or learner] is to situate knowingly in one's own life and interact with full unknowingness about the other's life.

—Dr. Patricia L. Munhall

Traditional teaching approaches in courses that primarily involve care for individuals requiring nursing interventions for health concerns typically include lecture, while integrating, at times, case studies or problem-based team approaches to learning. Learner strategies that are frequently used include memorization of specific assessment techniques for identifying diseases, treatment for specific disease processes, and identification of specific medications most frequently prescribed. During these "nuts-and-bolts" courses in which nursing care of individuals across the life span is taught, learners develop critical reasoning to determine what assessment findings are pertinent in various situations, what pathological processes are occurring, what impact these processes have at multiple levels, what the appropriate pharmacological or nonpharmacological interventions are, and why. Specific examples of transformative learning activities that can be used in courses involving nursing care concepts for those experiencing either acute or chronic conditions across the life span are presented in this chapter.

In a nutshell, nursing education's goal is development of nurses who provide quality and safe care for individuals, based on the best evidence and client preferences. Foundational courses such as those discussed in Chapter 3 provide background from which further knowledge is developed. Corequisite or subsequent courses involving nursing care provision build on these foundational courses. Although the names for courses (i.e., medical-surgical nursing, critical care, etc.) and content have changed throughout the years, nurse educators in practical, associate, baccalaureate, and graduate programs have a common goal of helping learners to understand the complex and various concepts involved in providing nursing care for individuals experiencing acute or chronic concerns.

We propose incorporating transformative learning approaches with other teaching methodologies to provide a framework for attainment of learner outcomes beyond those that are course-specific. Learners can be empowered to seek answers to questions such as:

1. Why should I care about_____?
2. What do I need to consider when I care for a person and their family who are concerned about_____?
3. On what evidence do I base my thoughts when considering various nursing actions?
4. Where can I find information based on high-quality evidence?
5. Can I state the rationale for potential nursing action(s) as I collaborate with the individual/family to plan care?
6. Can I discuss potential risks from nursing actions or anticipated benefits?
7. Am I able to determine patterns from individual responses from which I can develop a basic reasoning for clinical judgment?

In Box 4.1 there are suggestions on how the questions above can be used to stimulate critical reflection and/or dialogue. We also demonstrate how transformative learning approaches can be integrated with other teaching approaches such as storytelling, unfolding case studies, learner blogs, or digital storytelling. Content that is highly empirical may not encourage learners to experience transformative learning but can provide a foundation for further reflection and transformation. Transformative learning principles and approaches can assist faculty to promote transformative learning during classroom and clinical experiences by encouraging assumption hunting, disorienting dilemmas, dialogue, critical reflection, and capitalizing on happenstance occurrences.

ESSENTIAL CONTENT FOR ACUTE TO CHRONIC NURSING CARE

Courses related to health promotion, disease prevention, assessment, management, and specific nursing interventions also include other concepts such as communication, collaboration, prioritization, delegation, professional behavior, ethics, morals, and safety issues. Thus, it is critical that the educator include these concepts to increase learner awareness of providing holistic and interprofessional care. For example, the concept of oxygenation cannot be separated from the concepts of safety, clinical judgment, and patient teaching.

BOX 4.1   Suggested Uses for Reflective Thinking Questions

1. Self-reflective journaling
2. Threaded online discussions
3. Group discussion prompts
4. Preclinical or post-clinical conference discussion prompts
5. Outline for learner activity to summarize or review content areas
6. Student blogs
7. VoiceThread discussions

Additionally, the concept of pain cannot be separated from the concepts of communication, advocacy, ethics, and clinical judgment.

In courses for care of persons experiencing acute or chronic conditions, health and illness can be considered along a continuum that is influenced by multi-morbidities and socioeconomic factors, in which nursing care involves assisting individuals to attain an optimal quality of life at a particular point in time. Nurses often interact with individuals and families at one point in their lives. A nurse must have the ability to integrate past history and the patient's goal of reaching the highest attainable level of health, realizing the client's goal may differ from the goal anticipated by the health care team. This entails constant surveillance by an astute nurse, with support of the individual and family.

Concepts should include providing nursing care for individuals and families at all ages, across health care delivery settings, for acute and/or chronic concerns, most likely with multimorbidities and various levels of health literacy. Empirical learning regarding health and illness is necessary. Teaching approaches to assist learners to become more aware of holistic concerns can be integrated with the presentation of empirical facts to increase learner understanding of possible health trajectories in which there is a continual, dynamic movement along the health–illness continuum and adaptation to complex situations where individuals and families develop new normals. A learning outcome example might include: learners will demonstrate knowledge to promote health, prevent or manage illness, prevent complications, and enhance coping with life changes. This involves awareness of physical, cognitive, psychosocial, spiritual, and developmental needs of individuals and anticipatory knowledge needed by nurses to continuously be alert for cues in surveillance mode. A five-finger approach can help learners in clinical settings to be cognizant of constant shifting of patients' status within these five assessment dimensions. Educators can encourage learners to relate each of the dimensions to one of their five fingers, then to image an overarching assessment of family/community/access to resources. Self-reflection, self-awareness, and a willingness to critically analyze, synthesize, and evaluate past experiences are necessary to develop or change thinking. When beginning nursing education, learners can be at a disadvantage due to limited experiences from lack of nursing practice or life experiences.

HOLISTIC ACUTE AND CHRONIC NURSING COURSES

Content specific to the needs of pediatric, adult, and geriatric clients requiring acute and/or critical care is often considered according to needs within the physiological, cognitive, psychosocial, spiritual, and developmental dimensions. Several years ago, during the development of a new curriculum based on recommendations from various nursing education organizations (Agency for Healthcare Research and Quality (AHRQ), Commission on Collegiate Nurse Education (CCNE), National League for Nursing (NLN), Institute of Medicine (IOM), Quality and Safety Education for Nurses (QSEN), John A. Hartford Foundation, etc.), we conceptualized presentation of concepts with inclusion of variations for the different ages or acuity levels. In the design of the holistic acute care across the life span course and holistic chronic care across the life span course, the overarching learning goal is providing quality care for individuals and families to manage acute or chronic conditions.

In these courses, content is divided into chunks to help learners organize complex facts and to provide meaning and understanding for learners. Content is presented in such a manner to broaden learner perspectives in developing a more holistic view of patient/family needs and/or interventions. Scaffolding from previous knowledge encourages discourse with an outcome of enhanced awareness of what is known and what needs to be known for anticipatory problem solving and application of knowledge (see Chapter 14, "Self-Regulated Learning"). Instructional design for these courses integrates clinical situations with classroom teaching to provide opportunities for nurse educators to model application of content through discussions and examples of clinical situations in which the content has been or will be used to assist in formation of clinical reasoning and judgment.

Traditionally, lecture had been the primary teaching approach in these courses, supplemented with case studies for application of rote facts. Faculty now encourage transformative thinking in learners by using teaching strategies that increase awareness of patterns from which prior knowledge and experience can be connected to new information. A problem may exist, however, when learners lack life experiences and/or prior knowledge on which to make connections. This may result from content having been taught as isolated facts, with little or no meaning or usefulness to the learner. The outcome is that content is learned long enough to complete course requirements, then the facts are forgotten, and learners are unable to apply the knowledge to actual situations. Additionally, learners with minimal life experiences or prior knowledge may have difficulty in linking nursing theory to practice; resulting in minimal motivation to connect isolated facts with situations in which these facts can be applied.

Learning activities and the placement of these activities within these courses is planned to help learners connect the content to important concepts. For example, learners are prompted by questions such as, "If an individual has a low blood sugar and a change in level of consciousness, what care should you, as the nurse, provide to improve patient outcomes?" Learners must draw from technical knowledge learned in anatomy and physiology and pathophysiology, related to hypoglycemia, along with communicative knowledge to identify possible causes and solutions to the problem.

In designing these courses, faculty members have realized that focusing teaching mainly on the highly empirical or technical content through lectures is not effective. Content for care of those experiencing acute and chronic conditions demands that learners develop a valuing of those for whom care will be provided, a valuing of the content that will enable the learner to transform to a practicing nurse, and a valuing of the best evidence for interventions that include skill performance. Transformative learning approaches can help learners to identify assumptions, prior knowledge, and experience through self-reflection and/or dialogue. From understanding gained during the critical self-reflection and discourse, new knowledge can be built.

TRANSFORMATIVE LEARNING ACTIVITIES

McGonigal (2005) describes six steps necessary for faculty to create a shift or change in perspective consistent with transformative learning theory (TLT). These conditions include:

- an event that allows learners to identify gaps in current knowledge,
- circumstances that allow the learner to identify and discuss their personal assumptions regarding the situation,
- analytical self-reflection where the learner discovers the premise of these assumptions and influences or limitations they present to understanding,
- discourse with other learners and faculty to investigate alternative views and methods,
- opportunities to practice and apply new perspectives,
- an environment that fosters and rewards intellectual openness.

Transformative learning activities can spark learners to engage in analysis of an individual/family-centered scenario. By situating the need for facts into a specific situation through such tools as video clips, problem-based learning, clinical scenarios, unfolding case studies, and/or storytelling, learners are able to identify patterns related to specific concepts. Then, through critical self-reflection, answers may become apparent to questions such as:

1. Why should I care about_____?
2. What do I need to consider when I care for a person and their family who are concerned about_____?

Dialogue with peers, faculty, and clinical experts fosters awareness of other points of view regarding the concepts presented in the scenario. Discussion can be encouraged by questions such as:

1. On what evidence did I base my consideration of alternative nursing actions?
   a. Following discussion, does the selection of the evidence for nursing actions change?
   b. Following discussion, are different nursing actions selected?

2. Can I state the rationale for potential nursing actions as I collaborate with the individual/family to plan care?
   a. During dialogue, does my interpretation of patient/family values or preferences change?
   b. During dialogue, do my rationales for nursing actions change based on other points of view or rationales?

3. Can I discuss potential risks from the nursing action and anticipated benefits?
   a. During dialogue, does my knowledge increase about potential risks or benefits?
   b. During dialogue, does my consideration of potential harmful effects compared to potential benefits change?

4. Am I able to determine patterns in various individual responses from which I can develop a basic reasoning for clinical judgment?
   a. During discussion, in what way do I relate the concepts to other situations?

    b. Can I determine the difference in a personal assumption and a pattern?
    c. Is my reasoning flawed on which I based my clinical judgment?

Critical self-reflection about the situation, the selected nursing interventions, evaluation of outcomes, and what occurred is necessary to make changes in thinking or behavior as needed for future situations. During this reflection learners should ask themselves question such as:

1. Why did I do or select _____?
    a. Do I have hidden assumptions that I have not realized?
    b. Do I have personal values that influence my preference for a particular intervention?

2. What did I not consider?
    a. In what way was my awareness increased by other points of view?
    b. How can I use what I learned about my thinking in future situations?

3. How could my assessment or intervention change in different situations?

Critical self-reflection also allows for development of attitudes that motivate future learning.

During critical self-reflection and dialogue, learners' personal and situational variables may influence the learners' perception of a threat to self-concept or perception of self-efficacy requiring awareness of what Mezirow (2000) describes as a disorienting dilemma. Although learners personal and situational variables are often beyond faculty control, support for various points of view or levels of understanding and thinking can be provided through an authentic and trusting environment. Learners may identify an area in which more knowledge is needed or in which their thinking is flawed or may disengage. The challenge for nurse educators is to link pertinent content to situations in such a manner that learners can identify variables and patterns that connect concepts, nursing actions, and desired outcomes. This can promote change in what is known and how it can be used, or what Cranton (2006) describes as re-learning. Learners need to realize that decision making regarding appropriate nursing interventions involves knowing how to assess for needs and compare assessment findings with standards.

Development of *clinically based scenarios* assists nurse educators to present opportunities for situated reasoning that includes consideration of holistic needs experienced by individuals/families and can be integrated when presenting information regarding nursing concepts. For example, a transformative learning activity can be designed in which learners are asked to identify the underlying problem in a scenario in which arterial blood gas (ABG) results are abnormal and to relate appropriate nursing interventions. By applying current knowledge to the situation depicted in the scenario, learners attempt to problem solve. Learners must use empirical knowledge about oxygenation as interpreted by ABG results, yet may not be able to connect the abnormal ABG to electrolyte problems or cardiopulmonary dysfunction. Critical self-reflection and dialogue can help learners identify deficits in thinking, possibly influenced by assumptions, beliefs, or missing information, which may have led to inaccurate answers. Further critical self-reflection and dialogue can help learners identify a valuing (or not) of how this information could impact a person's life.

Another activity to promote awareness of client/family concerns can occur through the teaching technique of a *lived experience* of illness symptoms. Before a class meeting, learners are asked to relate clinical situations or anonymous experiences of family members or friends in a creative way to help others in the class identify how changes in oxygenation, for instance, can affect the person and family. One learner responded to this assignment by coming to class with a poster board around her chest/abdomen with ribs drawn to illustrate development of barrel chest and brought a model of a portable oxygen tank. She related the difficulty of life goal attainment, including inability to plan times for activities and the intrusion on relationships when chronic obstructive pulmonary disease (COPD) precluded ability to function as desired. She concluded by stating that she had lived with her father throughout development, health fluctuations, and subsequent death from COPD. Faculty and other learners had an opportunity to expand personal awareness and points of view from her visual representation of the effects of the disease and her sharing of personal experience. For some learners this experience led to further self-reflection and development of determination (emancipatory knowledge) to provide appropriate nursing care in similar situations.

Analogies and narrations of stories can be helpful for learners to connect what is known with what is yet to be known. Prior knowledge of facts can be applied differently in various situations to identify both root cause and best action. Past empirical, aesthetic, ethical, and personal experiences may need to be evaluated, validated, or re-learned to make sense of various situations. As learners progress from basic recall of facts to application and analysis, they can distinguish what they know and do not know to discover a new understanding (Forehand, 2005; McGonigal, 2005; Roland, n.d.; Wilson, 2006). For instance, learners are taught that persons experiencing hyponatremia are likely to experience cognitive changes. Narration of a story based on faculty member experience caring for a patient can encourage learners to build on emotions (aesthetic knowing) to better understand the person's experience.

One example is the story of Mary, an 80-year-old, who was admitted to the hospital with chest pain and subsequently developed severe hyponatremia. As Mary's sodium dropped, her orientation decreased as well. Mary's family had to stay with her 24 hours a day to prevent the use of restraints as she was unaware of her surroundings. An increased awareness of how difficult it is to maintain safety for someone who is disoriented to place and time became more obvious during the recounting of the family member's experiences of keeping Mary in the bed throughout the night. Mary's constant request for "just a little water" during required fluid restriction was described; learners were asked to recall feeling thirsty but unable to drink and how this would impact providing nursing care.

An unfolding case study can be used to demonstrate the pattern of unknowing as well as to illustrate empirical, aesthetic, and ethical knowing. Consider the example of Nana, a 92-year-old who has recently relocated to an assisted-living facility following a broken hip. Educators can provide a weekly update on Nana, and her physical, social, psychological, mental, behavioral, and family characteristics can expose learners to the effects of chronicity. Discussion could include possible risks due to age, life situation, coping with losses related to self-concept, changes in roles, transition in relationships from selective interpersonal relationships to dependency, and changes in social and living environments. Opportunities for critical reflection and dialogue can be incorporated into the weekly updates to encourage deeper understanding of factors involved in chronicity, transition across health care settings, and how this can affect health along the continuum.

This unfolding case study provides opportunities to integrate content learned in prior courses or levels of education. Developmental considerations are brought to light during a discussion of Erickson's ego integrity versus despair stage as Nana experiences loss from perceived inability to leave her desired legacy. As the case study unfolds, Nana experiences anxiety from her awareness of limited time, energy, and opportunity for leaving something meaningful to those she loves. As Nana's unfolding case continues, faculty members may model unknowing when students question the information provided. For example, a student asked if Nana's desire to leave a legacy could possibly lead to experiencing spiritual distress. The faculty member acknowledged unknowing related to connections between desire for leaving a legacy and possible spiritual distress. Modeling of unknowing by the faculty member during discussion of the case demonstrated authenticity. Through this modeling, learners observed the importance of self-reflection and dialogue about their own thinking and what information may be needed in clinical experiences.

The suggested transformative learning strategies and activities previously discussed above were all planned and primarily included empirical knowing. However, educators should be aware that happenstance learning opportunities may occur whereby learners reconsider or revise current meaning perspectives. Emancipatory thinking is the ultimate outcome of incorporating transformative learning approaches within teaching strategies.

CONCLUSIONS

Nursing practice necessitates an ability to use various types of knowledge to provide quality and safe care. Courses regarding nursing care of client/family units across the life span include pertinent information about physiological, cognitive, psychosocial (including cultural and life span factors), spiritual, and developmental needs, which provide the foundation for further learning. Faculty must build on this foundational knowledge to assist learners in developing the thinking skills to determine pertinent information and consider plausible interpretations, leading to collection of relevant evidence to select the best course of action (Tanner, 2008). This involves critical and self-reflection to deepen the breadth of situated learning required for nursing practice.

Educators help learners build a foundation for becoming a nurse by creating authentic transformative learning environments. However, educators must realize and be prepared for isolated or cumulative events to be the impetus for individual students to self-reflect, question past habits of mind or points of view, or to engage in meaningful dialogue that provides additional insights about disorienting dilemmas. Cognitive dissonance may have to occur for learners to question past self-concept, develop intellectual humility, or question assumptions and to develop new perspectives. Nursing educators must strategically and intentionally set the stage for reflection and transformative learning. Individual educators, in effect, add a drop of water to learners' buckets (of understanding), capitalize on the fact that each learner is different, and the filling of the bucket will occur at unpredictable times.

Throughout this chapter, we have offered a number of strategies and activities that can stimulate transformative learning in providing care for clients with acute and chronic conditions. See appendices for further learning activities.

REFERENCES

Cranton, P. (2006). *Understanding and promoting transformative learning: A guide for educators of adults* (2nd ed.). San Francisco, CA: Jossey-Bass.

Forehand, M. (2005). Bloom's taxonomy: Original and revised. In M. Orey (Ed.), *Emerging Perspectives on Learning, Teaching, and Technology.* Retrieved from http://projects.coe.uga.edu/epltt

McGonigal, K. (2005). Teaching for transformation: From learning theory to teaching strategies. *Speaking of Teaching, 14*(2). Retrieved from http://www.stanford.edu/dept/CTL/cgi-bin/docs/newsletter/transformation.pdf

Mezirow, J., & Associates. (2000). *Learning as transformation: Critical perspectives on a theory in progress.* San Francisco, CA: Jossey-Bass.

Roland, M. H. (n.d.). Classworks and Bloom's revised taxonomy. *Classworks by Curriculum Advantage.* Retrieved from http://www.classworks.com/pdf/Blooms%20Revised%20Taxonomy.pdf

Tanner, C. A. (2008). The future of nursing education: A collaborative perspective. Oral presentation at *2008 NCSBN Faculty Shortage: Implications for Regulation Symposium.* Retrieved from https://www.ncsbn.org/2373.htm

Wilson, L. O. (2006). Beyond Bloom—A new version of the cognitive taxonomy. *Leslie Owen Wilson's Curriculum Pages.* Retrieved from http://www.uwsp.edu/education/lwilson/curric/newtaxonomy.htm

5

Transformative Learning in Specialty Courses

Marilyn K. Rhodes, Ginny Langham, Arlene H. Morris,
and Debbie R. Faulk

We change our point of view by trying on another's point of view.
—Jack Mezirow

In population-based nursing courses, teaching involves how and why to provide nursing care for individuals, families, communities, or aggregated populations. Population-based courses in nursing curricula include maternity and newborn, pediatrics, geriatrics, mental health, and/or community health. Some learners will come into contact with the above populations for the first time during nursing school, or interactions with these populations during nursing education may be quite different from past contacts. Learners most likely will not have had any firsthand knowledge of the intimacy involved in providing maternal/women's health care, interacting with those experiencing mental health concerns, with those living in poverty or with the very young or old. However, learners may have developed habits of mind about these populations from either assumptions, exposure to media, or from personal background knowledge that contribute to their points of view. Nursing students must learn how to assess for individual variations within these populations and how to effectively interact within larger systems (i.e., environment, socioeconomic, or heath care delivery systems) in addition to empirical knowledge about pathophysiology and nursing interventions required to care for populations with shared characteristics.

In Chapters 3 and 4, transformative learning activities were presented that specifically address course concepts and content. However, in this chapter, overarching content areas that are core to providing nursing care for population groups or individuals that share similar characteristics will be discussed in light of transformative learning according to instrumental, practical, and emancipatory types of knowledge (see Chapter 1, "Types of Knowledge Foundational for Transformative Learning"). Population-based courses must include technical content (theoretical/empirical knowledge that allows manipulation and control of one's environment) specific to the courses, yet much of the learning includes practical (communicative—knowledge required to understand another person through language) and emancipatory (knowledge that comes from questioning instrumental and communicative knowledge and depends on adult learners' self-knowledge, self-determination, and self-reflective skills). By considering these types of knowledge, some overarching concepts are similar in what at first may seem to be very different courses.

OVERARCHING CONCEPTS IN SPECIALITY COURSES

Nursing care of individuals, families, or groups must include consideration of the impact of cultural beliefs and values on health behaviors, the establishment of trust with those providing health care, sources for obtaining health information, and the influence of each of these on level of health literacy or current health-promotion behaviors. Development of nursing students' skills in authentic listening to consider internal and external factors that influence clients' behaviors is a beginning component for teaching learners how to anticipate potential needs for assessment or interventions. Internal factors include clients' values, beliefs, motivation, self-efficacy, and so on. External factors include personal financial resources, social resources such as family or community support, access to care, number and power of competing stressors, etc. Teaching strategies in which learners identify similarities and differences among individuals and groups are helpful, yet educators must avoid stereotyping by encouraging learners to identify hidden assumptions or to consider others' points of view.

Experiential learning to promote perspective transformation can include working with the public health department, outreach organizations, senior centers, or any agency that cares for people outside acute care health centers. Planned or happenstance occurrences of dialogue can create a setting to begin exploring hidden assumptions. For example, students had an impromptu meeting with a faculty member about a teaching project for residents of a community home for behavioral rehabilitation. The students explained that their selected topic for teaching was adherence to prescribed medications and outlined progress made on the project as: "We will begin by talking with the residents, then share information about several common medications." When asked why they were teaching this particular content, they responded that those with mental concerns usually stop taking their medication when they feel better because their symptoms decreased. When asked how they knew this, the students responded, "They just do." Through this dialogue, the students came to realize that assumptions were guiding their nursing actions when the faculty member asked the question, "How do you know that?"

After admitting that their plan was based on assumptions, the students responded to the request to consider other possible reasons that medications might not be taken: no money to purchase, inability to get or maintain a job, or separation from family or other support. The students further reflected upon recent class content that possible auditory hallucinations were preventing residents from taking the medications. Other possibilities identified included that the side effects of the medication could be more undesirable than the desirability of the intended effects, that residents might not have hope for improvement from the medication, or that other substances may be substituted for medication.

The students then created a different plan for the teaching project, stating that they would have to find out the residents' motivations, or the residents might never adhere to their medications, no matter what the students taught them. Once the students realized that their project was less about their performance and more about the residents, they realized that they needed to be authentically present, to listen and then to individualize teaching according to the resident's needs.

The guided dialogue in this situation prompted the students to critically think about their project in terms of valuing the residents, rather than only completing the assignment. The students realized that they had assumptions about the residents in this instance and understood that they may hold assumptions about other populations as well.

STRATEGIES FOR TRANSFORMATIVE LEARNING IN SPECIAL POPULATIONS

Men and Women's Health Course

Although content and concepts may be clustered differently in various nursing curricula, issues regarding men and women's health are presented at all levels of nursing education. However, within nursing curricula and heath care delivery settings, there is a need for educators to guide learners in developing awareness of pertinent health-promotion behaviors, specific assessments, and specific health concerns and interventions to manage those concerns. A balance is needed when considering individual needs and anticipating needs of groups sharing similar characteristics. For example, a young homosexual male will need to be assessed for HIV, but HIV cannot be assumed because the client is a homosexual. Another example is that all young pregnant women are not anemic, although they should be screened for anemia.

Maternity and Newborn Population

The teaching strategy of an inclusive, unfolding case study will be discussed here as the case is applied to concepts taught in a course on maternal and newborn nursing, then applied to different population-based courses. Transformative learning approaches are integrated throughout the case study to foster application of clinical reasoning and ethical comportment in actual settings of care. Through the use of guided or unguided critical reflection, critical self-reflection, and dialogue, educators can encourage learners to "try-on" perspectives different from their own.

The inclusive unfolding case study involves a young, unmarried gravida, who lives in a nuclear family in a working-class neighborhood:

> Sue is a 16-year-old, Caucasian, unmarried female who is a junior in high school. She presents to a community clinic at 35 weeks gestation, Gravida 1 Para 0. To date, she has gained 18 pounds. Her vital signs and OB checks are normal. The fundal height reveals appropriate growth. Fetal heart rate (FHR) is 150. She states the baby, "still moves all the time."

After students in a maternal/newborn course are introduced to "Sue," the nurse educator may begin asking questions about Sue's physical well-being to discuss specific instrumental maternity nursing knowledge such as:

1. What are normal vital signs and OB checks?
2. Where should the fundus measure at 35 weeks?
3. Is 18 pounds appropriate, based on her pre-pregnant weight, which was ____?
4. Is the FHR normal?
5. What are potential complications for an adolescent pregnancy?
6. What is the teen pregnancy rate in this area?

Next, the educator can incorporate critical self-reflection to allow students the opportunity for examining personal perspectives and to determine if their perspectives promote or impede person-centered care. For example, questions that might be used to stimulate critical self-reflection include:

1. Is 16 years old too young to be having a baby?
2. Is this an intentional pregnancy? Why would this matter?
3. Does Sue have family or community support?

As the case unfolds, students learn that this was an unplanned pregnancy, although Sue had been dating her boyfriend (Joe) for over a year.

Joe and Sue had always talked about getting married after graduation, but when Sue learned she was pregnant, Joe and his family moved out of town. She does not know where he and his family moved. She tells you (the nurse) she plans to keep the baby and bring the baby to daycare that is sponsored by her high school. Sue lives with her mother and dad who, although not happy about the pregnancy, plan to help her raise the child and help her complete high school. Sue is receiving resources from Women's Infants and Children (WIC), and her parents' health insurance will cover her expenses. She recently applied for further government assistance (Medicaid) for her baby.

At this point in the case, a faculty member asks students how they would respond if someone made the statement, "Great, more people receiving government assistance!" The educator can guide dialogue to allow students to "try-on" other perspectives. This dialogue prompt will likely evoke emotional responses from learners. Faculty members ask learners to self-reflect to understand communicative knowledge by describing how they would feel if they were Sue, if they were the person making the comment, or if they currently receive government assistance in some form. The anticipated learning outcome is development of emancipatory knowledge as learners question both past and recent insights and possibly transform perspectives.

Later in the course, after students have rotated through labor and delivery, the faculty use Sue's case to continue the discussion. Using the following information, learners are asked to create a concept map for providing care to Sue:

Sue was admitted to labor and delivery at 37 2/7 weeks with premature rupture of membranes x 6 hours. She is accompanied by her mother and maternal aunt. Her admission exam reveals that at 0700, she was 4 cm dilated, 100% effaced, Vtx at 0 station. Her contractions are occurring every 3 minutes lasting 60 seconds, FHR rate 140–150, + accels, + variability, no decels. VS normal. At 0800, Sue's pain was 7 on 0–10 scale, Sue whimpered with contractions; her mother and aunt were sitting in chairs close to her, but did not talk to Sue or try to comfort her during contractions. Sue's mother said she may not have an epidural because she must feel the pain of labor to discourage more babies. A nurse stays with Sue, helping her with relaxation and breathing techniques for labor. Sue's progress is normal for a nullipara. She receives two doses of IV narcotics; each time her pain decreases to 2 on 0–10 scale for one hour following the medication. Sue pushes for 50 minutes. At 1412, Sue delivered a baby boy with Apgar scores 8/9. The placenta delivered at 1417 intact. The baby weighs 6lb. 2oz, cries loudly and was brought to Sue and placed skin to skin. Sue has a 1st degree perineal laceration which is repaired by the midwife. At 1430, the mother helps Sue to breastfeed her infant. The mother and aunt praise Sue for being a strong young woman and delivering a healthy baby.

Students can create concept maps by discussing the progress of labor, physical care, and emotional support provided during Sue's labor and delivery as well as social, economic, spiritual, and mental health domains. The faculty ask the students if they believed that Sue's mother was "being mean" when she refused epidural anesthesia for Sue. Students may discuss intense emotions if they believe that Sue's mother was "being mean," if they believe pain would be a deterrent to future pregnancies, or if any of the students had similar personal experiences (including male students who may have been denied medication for pain).

As dialogue regarding the unfolding case continues, the educator can promote transformative learning by guiding learners to explore perspectives about adolescent pregnancies and how one's perspective affects the ability to provide quality, person-centered care. Critical self-reflection is encouraged to continue after class dialogue ends.

Mental Health

Nursing students may have expressed concern, perhaps including fear based on limited points of view, about their ability to provide care for persons who experience mental illness, possibly developed from exposure to stories or media portrayal of mentally ill persons. Transformative learning approaches can assist these learners in the development of practical reasoning, situated cognition, and ethical comportment. Experiential learning allows interaction of learners and persons living with mental illnesses. Educators must ensure experiences where the students feel physically safe and create a safe environment in classroom and clinical conference settings that encourages students to explore their perspectives. Sue's unfolding case study can be used to introduce a previously known "person" to the students in a mental health course or a course in which mental health issues are integrated.

Sue returned to high school when the baby was 2 weeks old. At first, she worked hard to catch up with her classes. She had always earned good grades, but now didn't seem to care about her studies. After only 4 days in school, Sue called her midwife, crying, and said she "didn't think she could do this." She didn't want to finish high school and she didn't feel like she could take care of the baby. The midwife suspected that Sue had postpartum depression and arranged community transportation for Sue to be seen in the office that day. Sue was treated with an antidepressive medication and began twice weekly group therapy. She also reduced her academic load and now attends high school half days.

The educator asks learners to consider potential contributing factors to Sue's development of depression: hormonal imbalance, increased stress from role changes or role overload, interpersonal relationship/family dynamics, grief over her lost role in her high school class, anger from Joe's departure and lack of support, and so on. Students are encouraged to develop assessment questions that they could ask Sue if they were the nurse (communicative knowledge). Learners are then asked to consider possible outcomes if Sue stopped taking the antidepressive medication or stopped participating in group therapy (potential suicide or abandonment of the baby).

Transformative learning educators must be aware of the potential that some learners will not want to participate in critical reflection of this unfolding case, in critical self-reflection to identify personal belief or similar past experiences that may be too painful at this time, or to participate in dialogue. Nurse educators who are mindful of the potentially painful reminders that such dialogue could provoke should not call on students to reply to direct questions, but rather ask for responses from the class as a whole. Educators should also be aware that there may be learners in the discussion who are currently experiencing similar situations and may look to the class content or to the educator for advice on how to manage their own health concerns. Self-reflection journaling activities can allow students who are uncomfortable with dialogue to examine their perceptions more privately.

This unfolding case provides an opportunity to explore family theory as well as decision making regarding life choices in addition to mental health concerns. Do students have an underlying assumption that because a person could have avoided the situation or made different choices, that nursing care should be any different? Transformative approaches can help learners appreciate how valuing the patient as a person can lead to greater practical reasoning and ethical comportment.

Community Health

In community health courses nursing students learn to provide care for vulnerable populations as determined by socioeconomic status, age, employment status, disease/state of illness, or events beyond the control of the persons, such as natural disasters. Nursing students, being considered persons of privilege, may have developed assumptions about these populations based on erroneous or incomplete information. Transformative learning approaches will help learners begin to reconsider or possibly change points of view, while increasing technical and practical knowledge with an outcome of developing a sense of civic responsibility.

Sue's story, as a transformative learning activity, can be continued or applied individually in a community health course. From the community perspective, Sue's case can introduce learners to concepts regarding promoting and protecting the health of aggregate populations. For example, Sue's situation can be explored in light of identifying internal or external factors that relate to vulnerabilities in the adolescent population, an unfolding development of Sue's need for family and community resources, and what the local, state, or federal community responsibility is for Sue. Additional unfolding case studies could be designed to help learners explore various ages or marginalized groups. For further suggested learning activities that can be used in community health courses see Box 5.1 and Table 5.1.

Unfolding case studies provide a teaching strategy that allows learners and faculty to be co-learners, sharing dialogue to consider how personal and other

---

BOX 5.1   Evidence-Based Practice Health Teaching Project

The purpose of this learning activity is to assist the student in implementing person-centered care emphasizing health promotion and disease prevention for individuals, families, and populations. In this learning activity the student will:

1. Self-select a small group of two to three students
2. Choose a health topic from options provided
3. Read the assigned content
4. Conduct research to locate best practice guidelines for the selected topic
5. Develop a health teaching PowerPoint presentation to present health information to college-aged individuals

Directions:

1. After self-selecting a small group of two to three classmates, choose a health topic from the following options:
   - Importance of Proper Nutrition in College
   - Dangers of Alcohol/Drug Use
   - Sexually Transmitted Diseases
2. Review the following content from the course textbook:
   - Chapter __: Evidence-Based Practice
   - Chapter __: Health Education and Group Process
3. Research the scientific literature. How is your presentation evidenced based? Use at least three current evidence-based articles from scientific journals to provide support for your project. Questions to guide your research: What interventions have been used with this population in the past? What do the authors say is most effective? What interventions are not necessarily effective?
4. As a group, develop a PowerPoint presentation (minimum of 10 slides) that is targeted for college-aged individuals. Creativity is encouraged in the design and development of the PowerPoint presentation, but the essential content includes:
   - Title page (including names of each group member)
   - Introduction and significance of health topic
   - Discussion of EBP articles
   - References in APA format
5. Submit the PowerPoint presentation to course faculty.

Table 5.1 Transformative Learning Activities

Transformative Learning Activity	Maternal–Newborn	Community	Mental Health
Clinical experience	No simulation that can replace the emotions or allow a nursing student to experience the intimacy of human birth	A community assessment of a vulnerable population is completed along with a health teaching intervention. Immersion experiences provide the learners with exposure to unfamiliar populations: soup kitchens, homeless shelters, senior adult day care centers, local health departments, outpatient and inpatient rehabilitation centers, hospice agencies.	Interaction with individuals experiencing a different reality Interpersonal communication Situated reasoning to assess and intervene as situations rapidly change
Extended pre-conference			Review of individuals' history Review of interprofessional team plan for care
Extended post-conference	Students are encouraged to express, in a safe environment, the impact of the experience as well as work through the nurses' responsibilities with rationales for this clinical area Students engage in interpersonal communication about the experience	In a familiar setting, learners engage in dialogue with peers and faculty regarding the immersion experiences. This provides an opportunity to discuss personal learning and explore previously held assumptions and beliefs regarding various populations.	Dialogue with peers and faculty regarding personal learning Discourse regarding differing points of view among learners, faculty, or health care team Evaluation of situational variables influencing the treatment plan
Reflection journal: Self-evaluation	The learner is expected to address the personal impact of the clinical experience, explore assumptions, and identify potential need for change in self.	Critical self-reflection regarding personal assumptions related to vulnerable populations may lead to a reevaluation and possible reformation of long-held personal beliefs.	Personal self-reflection regarding listening skills Personal self-reflection regarding effectiveness of therapeutic communication Personal self-reflection regarding assumptions/points of view and any emancipatory learning that occurred

(continued)

Table 5.1 *(continued)*

Transformative Learning Activity	Maternal–Newborn	Community	Mental Health
Simulation	Cath triad is employed during "OB Station Rotation" before the learners' clinical experience. The learner experiences urinary catheterization from the learner, patient, or instructor perspective Learners practice relaxation and breathing techniques	A disaster simulation provides the opportunity to enhance the learners' clinical judgment and knowledge before an emergency situation occurs. An acute situational simulation in a group setting is utilized to reinforce and strengthen CPR skills.	Opportunity to determine needed instrumental knowledge before actual clinical experience
Media	Movie: *Babies* Portrays childbirth and early childrearing in several cultures Stimulates discussion on similarities and differences in cultures as well as assumption hunting	Movie: *Unnatural Causes* Portions of a television documentary series are shown to raise awareness, reexamine personal convictions, and promote dialogue regarding the social, economic, and racial inequalities in health. "Community in the Arts" is designed to reflect the learners' perception and understanding of the terms "community" and/or "population." Learners are required to find and present any form of art (literature, poetry, painting, movie clip, etc.) that represents "community." The learner must facilitate classroom dialogue related to his/her perception of the term(s).	Movies: *Wit, A Beautiful Mind, One Flew Over the Cuckoo's Nest* Learners identify and discuss the experiences portrayed by individuals, families, groups, and various members of the health care delivery team. Further group dialogue provides opportunities for learners to discuss internal or external factors and determine the effectiveness (or lack) of the health care interventions.

| Collaborative learning | Learners are divided into small groups and provided with a list of health topics. Each group is expected to research, develop, and implement an evidenced-based health teaching project. Additionally, appropriate adaptations for populations across the life span are required. | Learner groups provide assessment for children in shelters for abuse, then plan appropriate play activities for developmental levels. |
| Guided assessments | Family assessment | Community assessment | In-depth assessment of a population group |

assumptions or points of view may influence nursing care. This teaching strategy is also very effective in helping students gain the three types of transformative knowledge needed to provide person-centered care. See Table 5.1 for other suggested transformative learning activities that can be used in specialty courses.

Pediatric or Geriatric Courses

We recognize that in some nursing programs, nursing care for pediatric or geriatric populations may be structured as independent specialty nursing courses. Nurse educators can design unfolding case studies similar to the case of Sue or use products that have been developed that promote situated learning through the use of computer software or licensing agreements for learners to access information similar to an unfolding case. Any of these products or faculty-designed teaching strategies can be modified to promote transformative learning by intentional addition of questions or activities that promote critical reflection and assumption hunting. Dialogue can occur in planned online or classroom environments, in clinical pre-conferences or post-conferences, or in informal discussion with faculty or other nurses. The anticipated learning outcomes are that learners will begin to consider the lived experience of individuals and families within age groups and the impact of internal or external factors on their lives. From these considerations, learners progress from technical knowledge to an increased awareness of practical knowledge and then develop reflection skills necessary for emancipatory knowledge. Additional learning activities, case studies, and examples of course modules can be found in the appendices.

CONCLUSIONS

Employing transformative learning approaches in teaching courses regarding special populations can increase students' awareness of people's needs beyond their scope of life experiences. The learning environment must be safe for learners to talk, question, and explore the concepts involved in providing care during a possibly unknown experience. The faculty must be authentic and comfortable with transformative learning activities as well as respectful of students and the individuals, families, and communities that are studied. Building on concepts from prior courses, learners bring technical/instrumental knowledge of health and wellness and professional nursing concepts. Studying special populations compels learners to consider past experiences and assumptions to be able to develop a level of comfort in these new environments of care. Learners must also evaluate if the extent of their previous knowledge is adequate as well as develop an awareness of their assumptions to understand to what degree these influence person-centered care.

Benner, Sutphen, Leonard, and Day (2010) commend the nursing profession for its effectiveness in experiential teaching. This style of teaching can be effectively utilized in the classroom using transformative learning approaches. Using case studies creates a safe environment for nursing students to learn together in teams or from each other as clinical situations provide exemplars of course content. This approach not only closes the gap between theory and practice but also promotes transformative learning by employing dialogue, critical reflection, assumption hunting, and co-learning.

REFERENCES

Benner, P., Sutphen, M., Day, L., Leonard, V. W. (2010). *Educating nurses: A call for radical transformation. The Carnegie Foundation for the Advancement of Teaching. Preparation for the Professions.* Stanford, CA: Jossey-Bass.

Mezirow, J. (1991). *Transformative dimensions of adult learning.* San Francisco, CA: Jossey-Bass.

6

Teaching Evidence-Based Practice Using Transformative Learning Approaches

Debbie R. Faulk and Arlene H. Morris

When you engage in reflection, you're working toward a goal: to thoughtfully consider the situation and determine problems that need to be addressed, skills that need to be strengthened, and perspectives that need to be changed. . . . In the classroom of life, reflection is a chance to review our decisions and behaviors and get ready for the next test that life provides us. We may not get a do-over, but we can think critically about our experiences to prepare for a do-better.
—Marilyn Asselin and Allethaire Cullen

Evidence-based practice (EBP) courses should be designed from the perspective of guiding learners to incorporate evidence into their nursing practice. Sounds simple, does it not? Unfortunately, as many nurse educators would attest, designing courses and creating learning activities that engage students in evaluating findings from research to begin the process of establishing a foundation for an EBP is a difficult task. Meeker, Jones, and Flanagan (2008) assert, "Many nurses fail to value or use research in practice" (p. 691). The literature abounds with suggestions on how to best pique learners' interest about research and EBP and how to help students make the connection between the two processes. Nurse educators must consider if their teaching/learning strategies are adequately preparing future nurses to provide the highest quality care for patients and families, in other words choosing actions from an evidence-base. In this chapter, we propose that the core transformative learning approach of critical reflection can facilitate learner valuing and understanding of EBP content, process, and outcomes. Teaching/learning approaches for EBP must enable learners to develop a solid commitment to providing care based on current, high-level evidence, which incorporates client/family values and health care providers' expertise.

FACTORS THAT INFLUENCE EBP COURSE DESIGN

Current methods in teaching EBP include a number of pedagogical considerations. One repeatedly identified issue in teaching EBP is how to help students value EBP content, thus resulting in a lifelong value in using findings from research studies in practice (Pravikoff, Tanner, & Pierce, 2005). Valuing EBP, as well as understanding the differences in the research and EBP processes, are vital as situations in health care become more critically dependent on evidence for the best care options to be readily retrievable by skilled nurses.

Various strategies are offered in nursing literature for teaching, learning, and valuing the EBP process. For example, Balakas and Sparks (2010) suggest a service-learning approach to teaching both the research process and EBP. Other suggested strategies include "acting as a research assistant" (Poston, 2002), using games (Lever, 2005), conducting small studies (Walsh, Chang, Schmidt, & Yoepp, 2005), and working in collaborative groups to conduct research projects (August-Brady, 2005). Rolloff (2010) questions specific strategies in teaching EBP and proposes using a constructivist model that leads to a learner-centered approach by considering individual learner goals. We agree with Rolloff that focus on individual learner needs and goals can engage learners in both EBP content and the valuing of its usefulness in lifelong practice.

Transformative learning principles (see Chapter 2, Box 2.1) and core transformative learning approaches (see Chapter 2, Box 2.2) can be used to design instruction that guides learners' development of thinking regarding EBP processes. Thus, a foundation for valuing the search and evaluating best evidence for practice can be formed for traditional nursing students or transformed for returning registered nurses (RNs) at baccalaureate and graduate levels.

Mezirow's (1991) three levels of reflection (content, process, and premise) are useful as a framework in designing transformative learning activities that can help learners understand the process and value of EBP. These three levels of reflection help the faculty in considering ways to design instruction by making pedagogical choices. Structuring learning activities to guide learners' thinking and reflection using the three levels can encourage development of a habit of mind in considering problems that occur in nursing.

FACTORS INFLUENCING LEARNER REFLECTION

When considering instructional design for nursing courses, specifically those necessitating evaluation of alternative ways of thinking such as EBP, educators must plan for all learners who bring unique characteristics and levels of prior experience, thus adding a complexity to the learner valuing and understanding of the content. The power of an individual's developmental level, emotional intelligence, and stress response and how these variables impact an individual learner must be considered when designing learning activities and opportunities.

Individuals view the world and daily occurrences through a habitual lens, often not realizing the view(s) they have, and often not completely understanding how developmental maturity, emotions, and stress can impact habits of mind and, therefore, development of points of view. These habits of mind are formed throughout childhood, experiences (or by having limited experiences), and vicarious exposure and reflection on others' lives through literature/drama/media. The very process of education involves helping learners identify their own habits of mind and expand or revise their points of view by identifying alternative thinking. To examine or reflect upon these habits of mind/points of view and alternative ways of thinking, a certain level of developmental maturity is required.

Developmental Maturity of Learners

To self-reflect Mezirow (2003) stated that both the developmental maturity to be critically self-reflective and the skill to exercise reflective judgment must be present. Nurse educators can promote critical self-reflection through an environment of safety for discourse, assumption hunting and consideration of alternatives, and provide guidance in development of skills for reflective judgment (prioritization of needs, effect-based reasoning, etc.). However, all learners will not be able, at the same time, to accomplish the necessary reflection—they may be in crisis mode, have narrowed perceptions, or not be intellectually and personally secure in self-reflection. Therefore, the faculty must know their learners' characteristics, maintain a hopeful view of potential for all to grow and develop, and structure content and learning opportunities that will assist learners to develop self-reflection. Kreber (2006) states:

> intellectual development occurs as frames of reference get revised as a result of reflection. . . . Transformation of one assumption may promote reflection on other assumptions. . . . Not in all cases, however, will reflection lead to a drastic change in frame of reference for, through reflection, we may also find our assumptions to be confirmed or validated. (p. 93)

The developmental maturity required for being open to self-reflection to consider thoughts not previously held can provide motivation for learning. For example, learners become aware that new information is needed because "what I know does not provide what I need to interpret this situation or make this choice of action." However, the process of examining self, thought processes, and personal identity characteristics can be potentially threatening to self-concept and/or self-efficacy. Although some learners may lack developmental maturity and thus withdraw from self-reflection and tenaciously hold to individual habits of mind, educators must not force self-reflection. Presenting self-reflective learning opportunities throughout the curriculum may allow these learners to develop emotional maturity to engage in the reflection process.

Stress Level and Coping Ability of Learners

Educators must encourage and stimulate skills for reflective judgment, which can logically be taught in EBP courses as a method for reasoning by using evidence on which practice will be based. Reflection requires effort and energy and usually must be prompted by the stress/crisis/cognitive dissonance of realizing there is a problem/need/stressful event/crisis. Lazarus and Folkman's (1984) stress appraisal and coping mechanisms can provide a framework to consider how stress/crisis impacts an individual's ability to think about or reflect upon information that may be unfamiliar or difficult to understand. Primary appraisal of a stressful event involves an attempt to cope with the event, problem, or crisis. In primary appraisal, an individual asks "What is happening? Is there a problem? Does it affect me? If so, how?" An analogy can best describe this phenomenon. When an individual encounters a bear in the woods, the person identifies a potential danger ("Is it harmful or is it benign?"). Primary appraisal continues when the individual considers "What will I do?" (e.g., "Will I run or climb a tree?"). Folkman and Lazarus propose that secondary appraisal includes an evaluation of the outcome of the current action ("Am I outrunning the bear? How long can I out run the bear? Do I have other options?").

Lazarus and Folkman's (1984) findings regarding how individuals attempt to cope with stressful events is similar to Mezirow's (1991) three levels of reflection. In content reflection, the problem is identified. In process reflection, an evaluation is made of the problem-solving efforts, and in premise reflection, the individual places a value of importance on the premise of the problem. To continue the bear analogy, content reflection identifies that it is a bear that has come out of the woods, process reflection is used to identify that the bear is coming and is large enough to be a threat, and in premise reflection, the individual determines that he or she is not running fast enough to avoid danger.

Additionally, in crisis mode, focus is narrowly directed to survival needs, causing limited openness to other thoughts, suggestions, or ways of thinking. If learners are overwhelmed by the educational process, they may be unable to be open to thinking/reflection beyond surviving the course. They may attempt memorization as a coping method, but this learning strategy will be ineffective in nursing because nursing is a situated discipline in which content must constantly be evaluated and actions selected for the best anticipated patient outcome. Learners must have a positive, hopeful approach that future nursing actions have potential to promote health, diminish suffering, or provide comfort through all areas of living and dying. This hopeful view can motivate learning and a desire for competence in nursing actions.

Emotional Intelligence of Learners

An individual's emotional intelligence is also a factor that influences self-reflection. Emotional intelligence is both genetically inherited and results from social influences experienced during the growth and development process. To assist learners in developing the skill of critical self-reflection, nurse educators must help learners consider their personal abilities to cope and manage personal feelings, as well as consider the feelings of others (Goldman, 1995). Nurses display a variety of emotions in health care delivery situations and in the decisions (sometimes life altering) that are made. Helping learners reflect upon emotions that will be experienced in care delivery settings and in learning situations and how to cope or manage these emotions is critical. In courses such as leadership, public policy, ethics, and EBP where content is somewhat elusive, but nonetheless highly valued in today's health care delivery systems, learners may experience stress, demonstrated through a variety of emotions when reflecting on what is known and what is not known and how available findings may be pertinent to current situation(s). The idea of becoming a leader who will be responsible for change processes can be overwhelming and may thus block or prevent understanding and valuing of concepts involved in EBP.

By first considering the impact that an individual leaner's level of developmental maturity, stress/coping abilities, and emotional intelligence have on learning, nurse educators can then encourage and stimulate self-reflective learning opportunities that will result in understanding specific content/concepts and valuing the information.

TYPES OF REFLECTION FOR TRANSFORMATIVE LEARNING

As King (2005) aptly states, "the roots of transformative learning are found in the critical reflection of the being and self" (p. 36). Critical thinking is at the core of transformative learning and is needed for critical reflection. Ard (2009) provides a background for evidence-based nursing education practices for critical thinking and critical reflection through summary of research-based literature in nursing and higher education; DiVito (2000) identified specific criteria for critical thinking and critical reflection; Forneis and Peden-McAlpine (2007) related how anxiety impacts critical thinking and how critical thinking develops sequentially; and Profetto-McGrath, Hesketh, Lang, and Estabrooks (2003) discussed a correlation between critical thinking abilities and research utilization.

Bart (2010) appropriately points out that the depth of information is often sacrificed for breadth where the primary goal of a course is to cover as much content as possible. With this teaching ideology, critical thinking goals may be lost in favor of more shallow learning outcomes. In courses with abstract concepts, such as EBP, nursing students need to be able to critically reflect to become engaged in the processes needed for EBP (i.e., analyzing and questioning). Learning opportunities for critical thinking and critical reflection must be the focus of any EBP course.

Reflective thinking in nursing and nursing education has gained attention in recent years as a goal for improving nursing practice. "Reflection is a conscious, dynamic process of thinking about, analyzing, and learning from an experience that gives us insights into self and practice" (Asselin & Cullen, 2011, p. 45). Reflection as a broad concept can further be described by using Mezirow's (1991) three levels or processes of reflection to provide a structured approach in encouraging learners to develop patterns of thought and action in using EBP. With traditional nursing students, the three types of reflection may help to develop a habit of mind in understanding, valuing, and using EBP. For returning learners, the types of reflection may be used to help identify current assumptions from which points of view are expressed along with behaviors in practice settings and to encourage reflection on how prior habits of mind may impact problem identification and use of EBP.

Content Reflection

Kreber (2006) acknowledges that Mezirow's (1991) description of content reflection may be confused with reflection on course content, instead of "a clear sense of and description of a problem to be solved" (p. 94). Cranton (2006) also interprets Mezirow's meaning of content reflection as the identification of a problem or concern. When using content reflection in an EBP course in an RN to BSN program, learners often identify a problem with a lack of knowledge related to differences in the EBP and the research processes. When learners determine a need for more knowledge regarding comparison of EBP to the research process, a visual model comparing the two processes developed by Finkleman (2012) is used to stimulate discussion and further reflection. Finkleman's comparison algorithm allows learners to identify which type of process will be needed to determine the most appropriate way to proceed after identifying a problem or issue.

Learners also identify difficulty with how to determine problems or issues in health care, administration, or education. Learners are taught how to identify clinical problems and issues by observing interventions and client outcomes in practice settings. Using dialogue prompts in post-clinical, simulation, and classroom settings can stimulate content reflection to identify actual and potential problems that may result in undesired clinical outcomes or how clinical processes could be improved. Learners then reflect on what knowledge they currently have about how to solve or prevent these client outcomes from occurring. From this content reflection, learners are then introduced to formulating a question in population, intervention, comparison, outcome (PICO) format. For graduate level learners, addition of the teaching method in the PICO(T) format can be taught in identifying problems in educational or administrative settings.

By using content reflection, a problem with how to search for appropriate evidence can be determined. This reflection often results in learners' expression of great frustration with the actual search process and then how to determine what evidence is "the best" for the particular problem/situation. Content reflection activities help teachers and learners identify problem areas related to a lack of knowledge. Following identification of what is currently known and unknown, asking learners to identify and reflect upon current habits of mind about the EBP process allows for less stress when completing course requirements.

Process Reflection

Process reflection involves the process of understanding specific problems/issues and what is going on. For example, in an EBP course, learners are asked to reflect on a clinical problem, including how they think the issue became a problem (root cause analysis). Learners are questioned about an increased number of patients in one long-term care facility who have experienced falls within the past month during the evening hours. Process reflection can overlap with premise reflection as the learner's first question could be: "Why would this matter?" Learners would then identify that increased falls can result in pain or fractures leading to other complications, such as pneumonia, fat emboli, pressure ulcers, and so on if the person who falls has comorbidities. Learners would be encouraged to reflect further about the increased fall rate, considering a possible link between staffing number and mix, cognitive functioning of the patients during the evening hours before falls, physical status, emotional status, or any environmental situation such as change in time for mopping floors. Process reflection uses these variables to reflect, "How did this situation come to be?"

A component of process reflection may include data collection regarding the variables to more clearly identify the root cause. From this reflection, learners identify what has been done in prior efforts to reduce fall risk and compare these efforts to findings from different levels of evidence. Process reflection also enables learners to look at their habits of mind and to self-reflect regarding the effectiveness of past approaches to problems/issues.

When assisting learners to use process reflection in EBP courses, learners are encouraged to reflect on how the PICO(T) question was formed and if it is accurate. Additionally, learners reflect on how information regarding the problem was obtained and, if it is the most appropriate information for addressing the issue. For example, a group learning activity within a traditional baccalaureate program is to compose an accurate PICO question. Following the formulation of the PICO question using process reflection, group members are asked to self-reflect on the level and type of involvement of group peers. After group dialogue each learner completes a peer review form to assess process reflection and to assess how the group as a whole used process reflection to identify the problem and the information needed.

Premise Reflection

According to Cranton (2006), "Content and process reflection may lead to transformation of a specific belief, but it is premise reflection that engages learners in seeing themselves and the world in a different way" (p. 35). Teaching premise reflection includes a valuing component and how to evaluate which alternative action is most likely to lead to desired outcomes, while valuing the desired outcomes and valuing the process itself. In this way, nurses can use the three types of reflection in practice for clinical judgment. Premise reflection is used by asking learners to reflect on the following questions:

1. Why is EBP important to me at this point in my education?
2. Why do I care about this information in the first place?
3. What difference does it make to me?

Additionally, learners are asked to specifically reflect on an EBP problem or issue by answering, "Why is this a problem, anyway"? Student reflections may be posted to threaded discussions in online courses, in journal postings, or during in-class dialogue.

Example of Using Three Types of Reflection

To determine problems, learners must focus on the desired outcomes to identify issue(s) not being met. Learners use the three types of reflection to consider and plan appropriate interventions and then to evaluate both the process of care and the outcomes of care. For example, learners use *content* reflection when identifying that the number of urinary tract infections (UTIs) have increased over the past 6 months. Content reflection occurs as learners identify the content of the problem to be an increased number of UTI occurrences.

Learners can further reflect on the problem in a different way by considering potential causes of UTIs, including what *process* is involved. Thus, using *process* reflection, learners begin to consider "In doing (cleansing of the perineal area), I wonder what would occur if I did (a different process of care) as compared to doing it the usual way." Learners consider the different steps involved in providing perineal care or catheter care to analyze potential root causes and link to results of urinalysis that reveal a presence of *Escherichia coli* bacteria. Through further process reflection, learners consider what the potential effect would be if the use of bath basins was discontinued for catheter or perineal care—perhaps there would not be as much *Escherichia coli* bacteria cultured in the urinalysis.

In *premise* reflection, learners identify increased UTIs as a problem because they value human beings and value decreasing suffering. It is in premise reflection that motivation is involved, and learners are prompted to look for alternatives to usual thinking or doing (habits of mind).

In using the levels of reflection (three different views for considering a problem) to teach EBP, nurse educators assist learners to use *content* reflection when identifying a problem by teaching learners to constantly be on the lookout in practice settings to identify problems and issues, while considering that outcomes for patients, students, or staff may differ from those that are desired. Learners also need to be aware that processes could be improved in nursing care, education, or administration. For example, when using content reflection in nursing education, educators focus on identification of learner outcomes or areas for improvement in teaching methods. In nursing administration, problems are identified in structure, process, and outcomes. In all of these areas, learners can be taught to identify the population, desired outcomes, current intervention, and possibly comparison intervention using a PICO(T) format. Content reflection is used to identify the population and outcome, whereas process reflection helps with identification of the intervention and comparison. Furthermore, content and process reflections are used to evaluate whether the EBP or research process is indicated. However, premise reflection is used when considering if the problem is actually a problem worth pursing with available resources and one that can have potential impact on outcomes.

REFLECTIVE TEACHING STRATEGIES FOR EBP

Various teaching strategies can provide a basis for the reflective thinking process (i.e., clinical situations, simulations, unfolding cases, classroom dialogue, journaling, etc.). Completion of EBP reflective learning activities can assist learners and teachers in assessing where more knowledge is needed. The first learning activity example involves an unfolding case study to demonstrate learner engagement in the three types of reflection for understanding and valuing the EBP process. The case study presents a situation in which traditional practice is shown to be ineffective or counterproductive in attaining the desired outcomes (see Box 6.1). After reading the case study, learners are paired and asked to use content, process, and premise reflections related to Ms. P's case (see Table 6.1).

Students are given two hours to complete the reflection activity. The faculty member then asks for volunteers to contribute to a group discussion. Risk taking is encouraged, rather than emphasis on providing correct answers. During the ensuing dialogue, the faculty as co-learner, with the group of learners, evaluates the process of this learning activity and determines if more information was needed to answer any of the questions. Additionally, learners compare any nursing practices that are based on personal assumptions or traditional

BOX 6.1   Sliding-Scale Insulin: A Familiar Tradition

Ms. P is a 35-year-old female who was first diagnosed with insulin-dependent diabetes when she was age 16. She takes Novalog insulin twice a day while carefully monitoring her blood sugars, although often ignoring when the readings are high (which occur frequently). She eats whatever she wants and self-adjusts her insulin dosage to her blood sugars. For 3 days now she has been nauseated, weak, experiencing a lack of appetite and high blood glucose (BG) levels. She is admitted to the hospital with a diagnosis of diabetic ketoacidosis. While in the hospital, a sliding-scale insulin (SSI) dosage for glycemic control based on her BG levels is ordered.

Interestingly, evidence indicates that sliding scale is an ineffective method for treating hyperglycemia after it occurs. In other words, sliding scale does not prevent increases in BG nor does it prevent recurrence of elevated BG levels. The evidence (Summary of Revisions for the 2010 Clinical Practice Recommendations) indicates that not only is use of SSI ineffective but also the practice may be dangerous. Ms. P's order for SSI prescribed on admission is unlikely to be changed or modified throughout her hospital stay even though the evidence indicates this approach exacerbates hyperglycemia and hypoglycemia caused by rapid BG alternations which could lead to the possibility of a poor clinical outcome or even death.

Source: Case study adapted from *Controlling blood glucose levels in hospital patients: Current recommendation* by DeYoung, Bauer, Brady, & Eley, 2011, *American Nurse Today*, 6(5), 12–14.

beliefs rather than on scientific evidence. This case can illustrate how changes in practice may be indicated, yet how the process of changing practice is difficult, especially if the previous practice has been long held. Goals for this transformative learning activity are twofold: (1) for learners to develop in self-reflection and critical dialogue and (2) for learners to value the process of EBP and continue the behavior of using it throughout other courses in the nursing curriculum and in practice.

A second example provides a student-centered learning activity focusing heavily on valuing (premise reflection). Learners are asked to work in self-selected teams of three to prepare an EBP-TEAM project (Faulk & Morris, 2008). In this particular learning activity, students are required to use a specific EBP model as a guideline for writing and disseminating findings. A formal report is submitted before presentation of the findings in a poster presentation to the class. Students are also encouraged to submit poster abstracts to an annual clinical workshop hosted by the state nursing association. Critical to the learning outcomes for this assignment is the assumption that students sometimes have difficulty understanding evidence for practice versus a traditional research question and proposed study. The purpose of this EBP-TEAM project is to use the principles and context of EBP-TEAM to evaluate a nursing practice, policy, or procedure in light of current evidence and make recommendations for change to improve practice. Content, process, and premise reflection are all used in the completion of this learning activity (see Box 6.2). This learning

TABLE 6.1   Questions for Reflection Regarding the Case of Ms. P

Questions to Stimulate Reflection	Type of Reflection
1. Is this case as presented important (Ms. P's need for care)? Why or why not?	Premise reflection
2. Clearly and concisely identify the problem in the context of this case.	Content reflection
3. What knowledge do you not have, but would need related to taking care of Ms. P?	Content reflection
4. Based on identification of what knowledge is lacking and what knowledge is needed, identify possible sources of knowledge needed to take care of Ms. P.	Content reflection
5. Using your personal digital assistant (PDA), search for a practice guideline related to this issue. Additionally, search in the Cochrane Database for at least one systematic review. Discuss how the findings relate to Ms. P's case.	Process reflection
6. Identify options for providing care for Ms. P.	Process reflection
7. One member of the dyad should pretend to be Ms. P's nurse. Identify potential risks/benefits of the options.	Premise reflection
8. One member of the dyad should pretend to be Ms. P. Identify your values/preferences.	Premise reflection
9. Self-reflect regarding your (as the nurse) level of expertise regarding the option(s) most acceptable to Ms. P. and most likely to lead to the desired outcome.	Content reflection
10. Self-reflect on how you can increase your expertise (if needed).	Content reflection
11. Identify interprofessional interventions that would be involved in the care to be provided for Ms. P.	Process reflection
12. Self-reflect on how this learning activity has increased your valuing of EBP.	Premise reflection
13. Identify any knowledge of which you were not previously aware regarding the EBP process.	Content reflection
14. Identify any knowledge of which you were not previously aware regarding comparison of current best practice recommendations to current care practices.	Content reflection

activity can be used in hybrid and online courses. For online students, WIMBA Live® Classroom can be used for a formal presentation of the reports. It is from this learning activity that valuing of EBP has been a persistent learning outcome. For example, students stated:

> I really learned about research this semester. I always used to cringe at the word. Now that I feel more confident in my abilities, I am eager to go dig up some super-valid and credible EBP in my field of interest (natural childbirth/pro-breastfeeding/non-circumcision) so I can back up my beliefs with facts and maybe help to educate and empower women of the United States.

> At the beginning of the semester, the EBP assignment was, well just another assignment to get through. After attending the classes and working on the [project] I not only learned from it, but also enjoyed (yes, I said enjoyed) doing it. It was a valuable learning tool and I gained so much more from [the] assignment . . . .

> I think [the] assignments were helpful in applying the [EBP] process, reviewing the literature (including how to analyze a research article), what to do with the information once you have it (how to incorporate the information into practice

BOX 6.2   EBP-TEAM Project Guidelines

In self-selected teams of four, use the PICO method described in your text to formulate a clinical question within one of the four clinical categories: therapy, diagnosis, prognosis, or etiology. Once the clinical question and category are developed and approved by course faculty, follow the directions below:

1. Conduct a search related to your clinical category and question.
2. Identify the database(s) used in your search, key words used in the search, and how many articles/reports are yielded from the search.
3. Select four (individual) research studies from your search that specifically address your clinical question/category and screen each study for relevance and credibility by answering the following questions:
   - Is the research report from a peer-reviewed journal? How did you determine this? Cite the journal using American Psychological Association (APA) style.
   - Are the setting and sample of the study similar to your question (i.e., would they apply to your practice and patient population?)?
   - Is the study sponsored by an organization that may influence the study in some manner? If yes, name the organization and state what you believe the influence may be.
   - Are the study findings positive or negative? For example, treatment results in better outcomes, treatment makes condition worse, or there is no difference.
   - Identify the level of evidence for each study.
   - State the setting, population, and sample number for each study.
   - State the sampling method used (i.e., random, nonrandom, etc.).
   - State the data collection method for each study.
   - State descriptive and/or inferential statistics used in each study (if applicable).
   - State how the findings (from the studies as a whole) could be used to impact patient outcomes and how this information could be incorporated into your practice setting.
4. Conduct a Cochrane review to ascertain if a systematic review related to your clinical topic has been published. If one (or more) exists, cite reference(s) using APA, and answer the following questions:
   What were the search strategies used by the authors?
   How was the data collected and analyzed?
   What were the main results?
   State in your own words, the author's summary.
5. Search for any Best Practice Guidelines that have been developed related to your clinical category and question. If no guidelines

(*continued*)

BOX 6.2 *(continued)*

> have been developed, state this. If guideline(s) are found, provide
> example(s) in the report.
> 6. Submit all information in a formal written report by assigned due
>   date.
> 7. Present findings in a 10-minute presentation, specifically address-
>   ing the following:
>   - How could the findings be incorporated into the practice setting?
>   - What changes would need to be made to incorporate findings
>   into practice setting?
>   - How would client values and preferences need to be considered?
>   - What were the assumptions, values, beliefs, etc., related to EBP
>   before completing the assignment?
>   - What were the assumptions, values, beliefs, etc., related to EBP
>   after completing the assignment?

and disseminate the information to other health care team members), the importance of research in evidence-based practice. We gained knowledge about topics
affecting our patients, and experience in working as a team. I thoroughly enjoyed
the class and would like to be a part of a research team or do some research on
my own.

CONCLUSIONS

In this chapter, we assert that the transformative learning approaches of using content, process, and premise reflections can assist the faculty in considering options for designing instruction in EBP courses. It is well established
that nurse educators are challenged to find the right combination of learning
activities that will encourage attainment of knowledge related to the EBP process and to help learners value the use of current, best evidence for practice.
Creating learning activities that encourage the three types of reflection can
stimulate learners' critical thinking and can enable learners to develop habits
of mind in considering how best to address the myriad of patient problems
that occur in providing nursing care throughout a career. Further research using these transformative learning activities in various levels of nursing education can enhance the evidence base for nursing pedagogy.

REFERENCES

Ard, N. (2009). Essentials of learning. In C. M. Shultz (Ed.), *Building a science of nursing education: Foundation for evidence-based teaching-learning.* New York, NY: National
League for Nursing.

Asselin, M. E., & Cullen, H. A. (2011). Improving practice through reflection. *Nursing
2011, 4*(4), 44–47.

August-Brady, M. A. (2005). Teaching undergraduate research from a process perspective. *Journal of Nursing Education, 44,* 519–521.

Balakas, K., & Sparks, L. (2010). Teaching research and evidence-based practice using a service-learning approach. *Educational Innovations, 49*(12), 691–695.

Bart, M. (May, 2010). Critical reflection adds depth and breadth to student learning. Instructional Design, Teaching and Learning. Retrieved from www.facultyfocus.com/.../critical-reflection-adds-depth-and-breadth-to-student-learning

Cranton, P. (2006). *Understanding and promoting transformative learning: A guide for educators of adults* (2nd ed.). San Francisco, CA: Jossey-Bass.

DeYoung, J., Bauer, R., Brady, C., & Eley, S. (2011). Controlling blood glucose levels in hospital patients: Current recommendation. *American Nurse Today, 6*(5), 12–14.

DiVito, T. P. (2000). Identifying critical thinking behaviors in clinical judgments. *Journal of Nurses in Staff Development, 16,* 174–180.

Faulk, D., & Morris, A. (2008). Valuing evidence-based practice: A student-centered learning activity. *The Journal of Nursing Education, 48*(4), 232–.

Finkelman, A. (2012). *Leadership and management for nurses* (2nd ed.). Boston, MA: Pearson.

Forneis, S. G., & Peden-McAlpine, C. (2007). Evaluation of a reflective learning intervention to improve critical thinking in novice nurses. *Journal of Advanced Nursing, 57*(4), 410–421.

Goleman, D. P. (1995). *Emotional intelligence: Why it can matter more than IQ for character, health and lifelong achievement.* New York, NY: Bantam Books.

King, K. (2005). *Bringing transformative learning to life.* Malabar, FL: Krieger Publishing Company.

Kreber, C. (2006). Developing the scholarship of teaching through transformative learning. *Journal of Scholarship of Teaching and Learning, 6*(1), 88–109.

Lazarus, S. R., & Folkman, S. (1984). *Stress, appraisal, and coping.* New York, NY: Springer.

Lever, K. A. (2005). Introducing students to research: The road to success. *Journal of Nursing Education, 44,* 470–472.

Meeker, M. A., Jones, J. M., & Flanagan, N. A. (2008). Teaching undergraduate nursing research from an evidence-based practice perspective. *Journal of Nursing Education, 47*(8), 376–379.

Mezirow, J. (1991). *Transformative dimensions of adult learning.* San Francisco, CA: Jossey-Bass.

Mezirow, J. (2003). Transformative learning as discourse. *Journal of Transformative Education, 1*(1), 58–63.

Poston, I. (2002). Stimulating enthusiasm for research in undergraduate nursing students. *Journal of Nursing Education, 41,* 186–188.

Pravikoff, D., Tanner, A., & Pierce, S. (2005). Readiness of U.S. nurses for evidence-based practice. *American Journal of Nursing, 105*(9), 40–51.

Profetto-McGrath, J., Hesketh, K. L., Lang, S., & Estabrooks, C. A. (2003). A study of critical thinking and research utilization among nurses. *Western Journal of Nursing Research, 25,* 322–337.

Rolloff, M. (2010). A constructivist model for teaching evidence-based practice. *Nursing Education Perspectives, 31*(5), 290–293.

Summary of Revision for the 2010 Clinical Practice Recommendations (2010). *Diabetes Care, 33*(suppl 1), S3. doi:10.2337/dc10-S003. Retrieved from www.ncbi.nlm.nih.gov/pmc/articles/PMC2797388

Walsh, S. M., Chang, C. Y., Schmidt, L. A., & Yoepp, J. H. (2005). Lowering stress while teaching research: A creative arts intervention in the classroom. *Journal of Nursing Education, 44,* 330–333.

7

Teaching Leadership/Management, Public Policy, and Ethical Content Within the Framework of Transformative Learning

Francine M. Parker and Debbie R. Faulk

A critical reflection process, perspective transformation is intended to create ownership of new knowledge and, ultimately, adaptation to and social construction of new knowledge appropriate to the context.
—Carol McWilliam

Nursing curricula traditionally burst with empirical and technical knowledge giving the student a false sense that this is the only knowledge critical to becoming a nurse. However, courses that include abstract or elusive concepts/content such as leadership, ethics, public policy, etc., are also critical to building the foundation for a nurse who is open to transformation. A daunting challenge for nurse educators who primarily teach in these courses is how to help students develop a valuing of this critical knowledge. In these times of rapid change, not only in health care delivery systems but also in nursing education, educators must explore new teaching and learning strategies that will stimulate engagement and potentially help learners to value leadership/ management, ethics, and public policy content. In this chapter, information is provided to support the following theses: (1) leadership/management, public policy, and ethical skills are critical to becoming a nurse and (2) transformative learning approaches can be effective in fostering learner valuing of these skills.

The need for the concepts and content that are taught in leadership, public policy, and ethics courses is established followed by examples of transformative learning approaches and strategies that can be used in these three courses. Although public policy courses are primarily offered at the graduate level, faculty teaching at baccalaureate and associate-degree levels are realizing the importance of this knowledge and either incorporating concepts into existing courses or developing separate courses. The learning activities that are suggested in this chapter can be adapted to associate, baccalaureate, and graduate courses.

Before reading further, consider the following scenario and how it illustrates the need for nurse educators to critically reflect on teaching approaches in courses that are not saturated with empirical content. In a senior level professional nursing concepts course, Jane was evaluating a student-led seminar. The focus of the seminar was generational differences and leadership behaviors of practicing nurses. At the conclusion of the seminar, Jane seized the opportunity to have the students respond to a question she had long pondered as leadership and management faculty. Jane asked the students to reflect on the leadership and management course from the previous semester. She issued this caveat, I want you to be "rigorously honest" in your response to the following question: "Did you value the content?" After what seemed like several minutes, one student hesitantly made the following statement, "I did not value the content because I had no prior experience as a leader; nothing to link the content to. Leadership theory and styles had no meaning for me. It would have been better if you had taught me how to be a good *follower*." Although no other student offered a comment, nonverbal behaviors indicated overwhelming agreement.

LEADERSHIP/MANAGEMENT

To facilitate development of a knowledge base related to leadership/management concepts that will translate to practice, nursing curricula must address health care delivery within complex health care systems. As health care delivery systems are reforming or transforming, leadership and management educators should consider following the recommendations from the Committee on the Robert Wood Johnson Foundation Initiative on the Future of Nursing at the Institute of Medicine (2010) and from Benner, Sutphen, Leonard, and Day (2010) in planning course delivery, using teaching strategies, and developing learning activities. For example, learning activities should be designed to stimulate perspectives related to how nurses assume leadership positions to lead change, advance health, increase individual competencies, and enhance collaboration to improve the practice environment (Committee on the Robert Wood Johnson Foundation Initiative on the Future of Nursing at the Institute of Medicine). The outcomes of using these initiatives as a blueprint for creation of learning activities can be a student who internalizes knowledge, transforms thinking, and models lifelong learning through reasoned decision making and behaviors in the professional arena.

We recognize that leadership and management content varies widely in scope and substance within nursing curricula as well as across levels of education. For example, in many associate degree programs, leadership and management content is often limited in scope and depth to principles and definitions. The knowledge base that students need as a foundation for leadership and management development continues to include theories, styles, and characteristics of effective leaders; the concept of followership; the management process; and what it means to be a *great* leader and/or manager at both microlevel and macrolevel. Content in any leadership course must include the importance of developing transformational leadership skills. As health care systems continue to experience profound and rapid change, students must learn how to think like a transformational leader. This includes embracing change, motivating and influencing followers to be self-confident, self-directed, and committed to the mission of the organization. Creating learning activities that include critical reflection, self-reflection, and dialogue encourages learners to become transformational thinkers.

Before considering the use of transformative learning approaches in designing leadership and management learning activities, it is important to first understand that transformative learning is a paradigm shift from teaching massive content (which is a task that cannot be effectively accomplished) to engaging students as active participants in the learning process (McCallister et al., 2006). Nurse educators should plan learning opportunities that will encourage students to critically examine and reflect on their "fit" in a leadership/management role. Do they see themselves as followers, managers, or future leaders? Is it unrealistic for nurse educators to approach a leadership and management course with the goal that every nursing student, no matter what the level of education, is going to be a "leader"? Likewise, is it unrealistic for nurse leaders and administrators to expect that a novice nurse can be an effective manager at microsystem/macrosystem levels without experience in real-world practice? Professional staff development educators must also consider educational offerings that link leadership role expectations when orienting nurses that are progressing from staff to leadership positions, and to provide consistent content for further development. Leadership principles, characteristics of successful leaders and managers, and the management process can be taught, but until students/nurses have practice experience, they are likely to have difficulty with linking theory to practice in a meaningful way. By not encouraging practical leadership and management experience during nursing programs and during orientation and preceptorships after graduation, educators may be setting students up for failure.

Transformative Learning Strategies

A simple transformative learning strategy that encourages learners to gain insight into feelings and thinking is a leadership/management reflective journal. In this journal, learners reflect on their strengths and weaknesses during clinical experiences, identify assumptions related to leadership and management roles and identify how alternative ways of thinking about roles can be a springboard for lasting change (Kirkpatrick & Brown, 2006). The reflective journal allows learners to reflect on the power that assumptions have on their thinking, valuing, and behaviors. Faculty feedback creates the learning environment needed for the activity to be transformative. Cranton (2006) emphasizes this by stating, "Educators especially need to be aware of learners' needs for supportive and challenging feedback during transformative learning" (p. 66). The following student comments illustrate the use of the reflective journal as an effective transformative learning strategy for valuing leadership:

> I hold several perceptions of myself as a leader and of the leadership role. I am aware that I have qualities that make me both a good leader at times and a bad leader at times. The qualities that hinder my leadership ability include a lack of patience, my preference for doing most things without the assistance of others, and that I have a tendency to be extremely sarcastic and often find things to be humorous when others do not. Before taking the Leadership and Management

class, I perceived that the "leadership role" was all about being born with a charismatic personality and making sweeping, dramatic decisions during critical moments. I now understand that leadership is always a work in progress that requires a variety of skills. It is about an ability to think critically, to make accurate situational assessments, to see other perspectives, to inspire trust and motivation in others, and to be willing to put forth your efforts and thoughts. These abilities allow the leader to have confidence in decisions and actions, which grants power to the leader. A good follower possesses self-awareness of their own values and thinking to accurately judge the leader's behavior before deciding to follow.

I am loving this preceptorship, I am so excited to go to the meeting tomorrow_____ is such a motivational leader. She truly inspires you to want more, be more, and work more. She instills in you to be a hard worker and to always strive to do your best. She does not even realize the impact she makes on the lives of those around her. I am interested in seeing how she performs at the meeting tomorrow and meet the rest of her team. Starting this preceptorship, my goal was to do what was expected of me and just get it done. I now find myself inspired to be a great leader and to help others also want to be a great leader. I want to do the extra things it takes to be great, instead of getting by with the minimum. I do find myself becoming more comfortable with the idea [of being a leader]. I have been trying out my newly learned skills at work and have found them to be helpful. I am motivating myself and those around me to be great. I can honestly say that I have seen the results of both good and mediocre leadership styles. I see many more positive outcomes from the positive leadership style.

Nursing students come to learning situations with prior life experiences, which contribute to assumptions and expectations about how the world works. Although many nursing students have never been a leader or manager in any work setting, they almost all come with some preconceived ideas of what a leader *looks* like or how a leader leads and how a manager manages. If we believe the assumption that learning is based on what we already know, then the student comment that learning about being a follower was more important at that time is very true, as it is likely that each of us has had experience as a follower.

Using transformative learning approaches to create activities that engage students in leadership and management courses may result in the development of a value for this critical content, instead of simply learning to pass a test. Furthermore, internalizing values may prevent future nurses from returning to preconceived ideas when entering practice settings. Additional transformative strategies for teaching leadership and management concepts are presented in the appendices.

Similar to leadership and management, policy advocacy is also an elusive concept and may not be a role that nursing students have considered as critical to nursing practice. In the next section, we discuss the need for policy content at all levels of nursing education and provide specific examples of transformative learning opportunities that have been successful in helping students to understand and value the policy advocacy role.

POLICY ADVOCACY

After many years of teaching public policy to returning RN students at baccalaureate and graduate levels, it is difficult to not sound cynical when stating that the majority of practicing nurses do not value policy content. This may be related to students' preconceived ideas of the political world. For almost 20 years, the nursing profession has recognized and expressed the need for students at all educational levels to develop political acumen (Bowen, Lyons, &Young, 2000; Buerhaus, 1992; Conger & Johnson, 2000; Porche, 2012; Reutter & Williamson, 2000). As the largest group of health care providers, the nursing profession is in a perfect position to influence policymakers and stakeholders. Shrinking resources, nursing shortages, escalating health care costs, advances in technology, globalization, and accessible and affordable health care for all citizens are just a few of the issues impacting the nation and the profession. Never in the history of nursing has the time been more right for nurses to accept the ubiquitous responsibility of becoming a significant force in health care policymaking. To meet this responsibility, the profession must increase its cadre of nurses who understand how the *game* of politics is played, points of entry into the policymaking process, and the behaviors or actions needed to enhance and safeguard the nation's health. Individual nurses in all practice settings can no longer be free riders, benefiting from the actions of others. Participative/collaborative roles in decision making at all government and health care organizational levels must become the norm, rather than the exception, incorporating policy development and analysis to shape health care delivery.

Transformative Learning Strategies

A senior level macrosystem leadership course will be used to illustrate how transformative learning strategies engage students in making meaning of the policy advocate role using critical reflection regarding values, beliefs, and assumptions with a resultant outcome of a more holistic understanding of personal and professional paradigms. These teaching strategies and approaches can be adapted to all levels of nursing education as well as used in professional staff development.

The macrosystem course addresses nursing practice in an evolving health care system with emphasis on the unique challenges in the macroenvironment (structures, settings, and organizations) of health care delivery. The role of the nurse as leader and manager of an organization that exists in a unique sociopolitical, cultural, economic, and technological environment is examined. Collaboration and communication skills are emphasized to address professional, organizational, historical, and social factors that affect a health care organization's role and function in society. Course outcomes are listed in Box 7.1.

The course content includes the role of the transformational macrosystem nurse leader including self, relational, system, and strategic thinking skills. These skills are needed to shape change and to improve quality through evaluation of the political, economic, social, and cultural forces that impact macrohealth care delivery systems. Through an emphasis on the influence of political forces, students learn that economic, social, and cultural factors cannot be examined in isolation. The structure and function of government at all levels, the policymaking process from a theoretical perspective, and examination of who gets what in a system where scarcity is the norm are examined through the lens of distributive legal and ethical issues. Health care reform is examined related to the impact on the nursing profession as a whole and the

BOX 7.1   Macrosystem Leadership Course Outcomes

1. Examine the attributes of leadership theory and style important in the macrohealth care environment.
2. Interpret principles of transformational leadership as they apply to quality of nursing leadership and management style.
3. Analyze the political, economic, social, and cultural factors that affect health care delivery in an organization.
4. Demonstrate basic knowledge of the policymaking process, health care policy, finance, and regulatory environments, including local, state, national, and global health care trends.
5. Examine the major methods for financing health care in the United States and how the management of fiscal resources and policy decisions influence macroenvironments.
6. Examine the roles and responsibilities of regulatory agencies and their effect on patient care quality, workplace safety, and the scope of nursing and other health professionals' practice.
7. Describe strategies for effective change in individuals, organizations, and the profession.
8. Identify options for the potential resolution of legal and ethical issues related to nursing leadership and managing health care.
9. Integrate new knowledge and innovation to impact quality improvement at the organizational level.
10. Support the functions of health care delivery in macroenvironments through organization, management, and evaluation.

individual nurse. Threaded throughout all critical dialogue is the role of the nurse as policy advocate and leader.

Transformative learning approaches have been successfully utilized to facilitate development of a professional perspective related to the policy advocacy role. Two student comments best illustrate this point. During a seminar where critical reflection and dialogue were encouraged, one student made the following comment in an email to the faculty member:

> After today's in-class discussion, I have deeply pondered the integration of politics with nursing; I have come to the conclusion that part of nursing's progression as a profession relies heavily on political involvement. I fully agree with [the] stance that nurses should be actively involved in politics. Mahatma Gandhi had it right when he said "the future depends on what you do today." I really wish that emphasis had been placed on the word "do." Today's seminar encouraged action, and it is apparent that there is a lot of work to be done by nursing in order to possess more ownership in what happens to and within our profession from a policy/political standpoint. Joining the state and national level nursing organizations, and contributing to their grand efforts of closely monitoring and influencing policy that could directly affect nursing on a professional as well as a political level are warranted. On a more personal level, I can honestly say that I was a person who used to be very "anti-politics." I lived in a fairly utopian existence where I "took life one day at a time" and made sure that the people under my roof were cared for. With politics, it can be hard to see how the global state of affairs, be they on a state level or national level, can have an effect on nursing.

Although nursing is one of the largest parts of the health care sector, it seems very minute in the grand scheme of all things governmental to the layperson.

In another learning activity involving questions for reflection related to political advocacy, a student stated:

> The assumption can also be made that everyone in politics is dishonest; I thought this for a while myself. Of course, this is not true. My eyes have been opened since taking this course. I realized that the problem was with me, I was not involved in the political process. This course has inspired me to get involved in the political process and let my voice be heard. I know there are dishonest politicians just like there are dishonest nurses, but that should not stop me (us) from getting involved. So, how do we change things? Simply, by getting involved; because change begins with me!

A very effective transformative learning activity designed to enhance critical reflection and promote dialogue in the macrosystem leadership course is the *Talking Points Memo*. The goal of this activity is to increase awareness related to current public policy issues impacting health care and the role of nurses as policy advocates, as well as to help learners see how their assumptions, beliefs, and values frame pro and con points of view. Each student writes a memo at a specified time during the semester to post online using a course management system. Once the memo is posted and read by peers, each student responds to the memo by agreeing or disagreeing with the writer's point of view. The educator guides reflective thinking by asking students to identify individual frames of reference and points of view and pointing out the power that points of view may have on behaviors or lack of behaviors. Students are also asked to reflect on the validity of alternative ways of thinking about the issue posed in each memo. In one memo, a student posed this question: "Should illegal immigrants be allowed access to health care in the United States?" The student's point of view was expressed as:

> I believe strongly that access to health care is a HUMAN right. Humans have a right to have their dignity preserved regardless of how they got here, or their personal situation. Denying health care to any population could prove more costly later. Nurses should advocate for the improvement of HUMAN condition in all cases. While we are trying to achieve affordable health care for ourselves, we should also advocate for health care for our immigrant population as well. We are trained to provide nonjudgmental, culturally appropriate care. Let's not contradict ourselves and the promises we made!

In response, a fellow student posted this comment:

> What an interesting and controversial topic. In response to your memo on whether illegal immigrants should be allowed access to health care, I would have to say that I am opposed to this issue. You mentioned the rising poverty level among illegal immigrants. The assumption here could be made that this is due to an injustice, but could this mean that there are more illegal immigrants entering the United States and adding to their poverty level? I am of the opinion that paying for health care is difficult enough for the average American. How then are Americans expected to take care of illegal immigrants? It is my assumption that illegal immigrants are given more rights and better health care

than American citizens and I feel that this is unfair. I agree with the point that you made that ILLEGAL immigrants are breaking the law. What picture does the government paint to the American people when our own citizens are not taken care of and [we] have to watch illegal immigrants receive health care at the expense of tax payers? There is a clear difference between legal and illegal immigrants. I can appreciate the fact that one would want a more secure and better life for themselves and their families, however, it should be done through legal channels.

Changes in perspective regarding the policy advocacy role are uniquely reflected in another student's Talking Points Memo posting:

I must say that this program has truly created cognitive dissonance as far as my level of involvement with politics in general. While I have always been opinionated, I like to think of the way Ralph Waldo Emerson values the process of becoming more politically engaged . . . "An ounce of action is worth a ton of theory." I probably would not have agreed with you in the beginning of this program, but with a bit of pride and a pound of excited enthusiasm, I wholeheartedly agree with the notion that nurses must develop their political acumen and become more involved in legislation related to the profession. I am one hundred percent sure that the reason my attitude has changed is because of the instruction I have received in my studies in policy and politics. Joining the American Nurses Association and the state nurses association and becoming a "lurker" of sorts has been the very first step in becoming involved for me. Without my enrollment in this program, I cannot readily say that I would have EVER joined. I've also been talking to other nurses who work in my department about their level of exposure to these organizations and explaining why it is important for them to gain knowledge of legislation as it relates to nursing, or in general. . . . I have learned to welcome cognitive dissonance, and use it as an opportunity to do several thing . . . such as examine my own opinions and attitudes, explore opposing views, and figure out exactly how to make my voice heard—whether through voting, lobbying, or writing/phoning/emailing representatives.

As one might surmise, the hot button political issue of health care for illegal immigrants engaged the students in a healthy debate. Many of the students commented for or against the issue, identified that their assumptions were flawed, and readily recognized how these flawed assumptions could influence behaviors related to taking care of an illegal immigrant. The purpose of engaging students in critical reflection and dialogue for perspective transformation was accomplished, thus meeting several course outcomes.

The macroleadership course also includes an application assignment. Students participate in a *Nurse's Day at the Capitol* activity where learners can observe the political strategy of lobbying in action. Student involvement in the event includes visits with state representatives to discuss policy issues affecting nursing, followed by participation in a rally where nurses, students, and stakeholders from throughout the state gather on the front steps of the state capitol to advocate for nursing issues. Short, but powerful, speeches are delivered by legislators and key leadership figures in nursing and state politics. Following this activity, students are required to address the following questions in a short paper: (1) What assumptions did you have about this event before attending? (2) How did your perspectives transform after attending the event? (3) If you experienced no transformation of perspectives, state why you believe this is the case, and (4) Identify three lessons learned and how the lessons can help in your role as a policy advocate.

A final transformative learning activity used in the macrosystem course is a *leadership case study analysis*. To enhance decision making as related to systems, students select and analyze two case studies from a list developed by course faculty related to social, economic, and cultural factors impacting health care delivery. Learners answer a series of questions for each case study. Answers must include sound rationales citing professional evidence-based literature. Students then post answers to a designated area within a course management system. Each student reads two other students' postings and responds by identifying assumptions in the posting and by offering alternative ways of thinking about the case. Several examples illustrate how this learning activity is successful in promoting student reflection about personal assumptions and enhancing thinking related to alternative ways of looking at an issue:

> One *assumption* in this case was that the nurse assigned to the case was capable of handling the patient. Graduate nurses should be ready for anything. Although this may be true, it is not always practical. I agree with . . . [the] assessment that she should have [been] placed [with] a more experienced nurse on this case. She also mentioned that a male nurse might have been more practical, too. Here, again, is another *assumption*. A new male graduate nurse might have been just as uncomfortable. I really like . . . alternative plans. Her reward system to motivate and retain nurses sounds great. Everyone needs a pat on the back now and then. Likewise, staff input is useful. Oftentimes, the people in the trenches know more about what is going on than the "higher ups." Finally, I would also suggest counseling for this patient. What is making him act out? If his behavior is so inappropriate that it runs off the staff, perhaps there is something going on that we are missing.
>
> I would agree . . . that one should not compromise personal beliefs in order to meet professional goals. However, I believe I would agree to speak and offer my clinical expertise. An *assumption* is made that your clinical expertise will . . . sway the legislators to pass the bill. In actuality, there are other possibilities. If you believe that physician assisted suicide is wrong, this gives you the opportunity to be in the position to possibly stop passage of the bill.
>
> An *alternate way of thinking* would be that you could sway legislators against the bill and still have the opportunity to meet a pivotal goal in your professional career. The governor may not like that you did not side with him but you could still offer your expertise and present the facts and consequences of the bill in a way that would allow you to stay true to your religious and moral beliefs. In addition, you would not have to be concerned about how your love ones would feel. You may not have another opportunity to be in a position to make a change in something you believe is wrong. This is a perfect opportunity to be a nurse advocate . . . standing up for what you believe is right for patients and families when faced with end of life decisions.

As one might surmise in any learning activity used to stimulate sociopolitical knowledge, and for that matter transformational leadership thinking, ethics or ethical decision making is involved. Development of ethical comportment is one of the calls for reform in nursing education and is critical to becoming a nurse to fulfill the profession's obligations to society. For examples of the leadership case studies referred to in the discussion above, see Appendix A.

ETHICS

Presentation of ethics content varies across programs and educational levels from being threaded throughout the curriculum to being taught as separate courses within the curriculum or being taught within philosophy departments. One outcome from the extensive studies regarding nursing education conducted by the Carnegie Foundation for the Advancement of Teaching (2007) was the recognition of three apprenticeships for professional development (cognitive, skilled know-how, ethical comportment) deemed as critical for nurses' ability to deliver safe and competent care. One of the apprenticeships identified has direct implications for teaching ethical, and to a degree, legal issues and includes concepts of ethical standards, ethical comportment, and social roles and responsibilities of the profession (Carnegie Foundation of the Advancement of Teaching, 2007). While it is important for nurses to have a working knowledge of ethical theories, principles, and standards, until and unless application occurs, the concepts will remain elusive in many students' view. Ethical behaviors are critical for nursing as a profession, and these behaviors must be practiced and demonstrated by every nurse in every practice setting. Ethical behaviors, which encompass ethical comportment, are attributes that should not be viewed as "nice if the nurse is"; rather, they should be expected characteristics of nurses (Polifroni, 2007).

There are no set of rules, tools, or skills that definitively label the traits one must have to be considered ethical. Knowledge of ethical principles, such as veracity, integrity, justice, and beneficence can translate to ethical behaviors resulting in application of the principles into a nurse's practice. There are those who would argue that a person cannot be taught to be ethical, to which we heartedly disagree. While teaching/learning is a process, a lifelong process, the foundational groundwork can be laid in nursing curricula, where ethical behaviors are not only expected in students but also role modeled by faculty. Fairness and justice are exhibited in faculty behaviors regarding student assessment and evaluation. Respect for each student is apparent in class and clinical settings. Any form, level, or degree of student dishonesty, including cheating, is not tolerated, from signing the attendance for an absent classmate to verified plagiarism. Faculty directness and openness with students regarding potential infractions in a caring atmosphere sets boundaries and the tone for an ethical environment, where principles are espoused and demonstrated.

Ethical situations and dilemmas abound in every health care setting and clinical specialty and require the nurse to be a part of a team that undoubtedly will face difficult decision making. Case study-based discussions related to patient care situations, current workforce issues, and relational challenges, such as those between nurse and physician, are an excellent faculty approach to promote critical dialogue and an avenue for students to explore feelings. An important beginning phase for the nurse in becoming an ethical practitioner is self-reflection regarding personal and professional values. When faculty members incorporate case scenarios in seminars, in which ethical and professional values are linked to practice, indirect valuing of the ethical content may be the outcome (Aiken & Catalano, 1994). Indirectly acquiring values occurs in the myriad of one's personal life and work experiences, which can present as lessons to be learned, decisions to be made, and encounters made in daily living. The process of value clarification for nursing students can begin with a simple faculty-selected tool from the numerous choices that are available. One such tool calls for a ranking of work values, such as satisfaction, competence, and working alone, from most to least important. Students reflect on personal values and become aware of how alternate value selection by peers might influence decision making and one's approach to resolution in the workplace.

It must be emphasized that most nursing students are going to enter the workforce with a level of insecurity and lack of confidence regarding how to approach true ethical dilemmas or when to take an ethical stand. The Code of Ethics for Nurses (American Nurses Association, 2010) provides guidelines for the nurse, delineating actions reflective of ethical behaviors and obligations of the profession. Confidence will deepen as ethical behaviors, rooted in these principles and standards, are practiced.

Transformative Learning Strategies

The move from teacher-dominated, lecture-focused delivery to a transformative approach involving interactive dialogue is appropriate for ethical content that is established as critically important knowledge for a nurse. However, this content can challenge educators who wish to actively engage learners in a learning experience that students may not value because of the somewhat complex and abstract nature of ethical principles. Park (2003) reminds educators that learners who actively engage in what they are studying tend to understand more, learn more, remember more, enjoy it more, and are more able to appreciate the relevance of what they have learned than learners who passively receive what is being taught (p. 183).

Based on the assumption that legal and ethical concepts might become lost in our integrated curriculum, the faculty created an *ethical seminar* utilizing transformative approaches. Junior and senior students attend the joint seminar; attendance at the seminar twice in the program emphasizes to the student the importance and value the faculty place on the presented concepts. Case scenarios and real-world patient care concerns are the backdrop for engaging students in critical reflection and dialogue. Initially, the students are together for briefing and are presented with scenarios, followed by placement into smaller junior- and senior-level groups. Senior students serve as facilitators and lead the group in a discussion of the scenario. A faculty member serves as a co-learner, role model, and provocateur by pointing out assumptions and how individual points of view may influence thinking and behaviors. Aiken and Catalano (1994) make the point that when case scenarios are used in group seminars in which ethical and professional values are linked to practice, indirect valuing of ethical content may be the outcome.

It is our position that ethical and professional behaviors are intricately linked, and one cannot exist without the other. Transformative learning approaches can also raise awareness of the importance of embracing what it means to be an ethical professional. One such transformative approach of critical reflection and dialogue is used by the faculty in a senior-level professional concept course to encourage students to examine past habits of mind and frames of references as well as current points of view related to their *self-concept of a nurse*. The faculty member realizes the challenge of creating a safe, trusting classroom environment to allow students freedom to honestly and realistically appraise nurse behaviors and characteristics, which have been observed during clinical rotations. Serving in the role of encourager, facilitator, co-learner, and role model faculty creates the environment where students are confident that they can openly voice their assumptions. Students' habits of mind may have been shaped at an early age by an encounter with a nurse through personal experience, a hospitalized family member, or through exposure to popular culture via television or other media.

Faculty begin the learning activity with dialogue, asking the students to identify what were their perceptions of being a nurse before they began nursing school. Typically, it takes the students a few minutes to collect their thoughts and begin sharing. Remarks have included descriptions such as genuine, hard working, knowledgeable, smart, compassionate, quick-acting and confident. The faculty then asks the learners to share behaviors of nurses observed in clinical settings since beginning clinical experiences. Positive behaviors associated with nurses included competent, caring, creative, and good organizational skills. However, negative nurse behaviors are often cited in greater numbers by the majority of students and include uncaring, tired, wasteful, rude, unsafe, bitter, sloppy, condescending, lazy, and bad attitude.

While it is critical for the learner to emulate professional nurse attributes, the faculty leads the dialogue regarding consequences of assumptions, which may be based on prior points of view. While these isolated behaviors may have been observed, faculty cautions students not to generalize and label the entire nursing workforce as unprofessional and, further, to choose not to emulate those behaviors. Alternative ways of thinking are offered by faculty and student comments. As dialogue about nursing professionalism continues, ethical behaviors and moral courage become part of the discussion. Students begin to question negative behaviors observed in the clinical setting. The question then becomes, which behaviors do the students want to emulate? Brookfield (2009) posited that one's assumptions are the "conceptual glue that holds our perspectives, meaning schemes and habits of mind in place" (p. 294).

The transformative nurse educator assumes the role of co-learner when challenging students to see the broad range of behaviors, encouraging learners

BOX 7.2   Ethical Case Study Analysis/Asynchronous Dialogue

To develop analytical skills and the ability to concisely articulate points of view related to ethics, each student is required to participate in two ethical case studies by:

- Responding to questions posed for each case study
- Supporting answers with sound rationales using evidence
- Reading two other student's postings (responses to case questions) and offering support and/or refute of responses in one to two paragraphs
- Posting responses in the appropriate discussion room by due dates and times

Responses to peers must include identification of possible hidden assumptions and a comment about how these assumptions might impact decision making related to the ethical dilemma.

to not consider identifying behaviors as the learning outcome but rather considering that desired behaviors provide impetus for decision making related to assuming the role of an ethical professional nurse. Ultimately, the goal is for each student to change meaning perspectives related to professional and ethical nursing behaviors. Examples of further transformative learning activities that are used in a graduate ethics course are found in Box 7.2.

CONCLUSIONS

Transformative nurse educators understand that transformative learning does not occur until there is a behavior change and must be aware that changes in behavior may occur suddenly or over time. The journey of transformation from a nursing student to a professional nurse is a process. Building nurse leaders begins with foundational knowledge of leadership and management principles, a respect for the importance of public policy, and practice of ethical behaviors. These critically necessary concepts are the cornerstone of professional nursing practice without which the nurse cannot have a voice at the table or the courage to navigate in today's complex health care environment. Transformative approaches of critical dialogue and self-reflective thinking are well suited to teaching these abstract concepts, which students often do not embrace as the "nuts and bolts" of nursing as no skill is being performed on a patient. Astute faculty will bring the concepts to life in a transformative environment with strategies that challenge students' assumptions and promote critical reflection embedding an appreciation and desire for continued learning and a lifelong path to becoming an ethical leader.

Further research is needed similar to the study conducted by Morris and Faulk (2007) in which findings revealed changes in RN to BSN student behaviors, specifically in leadership and policy advocacy roles after using transformative learning approaches. These studies will add to the body of evidence regarding transformative learning as pedagogy in nursing education. For additional examples of transformative learning activities for teaching public policy and ethics, see Appendix A.

REFERENCES

Aiken, T. D., & Catalano, J. T. (1994). *Legal, ethical and political issues in nursing.* Philadelphia, PA: F.A. Davis.

American Nurses Association. (2010). *Code of ethics for nurses with interpretive statements.* Silver Spring, MD: Author.

Benner, P., Sutphen, M., Leonard, B., & Day, L. (2010). *Educating nurses: A call for radical transformation.* San Francisco, CA: Jossey-Bass.

Bowen, M., Lyons, K. J., Young, B. E. (2000). Nursing and health care reform: Implication for curriculum development. *Journal of Nursing Education, 39*(1), 27–33.

Brookfield, S. D. (2009). Engaging critical reflection in corporate America. In J. Mezirow & E. W. Taylor, & Associates (Ed.), *Transformative learning in practice: Insights from community, workplace and higher education.* San Francisco, CA: Jossey-Bass.

Buerhaus P. (1992). Teaching health care public policy. *Nursing and Health Care Perspectives, 13*(6), 304–309.

Carnegie Foundation for the Advancement of Teaching. (2007). *Study of Nursing Education*. Retrieved from http://www.carnegiefoundation.org/nursing-education

Committee on the Robert Wood Johnson Foundation Initiative on the Future of Nursing at the Institute of Medicine. (2010). *A summary of the February 2010 forum on the future of nursing: Education*. Retrieved from http://www.nap.edu/catalogue/12894.html

Conger, C. O., & Johnson, P. (2000). Integrating political involvement and nursing education. *Nurse Educator, 25*(2), 99–103.

Cranton, P. (2006). *Understanding and promoting transformative learning: A guide for educators of adults* (2nd ed.). San Francisco, CA: Jossey-Bass.

Kirkpatrick, M. K., & Brown, S. T. (2006). Leadership development in geriatric care through the Intergeneration Makes a Difference project. *Nursing Education Perspectives, 27*(2), 89–92.

McCallister, M., Venturato, L., Johnston, A., Rowe, J., Tower, M., & Moyle, W. (2006). Solution focused teaching: A transformative approach to teaching nursing. *International Journal of Nursing Education Scholarship, 3*(1), 1–13.

McWilliam, C. L. (2007). Continuing education at the cutting edge: Promoting transformative knowledge translation. *Journal of Continuing Education in the Health Professions, 27*(2), 72–79.

Morris, A. H., & Faulk, D. R. (2007). Perspective transformation: Enhancing the development of professionalism in RN to BSN students. *Journal of Nursing Education 46*(10), 445–451.

Park, C. (2003). Engaging students in the learning process: The learning journal. *Journal of Geography in Higher Education, 27*(2), 183–199.

Polifroni, E. C. (2007). Ethical knowing and nursing education. *Journal of Nursing Education, 46*(1) 3.

Porche, D. J. (2012). *Health policy: Application for nurses and other health care professionals*. Sudbury, MA: Jones and Bartlett Learning.

Reutter, L., & Williamson, D. L. (2000). Advocating healthy public policy: Implication for Baccalaureate nursing education. *Journal of Nursing Education, 39*(1), 21–26.

8

The Road to Professionalism: Transformative Learning for Professional Role Development

Arlene H. Morris and Debbie R. Faulk

> *To learn to be a nurse, one needs to think like a nurse, perform like a nurse, and act like a nurse.*
>
> —Authors

"Being professional" calls us to be our "best selves." The way we teach will form professional behaviors. Professionalism is an elusive concept and is often defined as a process that is dynamic, unpredictable, and highly individual based on personal characteristics, background, and life events. Professionalization, or professional socialization, is the process that manifests as the acceptance of a discipline's attitudes and values and is demonstrated through behaviors (Faulk, Parker, & Morris, 2010). Professional socialization involves two components: primary socialization, which occurs during childhood as a person learns the norms of the family and society, and secondary socialization, which occurs as a process that a person experiences throughout adulthood to meet the demands of social and workplace needs (Howkins & Ewens, 1998). Nurse educators are concerned with secondary socialization and resocialization of students in the development of a professional role identity. In the socialization process, the student has had little to no prior experience with the occupational genre and actually begins initial exposure to knowledge, values (attitudes), and behaviors (skills) through education, thus providing opportunity for decision regarding whether to integrate these values and behaviors into the individual's worldview and life choices.

In resocialization, a person brings a prior background of experience and substantive exposure to the profession, perhaps in differing roles. Then, through education, life, or work events, the person chooses to take on further knowledge, values, and behaviors over a period of time or in response to a triggering event. Hinshaw (1977) and Price (2008) suggest that socialization and/or resocialization can occur throughout the professional life of a nurse when assuming new positions and/or roles or when continuing education. We believe that the process of becoming (socialization) and transforming (resocialization) can be facilitated through learning activities using transformative learning approaches and will take a different *road* to professionalism by considering individual professional development in light of Shulman's (2002) way of looking at learning to encourage development of a professional role identity.

The following example demonstrates progression toward a professional role, leading to a commitment to a newly understood behavior:

> Noel had a dream—a dream of returning to school to obtain a master's degree in nursing. After ten years of practicing as a nurse on an oncology unit, her dream became a reality. She applied and was accepted into an RN to MSN completion program. She was determined to have an open mind as she engaged in the learning journey. Noel was aware that engagement was important to her learning, and began almost immediately to self-reflect on prior learning and understanding. Her most profound understanding occurred during a seminar on end-of life issues. During this seminar, Noel discovered Betty Neuman's Nursing Theory (1995), and desired to apply the concepts in providing care for patients who experience chemotherapy. Noel began to look at the lines of defense of the individual patients and assess for ways that the treatment for their cancer was threatening these defenses and possibly exceeding the clients' resources. However, she noticed that some individuals responded in vastly different ways to the stressor of chemotherapy, seemingly refuting her new knowledge about stress and adaptation. She reflected on her actions, the responses of those in her care, and on various content that she had learned in her nursing program. In her reflection, she identified that some of the clients had discussed with her a strong support system, and she began to consider how systems theory might also impact the outcome of those in her care. She determined to assess individual and family roles and responsibilities, adaptation to changes secondary to the illness and treatment, and to explore other resources for the family system.

SHULMAN'S TABLE OF LEARNING

In his work related to professional development, Shulman (1999) articulated that professional education must have at its core the thought of ongoing "individual and collective learning." Professional development begins with foundational knowledge but continues as an individual constantly engages, understands, and acts on knowledge, thus allowing the individual to continually be developing a professional role identity. As individuals participate in conversations about what is being learned, new insights arise. These insights may be related to existing theory, refute existing theory, or lead to new theoretical propositions. From discussions in larger circles of the discipline (or professional academy), the collective knowledge of a profession is ever growing and expanding.

Learning to be a professional, according to Shulman (2005), involves more than cognitive resources or understanding alone:

> It [professional development] is preparation for accomplished and responsible practice in the service of others. It is preparation for "good work." Professionals must learn abundant amounts of theory and vast bodies of knowledge. They must come to understand in order to act, and they must act in order to serve. (p. 53)

Learners must perform the skills pertinent to the profession, as well as understand the rationales in how to practice or act within the values and established standards of the professional discipline. Action implies the development and internalization of a set of values and commitments. As nurses begin to take on or transform a professional role identity, they integrate ability and character to create a direction for practice.

Shulman (1998) suggests that "the professional educator's challenge is to help future professionals develop and shape a robust moral vision that will guide their practice and provide a prism of justice, responsibility and virtue through which to reflect on their actions" (p. 516). Teaching an individual to be a professional is difficult at best, and some may even say impossible. However, working from the belief that professionalism can be taught, nurse educators can address the challenges of teaching professional behaviors within the framework of Shulman's (2002) Table of Learning. Shulman conceptualizes six elements of learning, which are visualized on a circle as pairs of educational ends (and means), suggesting that learning is situational rather than a lock-step process. According to Shulman, information can be obtained from others or from technology but remains only in a person's mind. Knowledge and understanding must be used and is refined in its application. Shulman further suggests that learners have the opportunity to engage with content in various ways and gain ownership over the learning and the outcome(s) of learning. Professional learning may begin at any stage within the dynamic cycle.

Shulman (2002) proposes as a possible initial stage in the cycle that learners must be active, or *engage*, in the learning process. This leads to the *understanding* of knowledge to the extent that a learner can restate the content in his or her personal words, thus "owning" the knowledge. Using the knowledge in an active manner may involve practicing the knowledge to perform psychomotor skills or *performing an action* to gain knowledge in another setting than that where the learning occurred. For example, nurses may use knowledge regarding hemodynamic balance in performance of blood pressure monitoring or may assess blood pressure to obtain knowledge of a person's hemodynamic balance or imbalance. This differs from memorization of actions to take in specific situations (such as the rule "sit and dangle prior to ambulation").

Action is related to *critical reflection*, including the knowledge of rationales, or why the particular action was selected, and what the anticipated results are. Thus, action is paired with critical reflection on the cycle of learning as critical reflection is necessary for selecting an action. *Judgment* is paired with understanding and is the appropriate application of knowledge in various settings, considering complex and shifting factors or standards, to determine a judgment regarding an action or situation. From the judgment, actions or interventions can be designed. Clinical nursing actions are based on judgment, leading to selection of a course of action (design of a plan for client care) and are continuously dynamic to assess for information or knowledge that would require an alteration in judgment. Judgment and use of knowledge can precipitate change in an individual's character, such that the learning becomes part of their identity. Learners then become *committed* to continuous learning and transformation of perspectives, thus leading back to commitment's paired element, *engagement* in new learning.

These elements of learning or educational means and ends can be combined with transformative learning principles and approaches to enhance design of learning activities and for creative methods for evaluating learning. The flexibility allows learners to demonstrate various elements in different settings or across the nursing curriculum throughout progression along a professionalism continuum.

ELEMENTS OF LEARNING FOR TRANSFORMATION WITHIN A PROFESSIONAL ROLE IDENTITY

Nurse educators, when considering Shulman's elements of learning (2002) in relation to development of professional role identity, realize that individuals may enter educational settings with some level of *commitment* to professionalism. Other learners may not begin their education with any commitment to professional behaviors but rather become *engaged* with nursing content and experience disorienting dilemmas that promote critical reflection and discourse. The discourse, either with peers, faculty, or other nursing experts, contributes to cognitive dissonance. From cognitive dissonance and reflection, learners must make a choice to engage in learning and change actions based upon new understandings. For example, learners may have observed nurses documenting before performing nursing interventions. Exposure to the Code of Ethics for nurses may trigger a disorienting dilemma and reflection involving questioning the values of the profession and their own values, leading to a decision to commit to behaviors more reflective of professional standards. Learners may then choose to revise behaviors or not. Learners' behaviors are observed through actions taken in practice settings. However, some learners will not commit to professional behaviors as a characteristic of their identity—professional actions or behaviors will not be observed in a nursing student or graduate. Again, the challenge to nurse educators is to guide learners to make judgments using technical and moral understanding to balance incongruencies between ideal situations and what is feasible in work environments.

Initial engagement with nursing concepts is where professional identity takes root and can occur at any point within nursing education or practice. Major events or small suggestions can stimulate critical reflection, which then develops into a personal commitment to professional behaviors such that professional characteristics become part of an individual's identity. The very individualism of learners contributes to the variability in what triggers the critical reflection and often relates to prior personal experience or consideration of personal points of view. The faculty and other observers cannot pinpoint a specific point in time that the commitment occurred but can only observe the behaviors.

THE ROAD TO PROFESSIONALISM IN NURSING

Professionalism from the nursing perspective has been debated for many decades, influenced by historical events and evolution of the scope of nursing practice. There are a plethora of books and articles that address the issue of professionalism from profession and individual perspectives. For example, professionalism is discussed as it relates to levels of education, pathways toward professionalism, conceptualization of the professional role, how professionalism is measured, or historical and system barriers to professionalism.

Controversy related to professionalization of nurses is rooted in a focus on differences rather than similarities. Brockett (1991) suggests:

> One way to work toward a common identity is to emphasize an approach to professional development that is not limited solely to mastery of the skills one needs in order to perform effectively. Instead, this approach would emphasize that each of us needs to understand both the "big picture" of the field and how each of us can make a unique contribution to it. (p. 5)

Cranton (1996) echoes this assertion by stating "the process of learning about practice is one that transcends many of our differences" (p. 162).

We conceptualize professionalism along a continuum, with cognition, skills, and attitudes involved in the development of habits of mind that result in professional behaviors. Huber (2000, p. 81) proposes categories of development from nonprofessional, to semiprofessional, to professional during the process of professionalization of occupations. However, we question categorization of individual nurses or learners with these labels. We suggest considering professionalization on a continuum, whereby individuals continuously develop professional characteristics, potentially lifelong. For example, a commitment to quality involves a desire to seek evidence for practice, which may include continuing education. Additionally, nurses must adhere to ethical principles, but the fluidity of application increases with further experiences and professional development. Awareness of responsibility to give back to the community may develop early or later in an individual's nursing career, as does growth and self-confidence in self-regulation and autonomy. These characteristics may develop separately, or may occur simultaneously, depending on individual backgrounds and situations. Lifelong learning necessitates continual commitment to develop in professionalism.

The road to professionalism in nursing often begins as learners engage in empirical content and participate in various learning activities that require reflection, judgment, and action to gain understanding for application in class and clinical settings. For example, students are socialized within nursing education to be aware of physical, psychosocial, developmental, and emotional client needs through using a holistic perspective. They are taught skill performance according to evidence-based practice guidelines, Quality and Safety Education for Nurses recommendations, National Database for Nursing Quality Indicators, The Joint Commission, Centers for Disease Control nursing innovations standards, and other guidelines as appropriate for content. Nursing students are taught to look for opportunities to address health literacy, health promotion, and illness management across the life span, considering family and community resources.

When students enter the workforce, they continue socialization. They may observe nurses who do not adhere to the practices they learned during nursing education, who take shortcuts that endanger clients, other health care delivery team members, or themselves. The challenge is for nursing graduates to develop a commitment to quality care, such that the commitment is part of their character or identity, and the learner continues these behaviors in spite of the temptation to compromise professional behaviors. In this manner, the new graduate can determine safe alternatives in specific situations or seek additional evidence on which to base their practice. The new graduate becomes a change agent within the health care delivery system.

As Shulman (1998) notes, "A profession is a practice whose agents claim is rooted in bodies of knowledge that are created, tested, elaborated, refuted, transformed, and reconstituted." (pp. 516–517). However, professional recognition in nursing does not occur only upon completion of a program of education, certification, or licensure. Rather, the road to professionalism continues daily, as choices in habits of mind, valuing, and professional behaviors are made. Awareness of the Code of Ethics and Standards of Practice are critical touchstones but not the only criteria for professionalization.

Instructional design for nursing education must balance values, understanding, and application of theoretical content as the basis for clinical behaviors, rather than rote memorization of a sequence of steps for clinical nursing skills. The dichotomy for educators and learners is to balance what is known as "best practices" with a spirit of inquiry to understand not only the rationales for the best practices but also to value identification of the underlying premises in efforts to continuously improve practice. For example, in a clinical setting, a student provides care for an older woman who recalls having a soft formed bowel movement everyday for the past 60 years. She is admitted to have assessments to rule out physical causes contributing to what she defines as chronic constipation. Her repeated straining has resulted in large hemorrhoids, which contribute to pain with defecation. She receives treatment for hemorrhoids as an initial approach. However, learners demonstrating a spirit of inquiry will also question hydration status and side effects of the medication she has recently begun to take for anxiety. Continued communication and interaction with the woman reveal fear of her body failing to function as it always did, then expression of fear of dying, then her expression of extreme spiritual distress. Therapeutic communication and resources to meet the woman's actual needs more effectively meet the underlying needs precipitating her anxiety for which she had been medicated, thus beginning the cycle. Professional nurses and nursing students with a spirit of inquiry are able to identify underlying issues rather than providing minimal quality of care by only carrying out orders for hemorrhoid treatment.

Professional development of nurses must include emphasis on the valuing of inquiry and reflection. In the socialization and resocialization process, nursing educators must design instruction to promote development of learner understanding and motivation, to facilitate the learners' commitment to then understand the underlying needs and motivations of those for whom care is provided.

TRANSFORMATIVE LEARNING FOR A PROFESSIONAL ROLE IDENTITY

The goal for learners in nursing is professionalization, which includes taking on the professional role identity through the process of lifelong learning, reflection, and transformation to commitment to quality in all actions. All learning experiences should be created with professionalization as the goal. Nursing educators must be mindful that situations beyond their control, influence learner reflection, and that critical reflection may lead to transformation in different dimensions of an individual (e.g., spiritual, relational, emotional, social, etc.). Transformation in any dimension influences the process of professionalization.

During planned learning activities for transformative learning, educators must be aware that some triggering events may be happenstance. For example, learners have expressed that a single sentence regarding nurse autonomy and personal accountability caused cognitive dissonance between awareness of the value of nurse autonomy and responsibility for clinical judgment compared to prior perceptions of the role of nurse as passive as portrayed in the media. Another example of a happenstance triggering event occurred when a visiting author stated nursing is not as much about caring as it is about intellect. This statement created a disorienting dilemma for a majority of junior- and senior-level nursing students at one school of nursing, leading to an opportunity to discuss the knowledge–caring dyad.

Learning activities that stimulate understanding within and among the various patterns of knowing (empirical, aesthetic, ethical, personal, political, unknowing; see Chapter 2, "Transformative Educator Roles Within the Context of Patterns of Knowing") can be planned to begin professional role identity. For example, identifying a nursing self-concept and philosophy of nursing in a journaling assignment or online threaded discussion often includes understanding in empirical, ethical, personal, and unknowing patterns, which leads to judgment required to complete the assignment. Problem-based or problem-directed learning activities such as case studies, simulations, or prioritization activities often necessitate use of empirical, aesthetic, ethical, and unknowing understanding for decisions and clinical judgments, which then contribute to professional socialization in various roles of the nurse. Understanding and application of concepts of leadership and management involve empirical, personal, ethical, and political knowing, resulting in judgment for clinical or institutional decisions required by a developing professional.

Activities to inspire learner reflection include exposure to nursing content and discussion with faculty or peers in various learning environments. Awareness of differences in points of view and habits of mind of individuals with whom learners learn, with whom they will work, and for whom they care includes empirical, ethical, personal, political, and unknowing patterns. The reflection regarding previously unconsidered possibilities may lead to cognitive dissonance, leading to further reflection until a point of view is determined. Action will occur based on the substantiated or new point of view and thus become a new habit of mind.

As educators and learners, we must keep our eye on the learning process and how the process relates to professional role identity. We desire that knowledge, which is inside learners, will move outward as displayed by professional behaviors/actions in all situations. We also strive for outside knowledge to become internalized. This inward and outward movement of knowledge (Shulman, 1999) is demonstrated through professional behaviors, further reflection, then commitment to professionalism, such that it becomes the very identity of a nurse.

Examples of Transformative Learning Activities

An example of a planned learning activity involves having students identify behaviors characteristic of the profession. After the discussion, students then self-reflect to identify their personal development along a continuum that represents each of the identified behaviors. The level of cognitive dissonance may vary among individual beginning students, among students with prior experience in nursing, or those pursuing graduate education toward a different nursing role.

In another planned learning activity, learners are asked to write their professional self-concepts in a beginning professional transition course. These are shared with other learners, who then identify assumptions or implied values within the professional self-concept. Identified assumptions and values are next discussed with a peer. The faculty make comments related to the identification of assumptions and values and offer alternative ways of thinking about professional self-concept. This learning activity is revisited during the final semester when students are asked to write another professional self-concept and compare to the initial self-concept by identifying any changes in values, beliefs, and behaviors. This is sometimes emotional for students who could initially not articulate a professional self-concept. For example, one RN to BSN student noted that the reflection about a professional self-concept resulted in an array of emotions when the student realized that prior nursing actions may not have been professional. This student also noted that many prior actions were based solely on rote memory and not on evidence-based rationales. In the words of two students:

> The "Perspective Transformation Journey" has changed my prior "habits of mind" in describing myself as a professional nurse in that I have developed a sense of the importance of being informed as a professional nurse in terms of research and EBP studies. I have also realized the importance of being politically active. I would summarize my professional self-concept to be the awareness of the importance of being informed on everything affecting me as a nurse professionally. It is important to not only closely follow the changes in [healthcare] but to also be informed on the political changes that affect the nursing profession at the state and national levels.

> The term professional takes on a whole new meaning for me. I have retrained my mind in thinking that not everyone in a profession is a professional. I still believe that being a professional comes from experience and not just a degree, but experience evolves with education. I have noticed a change in myself since nearly completing this program. I believe that I am more prepared now to present myself as a professional.

An additional planned learning activity involves individual learners identifying their personal values through a value clarification activity. Individual values are then compared with the National League for Nursing (NLN) and Commission on Collegiate Nursing Education (CCNE) values identified as essential for nurses. The activity generates tremendous critical dialogue as learners find it difficult to discern that, many times, their identified values are the same as NLN and CCNE, although stated in differing verbiage. Faculty initially function in the roles of expert in introducing NLN and CCNE websites and background to learners, then transition to the roles within the ethical pattern of knowing: facilitator, prober, encourager, dialogue prompter, and provocateur (see Chapter 2, "Transformative Learning Through the Lens of the Teacher"). Cognitive dissonance occurs in some learners if they identify personal discrepancy with or a lack of awareness of the essential nursing values. Further reflection may lead to identification of personal or nursing values that have conflicted with the learners' own past behaviors. This value clarification activity can also be used by professional staff development educators as potentially an annual event during which all employees reconsider personal and professional values compared to values essential in nursing.

An example of a planned transformative learning activity within the ethical pattern of knowing involves the use of case studies, brief scenarios, simulation events, or post-clinical conference discussions to create opportunities for critical reflection and dialogue about situations in which ethical decisions are involved. Faculty function in the role of expert, guides discussion regarding the Code of Ethics for Nurses as a basis for decisions and in the use of ethical decision-making models. Faculty members then transition to other roles as learners are encouraged to engage in self or group dialogue to identify personal assumptions, potential effects of those assumptions on patient outcomes, and then determine alternatives to prior thinking. From these reflections, best options for ethical resolution to the situation may be considered. Again, this type of learning activity can be used in professional staff development to keep ethical comportment in the forefront of practice.

In yet another planned example, RN students are asked to complete a *Perspective Transformation Portfolio* whereby they reflect upon progression of professionalization by identifying specific examples that demonstrate each phase of perspective transformation (see Chapter 1, "Phases of Perspective Transformation") and to link specific learning activities to the resocialization process. Several students stated:

> From a professional standpoint, I see myself as an ever-evolving person. I believe that because of my capacity to possess an open mind and learn new things, even at the expense of my current way of thinking, I have the capacity to change and create change in my immediate surroundings as well as my world. I believe that as a result of the . . . program, I have become an effective agent for change in my facility as well as my profession, and I plan to exercise my voice as well as my rights. I believe in empowerment; empowering coworkers, clients, and families helps to shape the health care world as we see it and helps it progress to new heights.

> A disorienting dilemma I personally experienced during this journey would be the [required] volunteer hours. I volunteered at a mission . . . that outreached to recovering drug addicts. It was heart breaking . . . to visualize and hear the stories of the recovering addicts. . . . This experience opened my eyes to the problem of substance abuse and made me realize that its destruction is alive and well in my local area. . . . This experience made me realize how important volunteer work and community outreach is and how many people it helps. . . . In undergoing self-examination, I did not realize how many assumptions I had about different topics or issues. The activities that helped me with this would be the portfolio project that we started in our first semester. Analyzing work experiences and identifying assumptions and alternate ways of thinking really was a "wake up call" for me personally. These activities helped me to see both sides of the issue. I believe the analyses have allowed me to identify my personal assumptions to allow me to be fairer when faced with similar situations in the future.

A blog is used in an online professional transformation course to enhance critical reflection and discourse and to increase awareness related to numerous current and future issues impacting health care delivery and the professional nurse. Faculty members begin the blog by posing a question or comment such as:

> In their call for radical transformation of nursing education, Benner, Sutphen, Leonard, and Day (2010, pp. 111–112) articulate that nurse educators must

develop teaching and learning strategies that promote motivation for lifelong learning. Reflect upon strategies used in this program. Which teaching/learning strategies have motivated you to be a lifelong learner?

Nurses are members of a professional discipline and are therefore obligated to support the profession. Do you agree or disagree with this statement? Why or why not? Your nursing responsibilities do not end when you "clock off" work or at the end of your shift. Do you agree or disagree with this statement? Why or why not? And if you agree, what do your responsibilities include?

Learning to be a professional, according to Shulman (2005), involves more than cognitive resources, or understanding alone:

It [professional development] is preparation for accomplished and responsible practice in the service of others. It is preparation for "good work." Professionals must learn abundant amounts of theory and vast bodies of knowledge. They must come to understand in order to act, and they must act in order to serve (p. 53). Respond to Shulman's statement regarding professional development.

Students then participate in the blog by making substantive comments such as:

I agree that the responsibilities of being a nurse do not end after clocking out. It was not until I began this program that I really believed that statement. It has become clear to me that nurses are responsible for their profession and the profession will be as strong as the work nurses are willing to put into it. This responsibility involves extra involvement while not on the clock at work. This includes fighting for legislation to improve nursing ratios, salaries and standards, pursuing higher education and professional certifications, and participating in nursing practice councils. While nurses are on the clock, they are usually taking care of patients and using every available minute to do so. It is the time off of the clock when nurses can improve their working environment by taking an active stand in their profession and fighting to make it the best it can possibly be.

The day that we took our very first nursing exam during a traditional nursing program, it served as just one marker of our alleged commitment to learning how, when, and where we could devote our minds and bodies to the profession. Many of us chose a nursing career for so many varied reasons; however, the main goal and idea behind declaring this professional field is to remain undivided in our attention to serving the ill. I believe that we are obligated as nurses to put forth the best effort to deliver safe and efficient care. I agree with the proposed statement because it all resorts to the notion of doing unto others as you would have them do unto you. . . .

All of the above learning activities were planned. However, as stated previously, happenstance events may trigger cognitive dissonance, critical reflection, and dialogue leading to transformative learning. An example of a happenstance triggering event that can be revised for a planned learning activity involves storytelling. During a discussion regarding application of nursing theories to actual clinical situations as a professional characteristic, the faculty in the role of expert related examples of various patients and how nursing theories help to identify roles of the nurse in providing care. The faculty transitioned to various roles as students identified personal assumptions about the clients described, the use of nursing theories to guide thinking and

BOX 8.1 **Transformative Learning Activities for Professional Role Identity**

Transformative Learning Activity	Questions for Reflection
Read the following article: Cutcliff, J. G., & K. L., Wieck (2008). Salvation or damnation: Deconstructing nursing's aspirations to professional status. *Journal of Nursing Management, 16,* 499–507. Reflect on the accompanying questions.	1. What assumptions do the authors make related to professional status? 2. Are there alternative ways to think about professional status? If yes, state alternative ways of thinking. 3. What professional status do you believe that the nursing profession desires to obtain? 4. What role does the nurse–client relationship play in relation to the concept of professionalism?
Reflect on current points of view related to the relationship between power and professional nursing practice after reading the following article: Ponte, P.R., et al. (2007). The power of professional nursing practice—An essential element of patient and family centered care. Online Journal of Issues in Nursing (OJIN). Retrieved from http://www.nursingworld.org/MainMenuCategories/ANAMarketplace/ANAPeriodicals/OJIN/TableofContents/Volume122007/No1Jan07/tpc32_316092.html "Meet" a peer of choice in WIMBA Live Classroom® to dialogue about the article and reflect on the accompanying questions.	1. What were your points of view related to power and professionalism prior to reading this article? 2. What role do your current professional values play in behaviors or actions related to power and professional practice? 3. What assumptions do the authors make related to the use of power in the practice setting? 4. How can the information in this article relate to your professionalization?
Reflect on this question.	What is the relationship of professionalism to roles, values and philosophy?
Reflect on the following statement by Dr. Teal McAteer, "Transformative learning focuses on the relationship between personal change and learning."	Articulate how your learning over the past semester mirrors this assumption (or not).
Reflect upon the nursing philosophy you wrote in *Transformation to the Professional Nurse Role* and answer the accompanying questions.	1. Has your nursing philosophy changed in anyway? If yes, how? If no, why not? 2. What assumptions did you have about a nursing philosophy prior to this course? 3. Have your assumptions changed? If yes, how? If not, why not? 4. Why is it important for a professional nurse to have a nursing philosophy? 5. How will you use your philosophy in the future?

(continued)

BOX 8.1 *(continued)*

Throughout this program, a metaphor of a journey has been used to guide you through the educational quest. During this journey you have experienced transformations in your thinking related to a plethora of issues impacting the nursing profession.	1. Give serious thought to one specific area or issue about which your thinking has been emancipated or liberated from old ways of thinking and identify your new thinking.
	2. Identify which learning activity or activities were instrumental in your change in perspective.
	3. In no more than one to two paragraphs, describe how the use of the *perspective transformation journey* metaphor shaped your attitude or thinking.
Use Mezirow's Phases of Perspective Transformation (1991) that describe the process for a personal perspective transformation to answer the accompanying learning activity.	Reflect on your learning over the past year and identify specific examples of changes in thinking or behaviors that you believe demonstrate each phase of perspective transformation. If there was a learning activity that you can link to the phase, identify the activity.

identification of patient needs and outcomes, and the use of nursing theories to guide nursing behaviors to attain the desired outcomes. Learners expressed the challenge of critically reflecting on situations through "new eyes," and discovery of unrealized assumptions, leading to making choices about professional identity and behaviors as a developing nurse. See Box 8.1 for a list of further learning examples for professional role development.

CONCLUSIONS

The road to professionalism in nursing is never ending. Nursing is a professional discipline, which involves more than just learning facts. Although cognitive learning is critical as a foundation, application of facts and commitment in using knowledge is critical for nurses to uphold standards and contribute to improvements in health care delivery. Transformative learning fosters reflection, reevaluation, and decisions regarding engagement and commitment, understanding and judgment, and reflection and actions and is therefore an effective pedagogy for professional role development. If, as Shulman (2005) proposes, professions have signature pedagogies, transformative learning as a pedagogy for nursing education can "form habits of the mind, habits of the heart, and habits of the hand" (p. 59).

In Part II, Chapters 3 through 7, transformative learning was situated within various nursing courses, and although not course-specific, professionalism was discussed within the context of transformative learning in Chapter 8. We now turn our attention to Part III of transformative learning as it relates to various nursing education experiences.

REFERENCES

Benner, P., Sutphen, M., Leonard, B., & Day, L. (2010). *Educating nurses: A call for radical transformation.* San Francisco, CA: Jossey-Bass.

Brockett, R. G. (1991). Professional development, artistry, and style. In R. B. Brockett (Ed.), *Professional development for educators of adults. New directions for adult and continuing education, 51.* San Francisco, CA: Jossey-Bass.

Cranton, P. (1996). *Professional development as transformative learning: New perspectives for teachers of adults.* San Francisco, CA: Jossey-Bass.

Cutcliff, J. G., & K. L., Wieck (2008). Salvation or damnation: Deconstructing nursing's aspirations to professional status. *Journal of Nursing Management, 16,* 499–507.

Faulk, D., Parker, F., & Morris, A. H. (July, 2010). Reforming perspectives: MSN graduates' knowledge, attitudes and awareness of self-transformation (MS #2052). *International Journal of Nursing Education Scholarship, 7*(1), art. 24. doi: 10.2202/1548-923X.2052. Retrieved from http://www.bepress.com/ijnes/vol7/iss1/art24/?sending=11080.

Hinshaw, A. S. (1977). Socialization and resocialization of nurses for professional nursing practice. *The 16th Conference of the Council of Baccalaureate and Higher Degree Programs, 1976* (NLN Publication No. 15-1659, pp. 1–14). New York, NY: National League for Nursing.

Howkins, E. J., & Ewens, A. (1998). How students experience professional socialization. *International Journal of Nursing Studies, 35,* 41–49.

Huber, D. (2000). *Leadership and nursing care management* (2nd ed.). Philadelphia, PA: W. B. Saunders.

Mezirow, J. (1991). *Transformative dimensions of adult learning.* San Francisco, CA: Jossey-Bass.

Neuman, B. (1995). *The Neuman systems model* (3rd ed.). Norwalk, CT: Appleton & Lange.

Ponte, P. R., et al. (2007). The power of professional nursing practice—An essential element of patient and family centered care. Online Journal of Issues in Nursing (OJIN). Retrieved from http://www.nursingworld.org/MainMenuCategories/ANAMarketplace/ANAPeriodicals/OJIN/TableofContents/Volume122007/No1Jan07/tpc32_316092.html

Price, S. L. (2008). Becoming a nurse: A meta-study of early professional socialization and career choice in nursing. *Journal of Advanced Nursing, 65*(1), 11–19.

Shulman, L. S. (1998). Theory, practice, and the education of professionals. *The Elementary School Journal, 98*(5), 511–526.

Shulman, L. S. (1999). Taking learning seriously. *Change, 31*(4), 10–17.

Shulman, L. S. (2002). Making differences: A table of learning. *Change, 34*(6), 37.

Shulman, L. S. (2005). Signature pedagogies in the professions. *Daedalus, 134*(3), 52–59.

III

Situated Transformative Learning

9

Transformative Learning in Simulated Environments

Cam Hamilton and Arlene H. Morris

Nursing education is in a time of dramatic change and challenge . . . filled with many opportunities . . . getting started with simulations or to take the next step in using simulations in nursing education . . . will lead to a new model for high-quality teaching-learning and clinical education.
—Dr. Pamela R. Jeffries

Use of transformative learning approaches in combination with patient simulation, a current popular technology-based tool, allows learners to explore assumptions, beliefs, and values. This, in turn, empowers nursing students to become independent, critical thinkers with a capacity to make clinical judgments that are necessary to manage today's complex health care problems. Developing activities that stimulate critical reflection/self-reflection and dialogue within simulation scenarios, allows educators to set the stage for learners to examine personal points of view and then to try on alternate perspectives of other points of view. Guimond, Sole, and Salas (2001) note that cues can be integrated throughout simulated activities to evoke dialogue. Additionally, learners' previous knowledge and assumptions can be assessed to encourage critical thinking and reflection as the learners seek alternative solutions to the situation. As nurse educators consider using transformative learning approaches in simulated experiences, they must be aware of and plan for learners who may experience disorienting dilemmas by including time for discussion during debriefing and time for interaction with learners if desired at a later time.

The following assumptions guide educators at all levels of nursing education and in professional staff development in the creation of specific simulated experiences for transformative learning:

1. Simulation is an effective teaching tool for transformative learning.
2. Simulation experiences are driven by educational outcomes and matched to the learner level of education.
3. Physical, emotional, and contextual realism is integrated into simulation to actively engage learners in the simulation experience.

4. Simulation environments must be encouraging, positive, acknowledging, responsive, and supportive to promote reflective analysis, dialogue, and discovery.
5. Debriefing in simulation can either stimulate or help resolve disorienting dilemmas as learners reflect on other points of view, thus providing opportunity for dialogue and reflection with resultant potential changes in perspectives and/or behaviors.

SIMULATION IN NURSING EDUCATION

The most common types of simulation used in nursing education include anatomical models, task trainers, role playing, games, computer-assisted instruction, standardized patients, low- and high-fidelity simulation, and virtual reality. All levels of nursing education are incorporating these teaching tools into the curricula (Suplee & Solecki, 2011). In addition to isolated experiences within nursing programs, many larger schools are partnering with other disciplines to create collaborative simulation experiences to improve understanding of each other's roles and responsibilities to cultivate interprofessional communication and cooperation. For example, Titzer, Swenty, and Hoehn (2011) discuss a collaborative simulation activity with nursing, radiology, occupational therapy, and respiratory therapy students. The activity permitted the learners to explore all possibilities or alternate viewpoints within the situation. These experiences led to improved problem-solving and teamwork skills. Interdisciplinary debriefing allowed for reflection and discussion of feelings, group needs, role clarification, communication, collaboration, and shared discipline-specific information. A second discipline-specific debriefing provided opportunities for each student to self-reflect and dialogue with others of the same discipline to communicate feelings and frustrations in working collaboratively with other disciplines.

Licensed practical/vocational nursing programs are utilizing simulation frequently due in part to increasing difficulty with locating suitable clinical sites (Suplee & Solecki, 2011). Simulation is also used at this level of nursing education to increase preparedness for safe practice (Schubert, 2010). Suplee and Solecki (2011) describe use of low- and high-fidelity mannequins along with standardized patients to facilitate the experience of a pediatric clinical. Schubert (2010) discusses altering any preprepared nursing scenario to meet the needs of learners in practical nursing programs to enhance practice regarding critical thinking and decision making related to patient safety.

In associate degree programs, benefits and barriers in using high-fidelity simulation have been discussed (Adamson, 2009), and suggestions for intentional placement of simulated experiences throughout the curriculum have been offered (Tuoriniemi & Schott-Baer, 2008). Tourineiemi and Schott-Baer describe several simulations developed for use in a community college setting where skills such as assessment, basic medication administration, and other interventions taught in fundamental courses are practiced on low- and high-fidelity mannequins. Scenarios are developed to include more advanced concepts as learners move through the program. In one example, learners are asked to care for a patient with pregnancy-induced hypertension in which they must assess the situation, communicate with the physician, provide emotional support to the patient, implement seizure care, and prepare the patient for a cesarean section. An example of a leadership and management scenario at the associate level requires learners to discover, manage, and collaborate with other health care team members in the care of a patient with tumor lysis syndrome (Tuoriniemi & Schott-Baer, 2008).

Simulation scenarios are strategically integrated into baccalaureate degree programs for clinical experiences or as adjunct tools to link theory to practice. Nurse educators in these programs utilize simulation to actively engage learners in the cognitive, psychomotor, and affective domains of learning. Leadership, communication, and teamwork skills are a part of the simulation experiences for baccalaureate programs. Interprofessional, patient, and family member roles are sometimes used within simulated experiences as scripted characters or standardized patients to enhance the learning situation. For example, during a simulated hospice home visit scenario, a faculty member assumes the role of the wife of the hospice patient. The patient is portrayed using a high-fidelity mannequin with breath and heart sounds, and voice projection. From a script, the wife questions students during the scenario, offers information if asked, provides distractions or cues as the scenario unfolds, thus adding realism to the situation. At the same time, the simulated patient is verbally responsive, offers assessment cues, and provides opportunities for decision making and skill performance of psychomotor activities. Critical thinking, decision making, and clinical judgment occurs when learners reflect on prior knowledge and dialogue with the patient, family, and other members of the interprofessional health care team.

Graduate nursing programs have adopted simulation to improve confidence levels of advanced practitioners in response to emergency situations and to develop enhancement of leadership skills (Bruce, Scherer, Curran, Urschel, Erdley, & Ball, 2009; Gordon & Buckley, 2009). The primary focus during simulated experiences for graduate learners is on leadership and management skills for transitioning to the role of the advanced practice nurse or in dealing with emergency situations (Gordon & Buckley, 2009). Some simulated experiences focus on skills related to specific practitioner roles such as the delivery of an infant as a midwife, the delivery of anesthesia as a nurse anesthetist, or advanced life support measures after cardiac arrest as a nurse practitioner.

Evidence suggests that simulation when used for development of knowledge for practice in specialty areas is more beneficial than enhancement of rote knowledge (Bruce et al., 2009; Gordon & Buckley, 2009; Kuhrik, Kuhrik, Rimkus, Tercu, & Woodhouse, 2008; Wayne et al., 2005). For example, a high-fidelity simulation involving a cardiac arrest scenario was described by Bruce et al. (2009) as including both undergraduate and graduate learners to demonstrate how knowledge, management, and confidence can be gained through simulation. During this clinical simulation activity, one graduate learner and four to five undergraduate learners were assigned to complete the advanced cardiac life support scenario. Leadership responsibilities of graduate learners included assessment, management, and evaluation, while undergraduate learners were to follow directives and initiate advanced cardiac arrest procedures. Reflections about the experience and openness to others' points of view during debriefing can lead to transformed new frames of reference, thus increasing graduate students' leadership skills and confidence in handling emergency situations (Bruce et al.).

Professional staff development educators can use simulated experiences to expand knowledge gained in education and practice. For example, staff development educators can identify knowledge utilized in one practice area (such as an orthopedic unit) and how and why that knowledge is needed when cross-training for another area (such as an oncology unit). Simulated experiences allow staff development educators to structure individualized learning opportunities based on typical client needs within each area, building new knowledge on the clinical judgments that are similar in both settings, and progressing to unit-specific needs. Additionally, professional staff development educators can partner with educators from academe to create scenarios that develop communication skills, orientation to various roles, or teamwork opportunities such as for a community disaster.

Creating Scenarios

Creation of learning scenarios using low- or high-fidelity simulation can be challenging and time consuming. Bruce et al. (2009) stated that approximately 32 hours were needed in preparation for a cardiac arrest simulation. These hours included the development and programming of the scenario, assignment of learners, and practice before implementation. Scenario development decisions include considering if the high-fidelity simulations will be recorded for review during debriefing. Learning outcome(s) must be clearly identified before writing a scenario. Consideration of learner self-assessment is also a critical component of a well-designed simulated activity. The self-assessment may occur either verbally or in writing, through threaded discussions, in clinical judgment rubrics (Lasater, 2007), or through reflective journaling. In creating the scenario for transformative learning, educators must be aware of unintended outcomes that may be positive, but may also evoke negative reactions from learners.

Hamilton (2010) developed two scenarios for use with high- or low-fidelity simulation in which learners respond to cues that lead to an experience of the death or recovery of a patient from a life-threatening situation. These two scenarios are also used to evaluate psychomotor skill performance. Both scenarios can be used to create intentional disorienting dilemmas through reflection regarding the reactions from family member(s) as role-played by the faculty and individual learner reactions to either the death or near-death experience. When using either of these scenarios, a nurse educator must be prepared for and understand how to react to learners who experience physical, emotional, spiritual, cultural, and/or developmental responses to the simulated situation. Learners who express prior experience with death or dying can be encouraged to dialogue with others who may not have had these past experiences. The dialogue may occur during debriefing or may occur at a later time when learners are more emotionally ready to consider other points of view.

Scenarios can also be designed to include intentional errors (i.e., wrong medication has been given) to provide an opportunity for learners to self-reflect regarding timely assessment of both patient and environment (Henneman, Cunningham, Roche, & Curnin, 2007). Unplanned disorienting dilemmas or happenstance opportunities may occur if learners' performance expectations are not met, leading to self-concept or self-efficacy dilemmas. Other intentional creations of scenarios that may lead to disorienting dilemmas include the following areas: ethical issues, prioritization, collaboration with patient and family, interprofessional roles, and communication, delegation, and leadership skills such as critiquing performance of another.

Debriefing

Debriefing includes discussion of what facts are known or not known and why, how clinical judgments are made, interpersonal and interprofessional interactions, ethical concerns, and psychomotor performance. Transformative learning as an outcome of simulation requires an environment of trust for critical dialogue to occur. Educators facilitate discussions during debriefing sessions and offer constructive comments. Dreifuerst (2009) presents examples of approaches to debriefing in which dialogue and self-reflection is blocked and suggests structuring debriefing for reflection. Poor facilitation of the debriefing process, such as the faculty devaluing the debriefing process or viewing it as a waste of time, openly blaming the learner(s) or forcing them to remediate without direction, or not leaving time for debriefing can prevent assimilation and accommodation of the experience.

Dreifuerst (2009) describes the components of a model for debriefing that includes the provision of a comfortable environment that allows time, reflection, and emotional release, and coaching to promote learner receptiveness to feedback through dialogue about alternative points of view. The nursing process can be integrated into debriefing experiences, promoting assimilation of the cognitive, affective, and psychomotor skills experienced during the simulation. Another outcome from integrating nursing process into the debriefing is to facilitate transference of clinical judgment into subsequent practice (Dreifuerst, 2009; Kuiper, Heinrich, Matthias, Graham, & Bell-Kotwell, 2008).

Planning for debriefing sessions must include opportunities for critical dialogue and for self-reflection at the time of the simulated event. Subsequent opportunities for critical reflection, self-reflection, and dialogue should be planned at a later date to allow time and opportunity for learners to engage in a deeper level of reflection needed to identify hidden assumptions, values, and beliefs that may drive personal decisions or behaviors. Planning for follow-up scenario debriefing in a class meeting can also allow for situated reflection and development of further clinical reasoning.

Debriefing presents the perfect opportunity for critical dialogue that is needed for transformative learning. Debriefing is an opportunity for reflective discourse, which Mezirow (2000) describes "Discourse in the context of Transformation Theory, is that specialized use of dialogue devoted to searching for a common understanding and assessment of the justification of an interpretation or belief" (pp. 10–11). The learner must critically reflect on their assumptions and weigh supporting evidence and alternative perspectives of others to arrive at a clearer understanding. Emotional maturity must be present in the learner in the form of understanding one's emotions, self-motivation, ability to recognize emotions in others, and clear cognition for transformative learning to occur from participation in discourse (Mezirow, 2000).

For the remainder of the chapter, the focus will be on teaching strategies that promote transformative learning through simulation. Specific simulation methods, potential learner outcomes, and barriers to selection of the method are showcased in Table 9.1.

TABLE 9.1   Types of Simulations, Learner Outcomes, and Barriers

Type of Simulation	Anticipated Learning Outcome(s)	Anticipated Barriers

Games
  Puzzles
  Computer games
  Jeopardy
  Bingo
	Development of decision-making skills through problem solving
	Understanding relationship of theory to practice
	Enhanced coping strategies
		Time consuming
		Difficult to design
		Learner competition may impede learning

Anatomical models
  Pictures
  Videos
  3-Dimensional models
  Computerized models
	Visual link to what is ordinarily not seen for development of technical knowledge	Provides information regarding only one anatomical area
		Limited connection between other body systems

Task trainers
  Orange or other types of fruit
  Injection pad or sponge
  Intravenous arms
  Chester Chest™
  Wounds
  Genitalia
	Promote single psychomotor skill development
	Skill competency
	Self-reflection
		Isolated skill learning without context
		No real-life interaction

Role playing
  Learners interact with each other or the environment
  Examples include:
  Virtual Dementia Tour™
  End-of-life decisions
  Management of emergencies
  Conflict resolution
	Interpersonal interaction
	Awareness of roles of interprofessional health care team
	Interprofessional collaboration
	Development of empathy
	Dialogue
	Socialization
	Use of communication skills
	Self-reflection regarding personal feelings and coping strategies
	Responding to clinical emergencies
		Unpredictable interactions
		Difficult to manage scenario progression without clear guidelines and expectations

Computer-assisted instruction Computer software or websites that allow for isolated learning of specific content area	Self-reflection about what is known or not known Discovery and situated reasoning Problem-focused experience with immediate feedback	Variable costs Learners must be self-directed Requires time commitment from learner

(*continued*)

TABLE 9.1   (*continued*)

Type of Simulation	Anticipated Learning Outcome(s)	Anticipated Barriers
Standardized patients Paid scripted actors Faculty actors Theater students	Identification of other's perspectives through dialogue Self-reflection of assessment and interviewing skills Clinical reasoning	Costs can range from $20 to $400 Training or preparation is required Some populations difficult to obtain or train (children or pregnant females)
Virtual reality Computer programs that portray real-life scenarios (i.e., Second Life©) Interactive video of unfolding case studies (e.g., The Neighborhood)	Real-world connections through perceptions of experiences Openness to alternative perspectives through questioning and reflection of knowledge and assumptions Interdisciplinary interactions	Costly Requires technical instruction, competence, and support for faculty and learners
Low-fidelity simulation Anatomically correct mannequins Basic Life Support (BLS) mannequins	Preparation for clinical practice Remediation practice Assessment and psychomotor skill performance in a laboratory setting	No real-life interaction unless simulated Scenarios and environment provide more realism, but time consuming to create and set up
High-fidelity simulation Anatomically correct mannequins with physiological reality and voice projection Examples include: SimMan® METI man® SimBaby® iStan®	Life-like practice Allows integration of holistic nursing concepts Collaboration, communication, critical thinking, clinical reasoning Self-reflection Critical reflection Dialogue Opportunity for discourse during scenario and debriefing	Costly Time consuming for development and integration Requires technology support and maintenance

SIMULATION SCENARIOS FOR TRANSFORMATIVE LEARNING

Various forms of simulated activities provide options for instructional design to enhance learning. Scenario creation that stems from identification of clear and concise learning outcomes and incorporation of planned debriefing opportunities enhance learners' abilities to "think on their feet." Selection of the most appropriate type of simulation to achieve the learning outcomes expands learner opportunities for exposure to variables that occur when functioning in multiple nurse roles. These carefully selected and created simulation scenarios can complement classroom and clinical experiences and, when created or selected with transformative learning as an overall outcome, can be an innovative, effective learning methodology.

Although the following scenario examples have been used in a traditional baccalaureate program, the scenarios can be adapted for practical and associate degree programs or revised to incorporate specific learning for graduate essential outcomes.

> Mr. Johnson is a 65-year-old gentleman admitted with atrial fibrillation, heart rate of 150 beats per minute (bpm). He has a history of coronary artery disease, diabetes, and hypertension. During his episode of atrial fibrillation, Mr. Johnson suffered a stroke (CVA) which currently has him paralyzed on the right side and his medications have caused him to have diarrhea. This is his second day in the hospital and he has converted to sinus rhythm with no signs of distress. Mr. Johnson was just moved to your telemetry unit for close monitoring. His vital signs are Blood Pressure 132/70, Heart Rate 75 bpm, Respiratory Rate 22, Temperature 99.1, telemetry sinus rhythm, and weight 300 lbs. The physical therapist comes to the nurses' station to report that she cannot do Mr. Johnson's range of motion (ROM) exercises until he is cleaned from a diarrheal stool in his bed. The primary nurse assigned to Mr. Johnson asks for help from another nurse and a patient care technician (PCT). The physical therapist follows behind to see if she can be of additional assistance.

The scenario is read aloud to learners as they receive a written copy for reference. Next, learners are assigned the following roles of primary nurse, staff nurse, physical therapist, and PCT. The scenario begins with the physical therapist arriving at the nurses' station to ask for assistance in preparing Mr. Johnson for his physical therapy.

> The primary nurse, staff nurse, and PCT walk into Mr. Johnson's room to prepare him for physical therapy. Mr. Johnson is on the floor.

It is at this point that there is an expectation that learners will experience a sense of urgency to assess the patient for a possible reason for being on the floor and remove him from the floor if indicated. This expectation would indicate use of problem solving by building on previous knowledge. Interestingly, during dialogue in the debriefing session related to this specific scenario, learners described this experience as thinking on their feet.

> As the scenario unfolds, the learners collaborate as questions arise, such as: What do we do?, Do we lift him to the bed?, Do we leave him on the floor? A solution is reached to leave him on the floor and begin an assessment. After log-rolling Mr. Johnson to a supine position, the learners observe that he is unconscious and without pulse or respirations. They now transition their thinking from a fall with possible injuries to an emergency situation during which decisions must be made quickly based on clinical reasoning in order to revive Mr. Johnson and to prevent brain damage.

Chaos often ensues as the situation continues, and learners rush to the crash cart and become somewhat confused as to which student should be responsible for respirations, chest compressions, and who should call the code.

One learner, acting as the primary nurse, calls the code while directing the PCT to perform chest compressions and the staff nurse to maintain the airway.

Although the learners functioning in the role of care providers are successful in restoring Mr. Johnson's respirations and heartbeat, they still have the problem of if or how to get him from the floor to the bed for further assessment.

The scenario ends, and learners are debriefed in a comfortable environment. Learners reflect on their behaviors, communication, and collaboration during the simulation experience. Learners identify strengths in critical reasoning for selection of interventions that revive Mr. Johnson. Learners identify weaknesses such as understanding various roles during a code and where supplies are located in the crash cart. The faculty member facilitates dialogue by using Socratic questioning regarding observations made during the simulation to spark disorienting dilemmas and to guide discussions.

For a second example involving low-fidelity simulation that involves minimal cost, Hamilton and Langham (2009b) describe a urinary cath triad in which learners are organized into groups of three. One learner assumes the role of patient, one accepts the nurse role, and the other becomes the evaluator. The expectation is that each learner will realistically play their role to provide a sense of authenticity to the simulation. In this scenario that involves insertion of an indwelling catheter before a planned surgery:

> The student who assumes the patient role answers and responds to the student in the nurse role. Simulated genitalia are placed on a fully clothed student in the role of patient as the nurse inserts the catheter.

Learning outcomes for the student in the patient role is to better understand potential patient vulnerability and to appreciate a variety of feelings including desire for privacy.

> The student who assumes the role of nurse performs the catheterization procedure. Appropriate sterile catheter insertion technique is followed on the mannequin genitalia.

Students in the role of the patient add a more realistic dimension for learners in the role of a nurse in that they communicate, display emotions and feelings, and behave cooperatively or uncooperatively, which does not occur when using a mannequin for catheter insertion. Learning outcomes for learners in the nurse role are to use critical thinking throughout assessment of the patient, communication, catheterization, and evaluation of the patient after the procedure. Additionally, learners validate the use of sterile techniques during catheter insertion.

> The student in the role of evaluator is responsible for evaluating if the catheterization procedure is done correctly, if time is appropriately managed, and if the student in the role of nurse demonstrated effective caring and communication. The evaluator then provides constructive feedback to the student in the role of nurse.

The student evaluator provides feedback based on printed evaluation criteria. Learning outcomes for the student in the role of evaluator are to make an evaluation about the skill performance as accurate or not, to evaluate caring behaviors of the student in the role of nurse, and to relate perceptions of patient advocacy during procedures. Additionally, students in the evaluator role learn to provide feedback in a constructive and positive manner. Each learner rotates through each of the roles to gain understanding of the experiences involved in being a patient, nurse, and leader.

Learner comments following the urinary cath triad simulation are usually positive. According to students, the patient role offers the most insight. By placing themselves in the role of patient, learners vicariously perceive emotions of vulnerability and potential embarrassment. Learner comments also indicate an increased awareness that nurses must be conscious of patients' potential vulnerability and the need for open, honest communication as a caring patient advocate (Hamilton & Langham, 2009b).

A third example of a low-fidelity simulation is called mock hospital. At least three mannequins are used to represent hospitalized patients. During this activity, learners receive a change of shift report regarding these patients' conditions. Each patient has a chart that includes admission diagnosis, physician orders, laboratory and radiology results, and history and physical findings. After the report, learners must assess and plan care for each of the patients for which they have been assigned. Clinical faculty members are present to facilitate and guide the learners. Learners must prioritize care for the three patients by providing assistance in activities of daily living, administering medications, providing treatments, and documenting care (Hamilton & Langham, 2009a; Gore, Hunt, & Hamilton, 2009).

Debriefing after the mock hospital experience, offers opportunity for self-reflection and group discussion to explore and share experiences with other learners. Alternative perspectives provide insight to transform thinking and planning for future experiences. Mock hospital experiences also allow for observation and evaluation of clinical adjuncts as well as an opportunity for clinical faculty and learners to form relationships before actual clinical experiences (Hamilton & Langham, 2009a; Gore et al., 2009).

A fourth simulation example that is used in a baccalaureate program incorporates a copyrighted activity (used with permission) called the Virtual Dementia Tour.™ This activity was created by P. K. Beville of Second Wind Dreams®. The Virtual Dementia Tour involves an experiential toolkit created for anyone seeking to understand challenges of those experiencing dementia. Learner outcomes include improved communication resulting from an increased understanding of the lived experience. Student comments have included how powerful the experience was, in that they perceived a lack of control over their environment and had learned about their personal response to perceptions of anxiety from inability to complete simple activities. Students have also stated that increased understanding of behaviors and possible reasons for those behaviors have led to increased therapeutic communication and patient advocacy when working with persons who experience trauma, developmental delays, mental disorders, or other cognitive concerns across the life span.

One final example of a high-fidelity simulation for junior- and senior-level student groups involves an environment staged to represent hospice care in a home setting. A high-fidelity mannequin depicts a patient who had a right lobectomy as result of bone metastasis. Senior-level students assume roles of the hospice nurse and PCT, while junior-level students assume the roles of student nurses. Based on information from the scenario, students provide appropriate care according to their roles. The patient's condition worsens, and care becomes more challenging. A standardized patient in the role of the patient's family member adds complexity to the scenario in that learners in their roles must respond to both the patient and family member needs. Faculty members must be flexible in making decisions to stop the scenario if learners are demonstrating inappropriate behaviors or if learners experience undue anxiety or other emotions from the scenario.

Much of the learning in this simulated activity occurs during debriefing in which dialogue results from learner reflection regarding providing person-centered care across settings. Additionally, debriefing can provide time for self-reflection during which personal awareness of feelings and assumptions that influence care and decision-making skills may become apparent. Critical dialogue among faculty and learners within a trusting setting can lead to further personal and professional growth. Dialogue "provides the context for making meaning within which [the learners] choose what and how a sensory experience is to be construed and/or appropriated" (Mezirow, 2000, p. 16) through discussion of assumptions and expectations revealing habits of mind.

CONCLUSIONS

Simulation can take many forms from using an orange to practice injections to a complex computerized virtual reality or high-fidelity mannequin. The goal of any simulation is to provide learning opportunities similar to actual experiences, but without the risk of harm to a real patient. No matter what the forum is, simulated experiences can motivate, engage, encourage knowledge retention, and transform thinking for learners to produce new knowledge or to consider alternative perspectives.

Simulated experiences are interactive tools for nurse educators that can engage any level of learner. Transformative learning can occur with each type of simulation. Mezirow (2000) explains that this transformation "may occur in one of four ways: by elaborating existing frames of reference, by learning new frames of reference, by transforming points of view, or by transforming habits of mind" (p. 19). Learners must intentionally assess meaning of the simulated experience based on previous knowledge and assumptions. Validation of the understanding is found through reflective discourse and dialogue with others (Mezirow & Taylor, 2009).

Nurse educators' role during these simulated experiences is varied. It is the educator's responsibility to create or to select the most appropriate type of simulation and to develop scenarios most likely to meet course learning outcomes and learning needs of individual students. Educators must be authentic in the development of a simulated environment and in providing a nonjudgmental atmosphere to preserve the learners' sense of self and induce trust. Most importantly, the debriefing session must be planned to encourage reflection and dialogue for transformation.

REFERENCES

Adamson, K. (2009). Integrating human patient simulation into associate degree nursing curricula: Faculty experiences, barriers, and facilitators. *Clinical Simulation in Nursing, 6*(3), e75–e81. doi: 10.1016/j.ecsns.2009.06.002

Beville, P. K. (1997). Virtual Dementia Tour®. Marietta, GA: Second Wind Dreams. Retrieved from http://www.secondwind.org/vdt

Bruce, S. A., Scherer, Y. K., Curran, C. C., Urschel, D. M., Erdley, S., & Ball, L. S. (2009). A collaborative exercise between graduate and undergraduate nursing students using a computer-assisted simulator in a mock cardiac arrest. *Nursing Education Perspectives, 30*(1), 22–27.

Dreifuerst, K. T. (2009). The essentials of debriefing in simulation learning: A concept analysis. *Nursing Education Perspectives, 30*(2), 109–114.

Gordon, C. J., & Buckley, T. (2009). The effect of high-fidelity simulation training on medical-surgical graduate nurses' perceived ability to respond to patient clinical emergencies. *The Journal of Continuing Education in Nursing, 40*(11), 491–498. doi: 10.3928/00220124-20091023-06

Gore, T., Hunt, C., & Hamilton, C. (2009). Mock it up: Mock hospital simulation unit as initial clinical experience. Presentation at *Technology Integration Program for Nursing Education and Practice,* sponsored by Duke University School of Nursing, Durham, NC.

Guimond, M. E., Sole, M. L., & Salas, E. (2011). Getting ready for simulation-based training: A checklist for nurse educators. *Nursing Education Perspectives, 32*(3), 179–187.

Hamilton, C. A. (2010). The simulation imperative of end-of-life education. *Clinical Simulation in Nursing, 6*(4), e131–e138. doi: 10.1016/j.ecns.2009.08.002.

Hamilton, C. A. & Langham, G. (2009a). *Mock Hospital Research Update.* Presented to Kappa Omega Chapter of Sigma Theta Tau International Honor Society of Nursing, Montgomery, AL.

Hamilton, C. A. & Langham, G. (2009b). Low impact simulation with high impact results. Presentation at *8th Annual International Nursing Simulation/Learning Resource Centers.* Conference, St. Louis, MO.

Henneman, E. A., Cunningham, H., Roche, J. P., & Curnin, M. E. (2007). Human patient simulation: Teaching students to provide safe care. *Nurse Educator, 32*(5), 212–217.

Kuhrik, N., Kuhrik, M., Rimkus, C., Tecu, N., & Woodhouse, J. (2008). Using human simulation in the oncology clinical practice setting. *Journal of Continuing Education in Nursing, 39*(8), 345–355.

Kuiper, R., Heinrich, C., Matthias, A., Graham, M. J., & Bell-Kotwell, L. (2008). Debriefing with the OPT model of clinical reasoning during high fidelity patient simulation. *International Journal of Nursing Education Scholarship, 5*(1), 1–14.

Lasater, K. (2007). Clinical judgment development: Using simulation to create an assessment rubric. *Journal of Nursing Education, 46*(11), 496–503.

Mezirow, J. & Associates. (2000). *Learning as transformation: Critical perspectives on a theory in progress.* San Francisco, CA: Jossey-Bass.

Mezirow, J., Taylor, E. W., & Associates. (2009). *Transformative learning in practice: Insights from community, workplace, and higher education.* San Francisco, CA: Jossey-Bass.

Schubert, M. (2010). Challenging practical nurses "on the fly." *Clinical Simulation in Nursing, 6*(3), e107–e126.

Suplee, P. D., & Solecki, S. M. (2011). Creating and implementing pediatric simulation experiences for licensed practical nursing students. *Clinical Simulation in Nursing, 7*(1), e127–e132. doi:10.1016/j.ecns.2010.01.001.

Titzer, J. L., Swenty, C. F., & Hoehn, W. G. (2011). An interprofessional simulation promoting collaboration and problem solving among nursing and allied health professional students. *Clinical Simulation in Nursing, in press,* e1–e9. doi: 10.1016/j.ecns.2011.01.001.

Tuoriniemi, P., & Schott-Baer, D. (2008). Implementing a high-fidelity simulation program in a community college setting. *Nursing Education Perspectives, 29*(2), 105–109.

Wayne, D. B., Butter, J., Siddall, V. J., Fudala, M. J., Lindquist, L. A., Feinglass, J., McGaghie, W. C. (2005). Simulation-based training of internal medicine residents in advanced cardiac life support protocols: A randomized trial. *Teaching and Learning in Medicine, 17*(3), 210–216.

10

Service Learning to Promote Social Transformation in Nursing Students

Ginny Langham and Michelle A. Schutt

Tell me & I'll listen.
Show me & I'll understand.
Involve me & I'll learn.

—Teton Lakota Indian Proverb

Experiential learning in clinical settings provides opportunities for hands-on application of newly acquired knowledge and skills while developing critical thinking and sound clinical judgment. Although traditional clinical experiences are a fundamental component of nursing education, service learning activities can further enrich learning through unique opportunities to link theoretical content with low-acuity encounters within the community. Nurse educators spend countless hours in curricular oversight and clinical planning in an effort to provide students with rich learning opportunities.

A transformative learning environment in nursing education can provide a plethora of occasions for students to challenge assumptions based on prior life experiences and personal values. Collaboration with nursing students, faculty, staff, and community partners can promote a lifelong interest and engagement in civic affairs, social justice, and cultural diversity, as suggested by nursing education accrediting bodies. In this chapter, we will explore the valuable teaching tool of service learning, describe numerous settings where transformative learning principles (see Chapter 2, Box 2.1) can be integrated into service learning activities, and offer examples of service learning activities that may promote not only professional and personal transformation, but social transformation as well. The following scenario provides insight into learner awareness of possible outcomes from participating in service learning activities.

Elizabeth and John attend a metropolitan nursing school. While returning to campus after completing six hours of health screenings at a rural elementary school in an adjacent county, the following discussion occurs:

Elizabeth: "I really wasn't interested in spending the day doing these health screenings. It seems like just one more thing to do on top of everything else we already have to do."

119

John: "I know, Elizabeth, I thought the same thing, too, yesterday; but, after spending time with these kids you get a chance to see how different things can be just twenty miles away from our own reality. I never considered that there were children that didn't have the same opportunities that I have."

Elizabeth: "What do you mean, John?"

John: "Well, I wasn't aware of the difference in availability of school nurses from one county to the next or the difference in access to health care. These kids had simple health problems that were not addressed because of lack of access—there is only one pediatrician in the entire county. I wouldn't have realized that if I hadn't participated today."

Elizabeth: "Well, now that we are talking about it, I see what you mean. I really just wanted to go and get it over with so I could get on to tomorrow's assignments. Sometimes it seems that we have to do all these things and I really don't get the reason why until much later."

John: "I know. I get so busy trying to get it all done that sometimes I don't get why we are doing what we are doing until several days later when I go to complete my reflection journal and actually have to analyze my learning. Sometimes I don't think I get anything out of it until that moment, then I have this epiphany and realize that even though I might not have gained a ton, I was able to do a lot of assessments, work with kids to see the difference between first graders and third graders, and get to talk with them and see the difference in maturity and communication. That makes all the growth and development content seem real."

Elizabeth: "Yeah. I think you are right. Maybe the faculty members are on to something here."

SERVICE LEARNING

Service learning can be defined as a structured learning experience that occurs with academic oversight in a community service setting, which integrates the activity with intentional learning and opportunities for reflection (Bassi, 2011; Cashman, Hale, Candib, Nimiroski, & Brookings, 2004; Cauley, Canfield, Clasen, Dobbins, Hemphill, Jaballas, & Walbroehl, 2001; Furco, 1996; Jacoby, 1996; Seifer, 1998). There are two anticipated outcomes from service learning experiences: (1) nursing students supply a needed community service, and (2) curricular learning objectives can be met. The American Association of Colleges of Nursing (AACN) (2008) advocates use of service learning projects as an active learning strategy to promote the development of the following competencies: critical thinking, creative problem solving, oral and written communication, application of evidence-based practice (EBP) concepts, health promotion teaching skills, and group processes. Additionally, the Pew Health Professions Commission (1993; 1995; 1998) continues to recommend that nursing education increase the number of community-based activities to promote competencies for various professional nursing practice settings.

Service learning activities differ from traditional clinical experiences in multiple ways. While most clinical learning objectives are based on student need and curricular outcomes, planning for service learning activities requires the faculty to partner with community organizations to determine population-based needs and to develop learning opportunities to meet the needs of both the student and the community. Through this collaborative partnership, the faculty can design learning activities that allow learners to apply foundational knowledge to real-life settings, to develop as nurses and citizens (Emerson,

2007), and to expand experiences into diverse communities (Nokes, Nickitas, Keida, & Neville, 2005). Intentional planning, implementation, and facilitation of service learning activities across the curriculum allows nurse educators to support professional development while also setting the stage for transformative learning.

Transformative learning nurse educators strive to produce caring, competent nurses who demonstrate values of the profession. This assumption begs the questions: (1) How does one teach another to be civic minded? (2) How can an appreciation for cultural diversity be developed? and (3) How can appreciation for volunteerism to meet professional nursing's social obligation be developed? Nurse educators have historically struggled with how to address these questions in curricular planning. We believe the use of transformative learning approaches and principles when structuring service learning opportunities may provide some answers to these questions. In the remainder of this chapter, we will discuss application of transformative learning principles within the context of service learning.

SOCIAL TRANSFORMATION

Underlying transformative learning principle: *Learning is driven by motivation to know, which may include attaining power to navigate through life's situations.*

The concept of *giving back* can be nurtured when students experience meaningful interactions within the community. In reaching out to help others, personal satisfaction and self-awareness can result. Through participation in community experiences, learners can engage in knowledge beyond the empirical pattern, such that new awareness becomes integrated into their personal identity. Service learning activities have been shown to increase one's self-esteem and to facilitate an advanced level of moral reasoning (Kraft, 1996). Consequently, involvement in such endeavors often leads to future civic participation (Meyers, 2009). When students are empowered by making a difference, the development of engaged citizenship and sustained involvement in public affairs can be fostered. College or university emphases on service or outreach endeavors provide opportunities for nursing students to interact with faculty, students from other disciplines, and community leaders. Various opportunities for service can motivate the student to identify areas of personal interest for continued participation.

Motivation of learners to participate in service learning activities can be increased with the awareness of possible outcomes from the experience, such as:

1. increased awareness of community needs;
2. increased awareness of the role of the nurse with individuals, families, and communities;
3. opportunity to interact with community or international agencies;
4. providing area communities with additional resources.

Strategic placement of community-based service learning activities throughout the nursing curriculum helps to meet the first transformative learning principle. For example, service learning can be a curricular progression requirement that is completed independently by students. Clinical courses can contain a component in which students are encouraged to seek opportunities, preferably involving an organization or agency of individual interest. Leadership skills and autonomy (empowerment) can be developed by having students contact the agency to make arrangements for date and time of service. Further development of autonomy can occur by having the student develop learning objectives for the activity, which incorporate and support the nursing program curricular outcomes and agency mission.

Social Transformation in a Local Community

Underlying transformative learning principle: *Learning approaches and activities promote identification of assumptions and critical reflection of individual meaning perspectives.*

The early phases of perspective transformation require well-thought-out planning and activity design. As Cranton (2006) points out, transformative learning requires exploration and questioning of assumptions and the reformation of thinking while providing the opportunity to function in a particular role. Deliberate staging of service learning opportunities in areas that expose students to unfamiliar populations or diverse cultures allows for a disorienting dilemma. For example, students may be required to provide health screenings in two opposing environments, a poor rural public school system and an affluent private college preparatory school. This activity can be used to facilitate perspective transformation in several ways. First, student nurses are afforded the opportunity to complete physical assessments and hone their assessment and communication skills in a safe environment. The evaluation of vital signs for multiple clients or the chance to view 30 tympanic membranes provides nursing students with numerous exposures. The repetitious process allows learners to increase comfort in the new role as a student nurse while developing competency in necessary actions that accompany the role. Additionally, faculty members can incorporate critical reflection and dialogue through various prompts. Students may be asked to compare and contrast the two school environments mentioned above:

1. How do the two environments differ?
2. How are the environments similar?
3. Describe the surrounding landscape of each school.
4. Is there a difference in how the hallways of the schools are decorated?
5. What type of overall atmosphere is projected in each school?
6. What is the demeanor of the teachers?
7. Did you observe any teacher/student interaction? If so, were they different?
8. How are the students dressed? Do they appear well fed and healthy?
9. What type of reception did you receive from school personnel?

This form of reflective exercise encourages students to consider numerous perspectives such as the impact of social conditions, economic challenges, access to and distribution of health care resources, issues related to cultural diversity, along with assessing community involvement and support. Comparative analysis is a helpful approach to reflective consideration and can promote opportunities for students to critically assess their assumptions.

The low level of client acuity encountered during health screening activities allows faculty to design learning activities that help learners to explore new roles and relationships in a transformative learning environment, as well as apply newly obtained knowledge and skills in nursing practice (Horton-Duetsch & Sherwood, 2008). Learners may enter the experience thinking "I do not understand why we have to complete this activity twice. What is the point?" Through the use of pointed reflection questions and dialogue with faculty and peers, learners can discover the advantages and disadvantages of the different school environments. Learners are then encouraged by strategic discussion prompts to identify and reflect on assumptions relative to the milieu in each area.

Social Transformation in a Group Setting

Underlying transformative learning principle: *Learning can be a shared experience.*

Collaborative learning or group projects can be effectively utilized as strategies that support development of transformative learning and critical thinking (DeYoung, 2003; King, 2005). When learners are clustered to accomplish a specific assignment or project, group members are forced to collaborate. During active engagement in team dialogue, agreement must be reached on the identification of a goal, the assignment of tasks, the details of the project, as well as the development of the final product. Through this shared process, various life experiences and opinions of others provide group members with an opportunity to appreciate and recognize perspectives that may be very different from their own. This meaningful group discourse can lead to self-reflection and questioning of personal assumptions and long-held beliefs. The ability to work effectively in a team setting is a worthy and desirable attribute of most professions. Accordingly, service learning activities have been identified by the AACN as a beneficial technique to develop competency in group dynamics (2008). Navigating the challenges of group dynamics can be complex for learners and faculty, but this strategy presents a strong potential for true perspective transformations to occur.

For example, in one nursing program, a large number of service learning activities involve a collaborative partnership with several county school districts to provide health educational teaching throughout the school system. Nursing faculty meet with teachers and counselors within the school system to foster an alliance to identify the most prevalent current health educational needs and to explore ways that student nurses can offer instructional support to varying age groups. This phenomenological approach allows the lived experience of school employees and children to guide the development and implementation of health-related interventions within the local school system. The expressed needs of the school system include topics such as smoking prevention, bullying, adolescent safe driving, eating disorders, sports safety, and proper nutrition.

For this specific service learning assignment, student nurses are placed into small groups and given a topic. Learners develop and implement a teaching project for elementary-aged children. Learner outcomes from completing this service learning activity include development of group organizational skills and teamwork, leadership and management, and time-management skills. Professional presentation and communication skills are required to effectively and appropriately communicate health information to the target audience. Furthermore, nursing students are afforded the opportunity to personally experience the perplexing issues facing public school children in a local area. There is also an increased sensitivity and awareness of the challenging obstacles that public school teachers and officials confront on a daily basis.

This community partnership example could easily be replicated by other colleges or universities with different populations of interest. The outcome of the partnership allowed for development of professional relationships across multiple disciplines and for networking several years past the initial contact. The personal growth and social transformation of nursing students did not go unnoticed. Consequently, the process has fueled faculty desire to continue to provide much needed health education teaching to children within the school district and has prompted the integration of this service learning project throughout the nursing curriculum.

Social Transformation in a Nursing School Setting

Underlying transformative learning principle: *Learning environments must be open, safe, and respectful of all.*

Community-based service learning activities provide low-acuity, low-stress environments for nursing students. In such settings, ample opportunity exists for repetitive performance of psychomotor skills, which builds confidence along with competence. Deeper understanding of specific growth and developmental content can be gained through repeated practice of communicating with various age groups. Such peer learning activities support King's (2005) assertion that an atmosphere of safety and trust lends itself to a transformative learning opportunity. When course content is linked to situations outside of the classroom, it allows learners a chance to make a connection between abstract concepts and real life. As a result, students can achieve improved academic performance as well as a more positive mind-set through a personal and social transformation (Meyers, 2009).

For example, one statewide initiative provides free annual health screenings to public school children in various counties by utilizing community partnerships among school leaders, community volunteers, and college nursing programs. Schools of nursing throughout the state provide manpower for these health screenings in rural and medically underserved communities. The program's overall purpose is collaboration among community partners to improve health care outcomes by providing health screenings, as well as health-promotion teaching projects to underserved public school children. The professionals involved include registered nurses, certified nurse practitioners, student nurses, public school counselors, public school nurses, public school administrative personnel, local dentists, and local ophthalmologists. The process includes collaboration with local public schools, performing physical assessments of individual children, documenting findings, noting irregularities/abnormalities, making appropriate referrals, providing follow-up information to the school nurse, and submitting all paperwork to local public school personnel. The anticipated results from these health screenings will produce aggregate data for the prevalence and trends of certain illnesses and/or conditions. Initial data collection has revealed several areas of concern.

This unique service learning example provided opportunities for nursing students to positively impact the health of public school children. In addition, the partnership allowed the modeling of service learning by nursing students to members of the rural community including students, staff, administrators, and community interest groups. The enhanced collaboration led to involvement with multiple interest groups. The service learning activity benefited all constituents by adhering to the principle of respect for all members of the community and for all learners (see appendices for other service learning opportunities).

Social Transformation in a Global Community

Underlying transformative learning principle: *Learning involves facts, feelings, ethical, intrapersonal, interpersonal, and social issues.*

Consider the example of a school of nursing that has made an international connection to another school of nursing in a lesser-developed country. Through collegial and student dialogue via the Internet, various ideas, assignments, and needs have been expressed. One of the positive outcomes of this endeavor is a joint effort of the United States school of nursing faculty and students to provide nursing journals and textbooks to the lesser-developed school of nursing. With the help of a neighboring church, periodic shipments of these needed materials are sent to the welcoming arms of nursing students halfway around the world.

This service learning activity promotes cultural, social, and educational awareness in both cohorts of nursing students. Through such partnerships, nursing faculty can foster and design transformative learning assignments, which allow students to become immersed in lifestyles and cultures unlike their own. When learners are encouraged to view an issue from a different perspective, they are more likely to develop a greater awareness and appreciation of diversity (Meyers, 2009). By addressing the expressed needs of a less fortunate nursing school, the U.S. student nurses are positioned to reconsider and possibly relinquish previous assumptions and/or biases to develop an increased level of acceptance, understanding, and compassion. For further consideration of global service learning opportunities, refer to Fitzpatrick, Shultz, and Aiken's (2010) text, *Giving Through Teaching: How Nurse Educators Are Changing the World.*

Providing learners with an opportunity to gain insight into cultural diversity through service learning activities creates an atmosphere ripe for perspective transformation. When learners are confronted with uncomfortable and unknown issues such as disenfranchised and diverse populations, extreme poverty, domestic abuse, and inequalities of access to health care, an opportunity is presented that allows the student to confront and grapple with some harsh realities of the world in which we live. It is as if the teacher lifts a veil from learners' views to disclose something that was previously hidden—an eye-opening experiential event. When established worldviews are challenged, and learners are empowered to advocate for social justice, a change begins to occur. Structured service learning activities can prompt kindness, caring, and personal engagement as well as provide a catalyst for social transformation and change (Meyers, 2009). This can result in decreased prejudice, increased tolerance, and a greater number of service-oriented individuals (Kraft, 1996). In this way, not only is the individual learner transformed; there is the potential for a much broader, societal transformation. Who does not want a more caring society?

Social Transformation in a Professional Setting

Underlying transformative learning principle: *Learning and relearning occurs throughout life.*

Another approach to the integration of service learning activities to support perspective transformation is the use of professional networking opportunities. For example, students may be required to research and develop EBP projects such as posters, PowerPoint presentations, or formally written papers. Critical dialogue can be stimulated and public speaking skills enhanced through various dissemination strategies that include in-class presentations, noon in-service programs for nurses in local hospitals, and formal presentations at professional workshops and/or organizations (i.e., the state nurses association and the local chapter of Sigma Theta Tau International Honor Society of Nursing). These activities meet the needs of local professionals for current and relevant information specific to the safe delivery of health care and disease management. Additionally, nursing students benefit from the opportunity to develop and present subject matter in a professional venue, thus emphasizing the importance of lifelong learning, promoting the value of collegiality, and advancing social integration into a chosen career. Students are exposed to the significance of professional networking and the exchanging of ideas, which can make a profound impression on a novice student nurse. These types of activities help cement the internal vision for the nursing profession and provide examples and suggestions regarding successful navigation of career development.

Furthermore, service learning activities within the professional setting can expose learners to a magnitude of social and civic engagement. Part of the professional nurse's role is giving back to the community through a service-oriented spirit. Community members, employers, and peers notice service-oriented endeavors. Community involvement reflects a personal trait that is often considered important for hiring and promotion (Katz, Carter, Bishop, & Kravits, 2004). Thus, lifelong and sustained social participation in activities that make a difference in the lives of others can result in many desirable outcomes, including career advancement and professional networking.

CONCLUSIONS

Acclimation to nursing includes examination, review, possible reformation, and integration of personal beliefs and values. In this chapter, numerous ways to integrate transformative learning principles into service learning activities have been explored in an effort to encourage development of nursing values and social responsibility. Service learning opportunities offer an excellent venue for learners to apply knowledge and to question personal assumptions related to a variety of issues, including socioeconomic concerns, cultural humility, and community involvement and support. The conceptualization and development of well-structured service learning activities that incorporate application of theory can promote professional and social development while simultaneously meeting community needs.

Service learning activities provide learners with an opportunity for personal, professional, and social growth. Learners may form connections with a variety of local organizations and agencies, or international associations. Participation in civic endeavors promotes a feeling of involvement, of belonging to something greater than self. When transformative learning principles and approaches are used in service learning activities, there is potential for increased personal and social awareness as well as the development of a responsible, civically engaged spirit of volunteerism (Mueller & Billings, 2009). Kouzes and Posner (2003) assert that an individual's authentic participation can enhance trust, cultivate partnership, and be perceived as "genuine expression of caring" (p. 29). A socially cognizant nurse promotes health and well-being for communities. A nurse's service-minded attitude provides an example to others, increasing potential for a more caring society.

Transformative learning principles can be used as a framework for structuring community service learning activities to awaken the ethical responsibility of citizenship within learners and faculty members. Transformative learning approaches of critical self-reflection and dialogue can enhance learner confidence, knowledge, and can be tools for becoming effective social change agents. When students recognize the impact of community social engagement and reap the rewards of personal satisfaction through making a difference, the practice is more likely to continue. Through critical self-reflection and dialogue, nursing students can experience a perspective transformation resulting in a change from an "I *have* to" attitude into an "I *get* to" attitude.

Forward thinking and creative planning can equip learners to be proactive in the creation of a better society. If students envision themselves as active participants in what "should be," a personal and social transformation occurs (Meyers, 2009). Freed and McLaughlin (2011) describe the cognitive skill of *futures thinking* that empowers student nurses to play a dynamic role in visualizing the future and experience a sense of obligation to be part of cultivating change. The types of service learning activities offered in this chapter may lead to personal perspective transformation and nurture a social connection with the local and global community. The strategic placement of service learning activities within the nursing curriculum can help poise the future nurses of tomorrow to make a societal difference within various populations. Known and unknown challenges of the 21st century necessitate a more diverse approach to nursing education and are more critical than ever to positively impact the health care needs of society.

REFERENCES

American Association of Colleges of Nursing. (2008). *The essentials of baccalaureate education for professional nursing practice.* Washington, DC. Retrieved from http://www.aacn.nche.edu/education/pdf/BaccEssentials08.pdf

Bassi, S. (2011). Undergraduate nursing students' perceptions of service-learning through a school-based community project. *Nursing Education Perspectives, 32*(3), 162–167.

Cashman, S. B., Hale, J. F., Candib, L. M., Nimiroski, T. A., & Brookings, D. R. (2004). Applying service-learning through a community academic partnership: Depression screening at a federally funded community health center. *Education for Health, 17*(3), 313–322.

Cauley, K., Canfield, A., Clasen, C., Dobbins, J., Hemphill, S., Jaballas, E., & Walbroehl, G. (2001). Service learning: Integrating student learning and community service. *Education for Health, 14,* 173–181.

Cranton, P. (2006). *Understanding and promoting transformative learning: A guide for educators of adults* (2nd ed.). San Francisco, CA: Jossey-Bass.

DeYoung, S. (2003). *Teaching strategies for nurse educators.* Upper Saddle River, NJ: Pearson Education.

Emerson, R. J. (2007). *Nursing education in the clinical setting.* St. Louis, MO: Mosby Elsevier.

Fitzpatrick, J., Shultz, C., & Aiken, T. (2010). *Giving through teaching: How nurse educators are changing the world.* New York, NY: Springer.

Freed, P. E., & McLaughlin, D. E. (2011). Futures thinking: Preparing nurses to think for tomorrow. *Nursing Education Perspectives, 32*(3), 173–177.

Furco, A. (1996). Service-learning: A balanced approach to experiential education. *In Expanding Boundaries: Service and Learning.* Washington, DC: Corporation for National Service.

Horton-Deutsch, S., & Sherwood, G. (2008). Reflection: An educational strategy to develop emotionally-competent nurse leaders. *Journal of Nursing Management 16*(8), 946–954. doi: 10.1111/j.1365-2834.2008.00957.x.

Jacoby, B. (Ed.) (1996). *Service learning in higher education: Concepts and practices.* San Francisco, CA: Jossey-Bass.

Katz, J., Carter, C., Bishop, J., & Kravits, S. L. (2004). *Keys to nursing success* (2nd ed.). Upper Saddle River, NJ: Pearson Education.

King, K. (2005). *Bringing transformative learning to life.* Malabar, FL: Krieger Publishing Company.

Kouzes, J. M., & Posner, B. Z. (2003). *Encouraging the heart: A leader's guide to rewarding and recognizing others.* San Francisco, CA: Jossey-Bass.

Kraft, R. J. (1996). Service learning: An introduction to its theory, practice, and effects. *Education and Urban Society, 28*(2), 131–159.

Meyers, S. A. (2009). Service learning as an opportunity for personal and social transformation. *International Journal of Teaching and Learning in Higher Education, 21*(3), 373–381.

Mueller, C., & Billings, D. M. (2009). Service learning: Developing values and social responsibility. In D. M. Billings & J. A. Halstead (Eds.), *Teaching in nursing: A guide for faculty* (3rd ed.) (pp. 173–185). St. Louis, MO: Saunders Elsevier.

Nokes, K. M., Nickitas, D. M., Keida, R., & Neville, S. (2005). Does service-learning increase cultural competency, critical thinking, and civic engagement? *Journal of Nursing Education, 44*(2), 65–70.

Pew Health Professions Commission. (1993). *Health professions education for the future: Schools in service to the nation.* San Francisco, CA: University of California at San Francisco Center for the Health Professions.

Pew Health Professions Commission. (1995). *Critical challenges: Revitalizing the health care professions for the twenty-first century.* San Francisco, CA: University of California at San Francisco Center for the Health Professions. Retrieved from http://futurehealth.ucsf.edu/Content/29/1995-12_Critical_Challenges_Revitalizing_the_Health_Professions_for_the_Twenty-First_Century.pdf

Pew Health Professions Commission. (1998). *Recreating health professional practice for a new century.* San Francisco, CA: The Center for Health Professions. Retrieved from http://futurehealth.ucsf.edu/Content/29/1998-12_Recreating_Health_Professional_Practice_for_a_New_Century_The_Fourth_Report_of_the_Pew_Health_Professions_Commission.pdf

Seifer, S. D. (1998). Service-learning: Community–campus partnerships for health professions education. *Academic Medicine, 73,* 273–277.

11

Transformative Learning in Clinical Experiences

Cam Hamilton and Arlene H. Morris

I hear and I forget. I see and I remember. I do and I understand.
—Confucius

Nurse educators can use transformative strategies to facilitate preparation of learners for nursing practice by providing opportunities for reflection and dialogue regarding assumptions, habits of mind, and patterns of behavior that may be incongruent with experiences in clinical settings (McAllister, Tower, & Walker, 2007). Nursing, a practice profession, incorporates clinical experiences within educational preparation to provide opportunities for learners to apply various theories in practice. Communication, collaboration, teamwork, problem solving, and psychomotor skills are components of the practice of nursing. Assessment, clinical judgment, interpretation and use of research findings, and leadership skills comprise professional components of nursing. At all educational levels, clinical experiences provide situations for nurturing professional behaviors. The learning goal of clinical experiences is development of competent nurses who provide safe care within each designated scope of practice.

Nurse educators can use transformative approaches in clinical settings. Encouraging learners to reflect during and after exposure to various clinical situations can guide learners to identify personal assumptions that influence understanding of clinical situations, possibly resulting in learners reconsidering their assumptions. From personal reflection and group dialogue, learners may realize other points of view that will influence problem solving, decision making, and behaviors during clinical situations. Educators cannot control the unpredictable, complex, specialized, and hurried clinical environments and must be aware that learners may identify assumptions or points of view in response to planned or unanticipated experiences. Therefore, educators must be flexible and astute when designing placement of content and when planning clinical experiences to equip learners to respond appropriately to challenges that arise (McAllister et al., 2007). Keen assessment, critical thinking, and ability to adapt or accept alternatives are needed to meet demands in practice.

The following assumptions guide the discussion in this chapter:

1. Clinical experiences provide learning opportunities for application of theories.

2. Learners must build on previous knowledge and experiences to provide actual nursing care in clinical settings.
3. Disorienting dilemmas may arise unexpectedly or may be anticipated within clinical experiences to spark critical reflection regarding previous knowledge.
4. Discussions before and/or after clinical experiences are critical for dialogue and sharing of experiences to promote reflection and awareness of others' points of view.

Before beginning the discussion related to transformative learning within clinical experiences, an example demonstrates how critical self-reflection during post-clinical conferences and after completion of clinical assignments can have profound personal and professional impact:

> During a post-conference following a clinical experience at a state-supported acute care psychiatric facility, Betty discusses her interactions with a hospitalized patient for whom she provided care during the past three clinical days. The instructor had encouraged students to interact with patients prior to review of charts in order to begin an independent assessment. Betty states how participating in a brief interaction prior to review of the chart was beneficial, "I met the young man, used my therapeutic communication skills, and learned about his goals for participating in his own health care and treatment management. When I later reviewed his chart, I read that he was a convicted serial rapist. I never would have talked with him had I known that. He is a real person, not just someone I would see on a news report. I think he wants to participate in treatment to not hear the voices anymore." Several weeks after the semester ended, the student told the faculty member, "I really had to search within myself after my inpatient mental health clinical experience. My older sister had a baby before she was married. My family believed this brought shame on us. I have been unable to talk with my sister because I realized that I had been so angry with her for the hurt my family felt. I realized that if I could talk with a man who had done very hurtful things to others and advocate for him to pursue his goals for getting and continuing treatment, then perhaps I could talk with my sister. During our semester break, I contacted my sister and we got together to talk. I am thankful for how this clinical experience actually worked out for my own personal benefit."

The above situation actually occurred and illustrates the powerful impact of critical reflection, critical self-reflection, and dialogue following clinical situations. In this situation, transformative learning occurred, both from planned learning activities and from happenstance occurrences.

LEARNING OPPORTUNITIES IN CLINICAL EXPERIENCES

Clinical experiences allow learners to interact with individuals, families, groups, or communities who have various health concerns, throughout the life span and in all health care delivery settings. The history of nursing education includes accounts of how actual experiences with individuals have provided rich opportunities for identification and reflection regarding the presentation and recognition of health concerns, nursing interventions, and outcomes from those interventions. War fields provided clinical experiences for Florence Nightingale, and Clara Barton's assumption hunting, industrial settings for

Linda Richards' reflections, while community settings were pivotal for Lillian Wald, Mary Breckinridge, and others. Current educators can reflect on how these nursing pioneers were able to transform personally and professionally, while influencing society and the development of the profession of nursing.

Recent changes in health care delivery in the United States have prompted a health promotion/disease prevention model of care, with earlier discharge from acute care facilities to home, rehabilitation, or long-term care settings. Faculty intentionally design clinical learning experiences for courses across the curriculum to expose learners to a variety of acuity levels and/or practice arenas. Learners are encouraged to reflect on their knowledge within clinical settings. When learners determine that additional knowledge is needed, or perceive a conflict in personal assumptions or knowledge with what is being experienced, they must critically reflect and discuss with the person or family being cared for and with faculty or other professionals. The dialogue enables learners to consider others' points of view and to discover applications or revisions of knowledge.

Jeffries (2009) points out that the issue for nurse educators may be in determining what learning experiences best occur in simulated environments and which outcomes can be better attained from experiences in clinical settings. As Scheckel (2009) discusses:

> The rationale that guides the design and selection of learning activities is reflected in the understanding that students should be educated for self-development and the various nursing roles in society. The selecting of experiences that enable curriculum outcomes to be met cannot be accomplished through a casual, hit-or-miss approach; learning activities must be thoughtfully designed to offer students the opportunities necessary to achieve the intended curriculum outcomes. [Clinical] learning activities are designed to engage students in listening to and interacting with others, observing, thinking, and doing in a manner that highlights the knowledge, attitudes, competencies, and skills to be acquired. (p. 154)

Thus, inclusion of well-designed learning activities within actual clinical settings provide opportunities for learners to reflect and acquire knowledge that would not be attained in other curricular settings (e.g., online or traditional classroom, simulation, viewing audiovisual recordings, computer-assisted instruction, etc.). Clinical experiences must also be designed to enable accomplishment of essential competencies for the level of educational preparation. For example, at the baccalaureate level, clinical experiences provide occasions for learners to practice quality, safe, holistic care that meets the needs of the individual, family, or community and to assess individuals and systems to provide leadership across settings of care.

Clinical experiences provide exposure for learners to encounter specific concepts related to health/illness/disease or professional behaviors within the curriculum. Experiences can assist learners to discover pertinent connections between theory and practice. However, experiences often vary among learners yet provide opportunity for similar outcomes. For example, nursing care for individuals encountering changes in circulation may occur throughout various health care settings (i.e., while checking blood pressures at a health fair or in the emergency department). Variety across the life span is shown by another example of a nursing student who must integrate knowledge of illness and its management for teaching regarding breathing techniques for asthma at both an elementary school and at an assisted living facility. Both examples encourage learners to use prior knowledge and to dialogue with individuals. During this dialogue, disorienting dilemmas may occur when learners are faced with different points of view from their own assumptions, leading to further critical reflection and consideration of rationales in the choice of specific interventions.

Experiences in health care settings provide opportunities for learners to develop cognitive and psychomotor (technical), or affective (communicative or emancipatory) learning. Clinical settings are selected based on anticipated stimuli for learning as related to course outcomes/objectives or competencies. During clinical events, faculty members monitor and facilitate learners' practice and professional behaviors. Nurse educators propose clinical expectations for learners that are appropriate to the course level within the curriculum. Learners begin with close supervision and become more independent in subsequent courses, with expected outcomes at higher levels. Motivation of learners can be increased through emotionally satisfying clinical experiences, and self-efficacy can increase, thus providing inspiration for further learning.

Early clinical experiences are geared toward increasing new knowledge by building on previously learned knowledge and skills. Close guidance and supervision is needed in these early phases (Emerson, 2007). As learners grow, they become more autonomous and begin integrating caring behaviors, which are nurtured and modeled by faculty throughout clinical experiences. Emerson states that

> instructional approaches in the clinical setting that enlighten the [learner] in regard to alternative ways of thinking and intervening, clinical questioning, and seminar or clinical conference activities such as debates and role-playing from the position of the patient of family members are examples of caring pedagogy. Caring pedagogies assist nursing [students] to learn how to care for their patients. (pp. 26–27)

Clinical experiences that support dialogue provide learners with an increased awareness of differing ways of knowing and an understanding of nursing roles in the context of personal and professional growth as a caring nurse (Emerson, 2007). For example, Jennifer provided care to a postoperative patient with a large abdominal incision. When Jennifer reminded him to use his incentive spirometer, the patient refused to do so, stating, "It is too painful." Later, the patient developed a fever, and a discussion ensued between Jennifer and the clinical faculty member regarding his use of the spirometer. Jennifer stated the patient would not use the device because it hurt too much. Dialogue between Jennifer and the faculty member provided Jennifer with an understanding of the need for lung expansion following surgery. The nurse educator encouraged Jennifer to consider ethical principles of autonomy, beneficence, and nonmaleficence. Further discussion and Socratic questioning allowed Jennifer to critically think through a solution to encourage the patient's use of the incentive spirometer.

Clinical situations create necessity for learners to engage in active learning, often problem-based learning that requires critical thinking, clinical judgment, and identification or articulation of what information is known as well as what information is not known or understood for providing safe nursing care. Learners' nursing role identity begins simply and progresses to providing care in more complex situations. Dialogue between learners, nurse educators, patients, families, and other members of the health care delivery team provide alternative perspectives of issues as complexity increases.

As students learn to unravel factors that influence health care management or health promotion motivation or behaviors, interactions between nursing students and patients become more complex. The influence of cultural aspects can be incorporated when planning clinical learning opportunities. Creative use of community settings provide transcultural experiences that effectively expose learners to diverse people, places, and resources as appropriate for the learners' level (e.g., beginning, intermediate, advanced). Transcultural experiences can include interactions with individuals, families, or groups from differing backgrounds, ages, socioeconomic levels, or motivation for health care behaviors. For example, nursing students can interact with older individuals in a nutrition center in a predominately poor rural community. During this clinical experience, students perform a holistic assessment, identify needed interventions, and present health promotion teaching. In addition, advanced nursing students interact with the older adults in reviewing medications and health literacy.

A second example of a transcultural experience is providing health care resource information for the homeless population within the community. This experience has resulted in learners identifying barriers to access and modifications that would be required for appropriate discharge planning. Learning outcomes that have resulted from this clinical experience are that faculty as co-learners have developed more awareness in the unknowing, ethical, sociopolitical, and empirical patterns of knowing. A third example of a community clinical experience is travel to another country to collaborate with a health care provider or nursing school. All of these are examples of creative design for rich clinical environments in which faculty and students as co-learners can critically reflect, self-reflect, and dialogue for transformation.

Within clinical situations, disorienting dilemmas are likely to occur when learners identify personal assumptions and points of view that are perceived to be inaccurate or inadequate during interactions. Faculty can encourage time for critical self-reflection and dialogue through integration of reflective journaling or discussion activities. For example, following a community hospice experience, learners are asked to journal what they learned, how they felt, and what they took away from the experience regarding nursing practice. Following this experience, one student commented, "One thing that is hard for me when dealing with hospice care is that the nurse isn't trying to help the patient to get well, but instead is trying to maintain the patient's quality of life as best they can while also maintaining the patient's dignity." The learner reflected on an assumption that nurses can help everyone to get well. The student realized that this assumption was in conflict with the reality of hospice nursing.

Clinical experiences in multiple health care settings can promote learner assimilation of how concepts interact and overlap. Overarching goals for learners in clinical experiences are to demonstrate application of knowledge in various settings and to gain an increased understanding of self as a future nurse. Identification of patterns and applications of content can result in greater retention of knowledge. The opportunity for learners to reflect, dialogue, and choose behaviors can promote commitment to actions and a nursing identity that can be applied in future situations.

PRECLINICAL AND POSTCLINICAL CONFERENCES

Transformative learning may occur during clinical experiences when learners engage in the performance of nursing care. However, an opportunity for reflection or dialogue may be difficult. For example, in the beginning a learner's concentration is task focused and may only consider if a task was performed accurately or not. The educator's focus may also be on ensuring that students perform tasks safely and in a timely manner. More advanced learner's can expand their focus to include not only if the tasks are completed accurately and safely but also to consider factors that affect care and if modifications may be indicated. Educators must interact with nursing students to guide them to develop a habit of self-reflection. Private discussions, pre-conference and post-conference, offer time for learners and faculty to openly discuss and reflect on anticipated or completed expectations of the clinical experience.

Pre-conference takes place in preparation for the clinical experience. Table 11.1 provides questions to prompt thinking in pre-conference regarding knowledge, assumptions, personal motivation, reflection, and disorienting dilemmas. The faculty member can discuss learners' personal learning goal(s) for the experience and remind learners of the expectations and anticipated outcomes of the experience. Learners reflect on previous knowledge in contemplation of meeting the necessary outcomes and may begin to identify some personal assumptions. Dialogue between faculty and other learners allows learners to identify gaps in knowledge or make changes in understanding to improve preparedness for anticipated learning opportunities. For example, a student is assigned to care for a patient with a recent stroke. The learner understands from previous nursing theory courses that it is necessary for patients to ambulate to prevent pneumonia, deep vein thrombosis, contractures, and muscle wasting, but the patient's condition prevents getting out of bed. Through dialogue, the learner reflects about how prior knowledge could be adapted for planning and implementation of nursing care (i.e., active and passive range of motion, repositioning every 2 hours, turn, cough, and deep breathing) to prevent these catastrophic events from occurring in a patient unable to ambulate.

Additionally, through self-reflection or dialogue, learners may identify motivators for applying what is previously known to what is currently needed, as opposed to concluding that past knowledge does not apply to the current situation. Learners may consider quality and safety initiatives, what would be desired if the person receiving care was a family member, model behaviors of a respected staff nurse or faculty, or desire positive affirmation for performance from staff, faculty, peers, or the patient's family. During self-reflection, learners may assume that the patient/family values are the same as their own. It is through interaction with patients, families, peers, faculty, and health care delivery team members that learners can identify conflicting points of view and thus reconsider their own assumptions. The reflection is likely to continue past the actual experience if the learner experiences a disorienting dilemma.

Faculty and learners readily engage in pre-conference discussions to adequately prepare for safe and effective clinical experiences. Post-clinical conferences occur following the clinical experience, allowing immediate recall of events and timely feedback. However, post-conferences can be rushed or omitted due to time constraints. Time for adequate reflection and dialogue should be allocated for post-clinical conference discussions, as these discussions provide opportunity for learner transformation when the pressure of performance is not a concern. Table 11.2 provides questions to prompt thinking in post-conferences regarding knowledge, assumptions, personal motivation, reflection, and disorienting dilemmas.

Faculty must establish a nonjudgmental culture during pre-conference and post-conferences to encourage and support honest and open learner reflection. The faculty facilitator must view each learner as possessing distinctive characteristics and values. All learners should have an opportunity to share and discuss concerns and experiences with faculty encouragement. The degree of faculty direction during clinical conferences will decrease as learners progress through the nursing program and are exposed to a variety of clinical experiences (Emerson, 2007).

TABLE 11.1   Preclinical Conference Questions for Transformative Learning

Category	Questions
Knowledge	What do you know about patients with _____?
	What skills are you able to do?
	How will you perform the task/intervention?
	What do you need to know before you _____?
Assumptions	What do you think the client expects?
	What are you expecting to find?
	What do you think is priority?
	What questions do you need answered to care for a patient with _____?
	Where will you find information on _____?
Personal motivation	Do you feel prepared for today's clinical?
	What are your goals for today?
	What do you think about caring for a patient with _____?
	What information do you need and why do you think it is important?
	Why should you seek alternatives for providing care for this person?
Reflection	What are some things you feel comfortable doing?
	Where do you believe you might need help?
	How have you dealt with similar issues?
	In what way have your classmates considered a similar situation in a different way than you have?
	In what way may the client/family values differ from your own and how will you plan for the differences?
Disorienting dilemmas	How will you handle _____ situation?
	You might observe one thing, but have been taught another, what should you do?
	What will you do if your values differ from those of the person/family for whom you are providing care?
	What will you do if the client's definition of health or motivation for health promotion/illness management differs from your own?
	What will be your approach if your priorities differ from those of the patient or other members of the health care team?

TABLE 11.2 Postclinical Conference Questions for Transformative Learning

Category	Questions
Knowledge	What was the most important thing to be learned from this situation? What problem(s) should you have foreseen? What did you learn? What did you learn about the individuals with whom you talked (cognitive/educational, physical/functional, psychosocial, spiritual, developmental)?
Assumptions	What was the priority(s) in the situation? Which patient do you believe that you learned the most from? Why? Describe a situation which was "eye-opening" for you. What did you learn from it?
Personal motivation	Were your personal goals for learning met? Describe how. Do you believe that your care was effective and efficient? Why or why not? What would motivate you to improve in another situation?

Reflection	How might you have handled the situation differently?
	In what area have you experienced the most growth (choose from communication, assessment, documentation, organization, critical thinking, or professional role)? Give one example of specific thinking or behavior.
	What would you do differently next time?
	Critical Thinking: what should you have known
	    In regards to preparation. . .
	    In regards to medication/treatment. . .
	    In regards to "putting the pieces together". . .
	    In regards to my patient's particular problem/needs. . .
	Communication: what should you have (or should not have) said
	    "I can't believe I said that."
	    "I didn't know what to say when he/she said. . ."
	    "My mind went completely blank when. . ."
	    "I didn't know where to go for help. I felt so stupid."
	Assessment: what won't you miss next time
	    "How could I have missed that _____finding(s)?"
	    "Why didn't I see that?"
	    "I can't believe I didn't assess_____!
	    "Maybe the next nurse will do it."
	    "I'm just not sure how to describe ____."
	Technical Skills: what do you need to practice
	    "I got discombobulated."
	    "I didn't have the supplies I needed."
	    "It wasn't exactly like in the skills lab."
	    "I know what to do. Why can't I just do it?"

Disorienting dilemmas	You are providing care in one way (e.g., doing a procedure or assessment) but being told to do it another way (e.g., by the textbook, procedure manual, another nurse). What is different about the two? Which way is right in this situation? Why? Why was this situation happening (e.g., drop in vital signs, patient vomiting, etc.)? What else should you have considered? How would either inductive or deductive reasoning have helped your thinking?

CONCLUSIONS

As suggested by Valiga (2009), in spite of many studies in nursing education, the state of the science remains weak. More nursing education research is available to evaluate learning outcomes and pedagogy with theoretically based studies. We offer transformative learning as one theoretical foundation for evaluating clinical learning experiences. In particular, questions related to learners' valuing of content from theory courses, learners' engagement in various types and locations of clinical settings in relation to variables of time, practical reasoning regarding the essence of the situation, and learners' integration to the role of the nurse are topics that need further research (Benner, Tanner, & Chesla, 2009).

Supportive learning, where acceptance rather than blamed is provided, is necessary for effective transformative clinical education to occur. In this type of environment, knowledge and responsibility is shared between learners and faculty (Benner et al., 2009; Case & Oermann, 2004). Dialogue fosters development of skills such as communication, collaboration, psychomotor performance, and so on. Benner et al. view one aspect of clinical learning as "[learners] need both theory and the opportunity to use and evaluate theory in practice, recognizing the limitation of theory in predicting particular patients' responses or specifying nursing actions" (p. 384). Reflection provides opportunities for assimilation of differing points of view through openness to transform personal assumptions and begin formation or reformation in nursing roles.

REFERENCES

Benner, P., Tanner, C., & Chesla, C. (2009). *Expertise in nursing practice: Caring, clinical judgment, and ethics* (2nd ed.). New York, NY: Springer.

Case, B., & Oermann, M. H. (2004). Teaching in a clinical setting. In L. Caputi & L. Engelmann (Eds.), *Teaching nursing: The art and science* (Vol. 1, pp. 126–177). Glen Ellyn, IL: College of DuPage Press.

Emerson, R. J. (2007). *Nursing education in the clinical setting*. St. Louis, MO: Mosby/ Elsevier.

Jeffries, P. R. (2009). Guest editorial: Dreams for the future for clinical simulation. *Nursing Education Perspectives, 30*(2), 71.

McAllister, M., Tower, M., & Walker, R. (2007). Gentle interruptions: Transformative approaches to clinical teaching. *Journal of Nursing Education, 46*(7), 304–312.

Scheckel, M. (2009). Selecting learning experiences to achieve curriculum outcomes. In D. M. Billings & J. A. Halstead (Eds.), *Teaching in nursing: A guide for faculty* (3rd ed., pp. 154–172). St. Louis, MO: Saunders/Elsevier.

Valiga, T. (2009). Ongoing development of the science of nursing education. In C. M. Shultz (Ed.), *Building a science of nursing education: Foundation for evidence-based teaching-learning*. New York, NY: National League for Nursing.

12

Transformative Learning in the Online Environment

Allison J. Terry and Debbie R. Faulk

Transformative learning can be fostered in an online environment ... through meaningful interactions among learners in which people feel free to express divergent points of view and feel supported and challenged by their peers and their teachers.

—Patricia Cranton

Transformational learning, particularly in nursing, is a unique form of relational learning. It requires the nurse educator to participate with students as he or she examines assumptions about teaching and learning as well as the various aspects of the student–teacher relationship. The process of developing learning communities through transformative learning can be easily implemented using online learning methodologies. In this chapter, we situate transformative learning within the online teaching environment. Students who have spent their formative years "twittering" and "tweeting" on various social network sites do not view an online community as impersonal and distant. Rather, they view these interactive networks as opportunities for interaction that can be nurtured during online instruction just as closely knit as face-to-face interactions.

Cranton (2010) articulates that a "community of inquiry" can develop in the online environment with a potential for engaging students in reflection and use of imagination. This environment sets the stage for "articulating, reviewing, and revising meaning perspectives" (p. 8). Thus, we believe that online instruction provides an excellent medium for the development of a caring community through transformational learning.

Southern (2007) notes that transformational learning encourages the creation of learning communities of care. These communities of care allow both students and teachers to participate together to shape the learning environment and create change. Ryman, Burrell, and Richardson support this assumption by stating, "Learning can be profoundly and personally transformative when it occurs within a community. Creating knowledge in learning communities can facilitate innovative solutions to increasingly complex problems in today's knowledge society" (abstract, 2010). The process of developing these care communities requires nurse educators to stretch the pedagogical boundaries so that students can navigate through the academic process in a way that is uniquely meaningful, while challenging students to expand their consciousness boundaries. When the learning community that is developed respects the unique qualities of each participant, the student as well as the teacher can develop a sense of belonging to a greater community that extends each participant's perspective globally.

ADVANTAGES AND DISADVANTAGES OF ONLINE LEARNING

Questions concerning differences in learner outcomes in online versus traditional environments continue to provide a rich research agenda. Synthesis of findings across various disciplines demonstrate no significant differences in learner outcomes and, in some cases, indicate that learner outcomes are better in the online environment (Glahn & Gen, 2002; United States Department of Education Report, 2009; Woo & Kimmick, 2005). As the use of technology and online learning increases and evolves, research related to differences in learner outcomes will continue to provide evidence for educator decision making. Nurse educators must continue to weigh the pros and cons related to the use of online learning when designing courses and learning activities. However, technology in education, though dynamic, must be incorporated into instruction because as Feeg (2004) stated, it is "now in our face" (p. 1).

Advantages

The advantages of online learning are approached from a universal perspective. Experts agree that technology has changed the way health care providers practice and how educators teach. Technology has widely impacted pedagogy in nursing curricula. Online learning can facilitate learning for those who learn through active, hands-on experimentation, yet also internalize the learning.

Synthesis of the literature indicates ample advantages to using online instruction to enhance the process of transformative learning. A major advantage of online instructional delivery is an increase in student interaction. Hanlin-Rowney et al. (2006) designed a qualitative research project that facilitated transformational learning in an online venue. They utilized an online group mediation to experience the group's multiple levels of connection. The participants reported experiencing a sense of engagement that was greater than any of the participants had previously experienced with face-to-face interaction in groups. Furthermore, the group participants reported that utilizing the online venue:

- Fostered dialogue between group members as well as a process of reflection,
- Made the process more meaningful because of the availability of all members' responses,
- Provided the opportunity of working with members globally, and
- Provided a record of all interactions by allowing field notes to be developed from online dialogue.

Another significant advantage of online instruction is its student-centered approach. Sherman (2006) found that the "Millennial Generation" will not tolerate being lectured to but, instead, expects the type of interactive engagement that can only occur through technology. Because this group of learners excels at multitasking as well as accessing information in a nonlinear manner, they expect to be instructed using virtual reality as well as simulation. The use of virtual reality allows users to absorb knowledge using all of the senses. Furthermore, as instructors no longer function as gatekeepers of information, students value them for their intellectual wellsprings as well as for their ability to guide learners electronically. Shovein, Huston, Fox, and Damazo (2005) found that online learning has a profound impact on learners by emancipation from the confines of schedules imposed by both work and personal commitments while providing the learner with a vast sea of data availability. Shovein et al. noted that technology literally allows the instructor to relinquish the role of the controller of information and instead assume the multiple roles of mediator, coach, and encourager as he or she guides the student to acquire knowledge.

An advantage of online learning for the educator is the promotion of the development of technology skills. Moon, Michelich, and McKinnon (2005) noted that the reduction in class time that occurs when learning is moved to primarily online venues forces the instructor to reexamine course goals and objectives for learner appropriateness, design online learning activities to meet the revamped goals and objectives, and acquire the technology skills needed to facilitate online discussions. In addition, Abel (2005) found that implementing a program of study online fostered teamwork within both academic departments as well as within various units of an academic institution. Usually, the faculty will have the benefit of instructional technology as well as classes in online technology to enhance their individual online toolkits.

An additional benefit to faculty members from the use of online instruction is the fostering of an increased level of engagement and commitment. Lautenbach (2008) found that instruction using technology is more effective when lecturers are fully committed, and this level of commitment, in turn, fosters engagement. Because engagement is inherently collaborative, this further promotes the use of collaboration and problem solving among the entire online community.

Disadvantages

There is no doubt that the advantages of technology in both practice and educational settings are invaluable, and with technology comes power. This power does not negate the fact that ethical knowledge is critical to the use of technology to prevent damaging oneself, others, and society as a whole. A full discussion of the ethical issues surrounding the use of online learning is beyond the scope of this chapter. However, suffice it to say that nursing educators teaching in online environments must apply the same ethical standards as those in the traditional classroom. Ethical standards such as fairness related to access must be considered in the online environment.

Another disadvantage expressed by many educators is that technology via e-learning is a cold and impersonal way to teach and can result in a lack of humanness in the instruction delivered. This human element can be engaged, however, through the ability of the learner to access a myriad of information and data. The human element of technology is further exhibited in greater student to student and student to teacher engagement (Shovein et al., 2005). This is crucial because at some point in the teaching/learning process, engagement is inevitable and imperative for all patterns of knowledge in nursing.

This brings us to another argument proposed by nurse educators—the assumption that aesthetic, personal, and ethical knowledge cannot be taught in the online environment. Whether engagement is through traditional face-to-face teaching/learning instruction or through online learning, varying the levels of engagement is a complex phenomenon. According to Shulman (2002), engagement comes first in the learning process and leads to knowledge and understanding. With e-learning, engagement depends primarily on the teacher's engagement with the technology. This engagement is exhibited through course design and development of learning activities to promote the uniqueness of nursing knowledge. Aesthetic, personal, and ethical knowledge can be enhanced through revolutionary technological innovations, which allow for human interchange or social interactions in the e-learning environment. For example, in an online senior-level transition to professional nursing practice course, a faculty led blog is used for the interchange of ideas related to current practice trends and the impact of future nursing issues within the context of professionalism. Students responding to the assumption: "Nurses with a powerful practice commit to continuous learning through education, skill development, and evidence-based practice," allowed for a lively interchange of points of view and for identification of the power assumptions have on behaviors. Several student comments included:

> I have also witnessed the fact that autonomy and research can make a nurse a more independent and professional individual. There have been many times when nurses ask the charge nurse for answers instead of looking for the answers themselves. This seems to lead to increasing dependence on others. Continuing education and evidence-based practice are part of a powerful professional practice.

> Without education, one cannot and almost should not continue delivering health care. Education of the nurse is crucial in learning the necessary means of health maintenance for self and the patient. The combination of education and evidence-based research and practice yield better forms of care and a well-read nurse.

> I agree 100 percent that knowledge is power, and I also think that an important component of knowledge is admitting when you are unsure or do not have the knowledge. A significant part of being a professional nurse is accountability. When I was a charge nurse, I felt much better about my nurses coming and asking questions versus those that never asked a question. Whether one has been a nurse for 20 years or 1 year, no one knows everything. This is especially true in the health care field where information and technology are constantly changing.

ONLINE LEARNING TOOLS FOR TRANSFORMATIVE LEARNING

There are a number of course management systems that allow for "housing" information in online courses, and decisions as to which system to use are most often based on university and school policies and, in some instances, teacher preference. Tools for teaching online continue to increase in number and in user-friendly capabilities. In making decisions as to which tools are most effective in the transformative learning environment, the educator must consider how the tools will promote use of transformative approaches, while not impacting self-directed, self-paced, independent, and individualized learning. It is also important for the nurse educator to note that, although there are numerous technologies that can be used to enhance learning and build online learning communities, technology can also block progress toward building these learning communities (Wicks, 2009). If we overwhelm the student with the technology or if the student lacks appropriate skills, the focus is on the technology and not the learning or community.

Probably one of the most familiar and simple tools for delivering information in the online environment is e-mail. In the transformative environment, e-mail can be used to stimulate student to student and student to faculty interactions. Critical dialogue can take place in this asynchronous venue. Faculty or students can self-reflect upon issues or questions that are posed in e-mails. Recchiuti (2003) studied the use of e-mail as well as instant messaging and online chat rooms by college students and found that specific groups of students are more drawn to each of these avenues than other students. For example, participants in the study extolled e-mail for its convenience and stated that they utilized instant messaging for its benefits of companionship and anonymity. Participants were more likely to take part in online chat rooms if they found interpersonal communication to be less rewarding. The findings also indicated that female students were more likely to use e-mail than male students and that those students aged 17 to 20 were more likely to use instant messaging than their older counterparts. Because of students' identified preference for specific online instructional delivery tools, this information means that specific populations of students can be targeted for marketing of an online instructional program based on their age and gender.

In contrast to the use of e-mail, instant messaging, and chat rooms is the use of video streaming as a tool to enhance online learning. Streaming video is considered to be the technique utilized in the transmission and viewing of video in real-time through the Internet. Hartsell and Yuen (2006) found that use of this technique as an instructional tool can effectively ensure that learners grasp the concept being taught if it is used to show a procedural demonstration. Video streaming allows the combining of video, audio, print communication, and software programs, as a means of feedback for students who are experiencing difficulties with a specific procedure.

In addition to video streaming, there are a number of web and screen casting systems that can be used to enhance learning in the online environment. These include WIMBA Live®, Camtasia®, Captivate®, or Panopto®. All of these tools can be used effectively in the transformative learning environment if used in combination with VoiceThread®. VoiceThread allows faculty and students to record text and audio related to uploaded images either through PowerPoints or videos. This digital dialogue tool encourages student engagement in the learning process and is less boring than e-mail and other asynchronous discussion boards or in just listening or watching slides either created by faculty or other students. VoiceThread allows educators to create transformative learning activities that encourage communication and collaboration with learners from all over the world. Consider the use of this online tool for dialogue with nursing students from other countries in examination of assumptions related to egocentricisms or in dialogue with nursing leaders and managers working in magnet institutions across the country. Students who have never worked in a magnet facility can vicariously experience this through these VoiceThread dialogues, perhaps transforming perspectives related to the relationship of magnet status to quality.

Another tool that can be used to present information and stimulate dialogue in the online environment is videoconferencing. Easily implemented using appropriate software, an affordably priced camera, and an Internet connection, this tool meets the learning style needs of a variety of students as it will appeal to both visual and auditory learners. This technology also allows for students in multiple classrooms in various locations to collaborate. Again, transformative learning approaches can be used with this technology. Videoconferencing encourages students to practice and improve presentation and communication skills because of being "on-camera" and hones research skills through preparation for upcoming conferences. This offers a great opportunity for more experienced students to mentor younger, less experienced students (Jobe, 1999).

Another tool that can be utilized to foster transformative learning in the online environment is WebQuest®. WebQuest is an inquiry-oriented activity in which learners interact with information from resources on the Internet that can be supplemented with videoconferencing. WebQuest can be used in the short or long term. The short-term WebQuest has as its goal for the learner to make sense of a new body of information. The long-term WebQuest allows the learners to analyze the previously acquired information, transform it, and demonstrate an understanding of the material by creating something that other individuals can respond to. Examples of longer-term WebQuests could be the interviewing of a simulated client online, an interactive case study created by learners, or the analysis of a controversial situation whereby students take a stand and then invite users to discuss their position on that stand (Dodge, 1997).

Open discussion in online forums can also be used to deliver online instruction. In these forums, there is a moderator who guides the discussion, while the audience has the freedom to raise issues, discuss various points that have been made, make comments, and ask questions. The online forum allows both the moderator, the subject-matter expert, and other speakers to participate in the discussion without having the expense and inconvenience of travel, while removing some of the barriers of the panel discussion and the formality of symposiums (Illinois Online Network, 2010). This tool can be used to engage online learners and allows educators to create learning opportunities using transformative approaches.

The various tools that have been briefly reviewed can fulfill multiple needs of the learner as well as the educator and can be used to foster transformative learning in the online environment. The use of such tools for online learning can also promote collaborative learning between students. Whether through small group work as mentioned previously or through brainstorming, case studies, simulations, or debates, the development of collaborative skills in students can prove to be invaluable to them later in their career. Employers now search for employees who are team players that can function as part of a larger group and as the group leader. Collaborative learning has been shown to be more effective than individual efforts at promoting cognitive development, student self-esteem, and the growth of positive, collegial relationships between students (Illinois Online Network). Finally, it should be emphasized that the responsibility for learning in the online environment is placed on the student, though the entire process is facilitated by the educator. The online instructional process will work most effectively with the proactive learner who is highly motivated and self-directed (Illinois Online Network). See Table 12.1 for a list of online tools and suggested uses.

RELEVANCE OF TRANSFORMATIVE LEARNING TO ONLINE LEARNING

For most educators, transformational learning will not be implemented in an online environment until its relevance has been established. The relevance to such an environment can be illustrated by a review of King's transformative learning opportunities model (2005). Implementation of this model serves to both empower and support learners while building a welcoming climate. Initially, the model postulates that an environment of safety and trust must be established for the learner. The student must believe that he or she can share ideas freely, that views will be respected, he or she will be given an equal

TABLE 12.1 Online Learning Tools and Suggested Uses

Online Tools	Suggested Uses
Email	Student to student and student to faculty interactions
Instant messaging	Critical dialogue in an asynchronous venue
Chat rooms	Encourage faculty or students self-reflection
Video streaming	Help learners grasp concepts through demonstration of procedures
Videoconferencing	Encourage collaboration in various locations Students practice and improve presentation and communication skills Offer opportunities for more experienced students to mentor younger, less experienced students (Jobe, 1999)
Web and screen casting systems, such as WIMBA Live Camtasia Captivate Panopto	Encourage student engagement in the learning process
WebQuest	Interaction with information from resources on the Internet Help learner to make sense of new information Allow learners to analyze previously acquired information, transform it, and demonstrate an understanding of the material Interview of a simulated client online Explore an interactive case study created by learners Analysis of controversial situations
Online forums	Raise issues for discussion Consideration of various points of view Participation in discussions without expense and inconvenience of travel

opportunity to participate, and confidentiality will be maintained. These are the same guidelines that must be maintained with any online discussion or online community that solicits participation from multiple members. For some participants, the fact that communication is occurring in an environment without face-to-face contact will encourage openness and honesty.

The second phase of the transformative learning opportunities model consists of determining learners' needs and expectations. The online environment is extremely conducive to implementation of this phase as learners' needs and expectations can easily be determined through the use of e-mail at various hours of the day or after traditional work hours. Again, students may be more open with teachers in discussing specific needs through an opportunity to express these without the potential embarrassment that may be associated with face-to-face contact. This can provide the educator with valuable information that might not be received otherwise.

The third phase of the transformative learning opportunities model consists of creating learning experiences for the student. This can occur through:

- *Engaging in critical reflection,* which more likely enable learners to examine their own assumptions and ask thought-provoking questions of classmates if an environment of safety and trust has been established.
- *Cultivating dialogue,* which results in learners who are well-versed in the intricacies of technology. For the most part, the Millennium Generation learners are more comfortable developing discussions online rather than face-to-face. They are accustomed to blog-type dialogue and social network interaction and, therefore, are more likely to be open and forthcoming in such an environment.
- *Envisioning and supporting application,* which occurs as learners share responsibility with the educator for the development of lifelong learning skills and experiences. This can easily be accomplished via an online discussion group where both students and educators participate and post regular comments as well as questions.

Finally, the transformative learning opportunities model culminates in revisiting needs, teaching, and learning. The online environment easily lends itself to implementation of this stage as blog postings can be saved and reviewed to determine how initial needs and the teaching learning process evolved throughout the length of the course.

STRATEGIES FOR FOSTERING TRANSFORMATIVE LEARNING IN THE ONLINE ENVIRONMENT

As presented in the previous section, there are many tools that can be used to deliver information in the online environment. Therefore, working from an assumption that transformative learning is based on the principles presented in Chapter 2, Box 2.1, and the key transformative learning approaches of critical reflection, critical self-reflection (including questioning personal values, beliefs, and assumptions), critical dialogue, and specific learning strategies and experiences can be created to stimulate changes in perspectives. A transformative learning strategy that is used in an online transformation to professional practice course provides an example of a learning activity that can be adapted for use by nurse educators at all levels. Student comments are also provided to illustrate examples of transformative learning outcomes.

Students in an RN to BSN completion program begin a *Perspective Transformation Portfolio* (PTP) during their first semester. The PTP is developed to enhance student critical thinking, perspective transformation, self-reflection skills, and learning over the course of the entire program. In addition, this learning strategy allows students to demonstrate knowledge, creative thinking abilities, and technological skills to future employers and graduate admission committees. Although there are numerous electronic portfolio programs on the market, to save money, students develop portfolios electronically by using a free wiki site of choice. The PTP is comprised of numerous transformative activities that students complete over the course of three semesters. A list of portfolio transformative learning activities within specific courses is presented in Table 12.2. To allow for adaptation of the learning activity to a specific course and/or educational level of preparation, Box 12.1 provides more specific directions related to the learning activities.

The following student comment illustrates a transformative learning outcome related to completion of a portfolio activity:

> The epiphany bells are ringing loud and clear. I now see my future. My weakness beginning this program and this semester was my thoughts of nursing management. My goal was to complete this program and assignment as quickly as possible to continue to move forward. Through the many talks that . . . and I have had, she has pointed out that I am needed in leadership . . . says that I have so much compassion for the bedside nurse, that it will make me a good leader. I believe that because of this course, I am inspired to be more. I want to be the difference. I want to learn more about leadership and managing in a positive way. I want others to want to be like me someday, and I want to always do good for someone else. I believe that what I have learned from my experience and from this course will make me a great authentic leader. I am self-disciplined and like to encourage others to do more and realize that there is more. I hope that I am able to begin and end a leadership career with these same thoughts. I really want to make bedside nursing in any fashion or facility a better place for all nurses. I want people to enjoy coming to work.

TABLE 12.2 Perspective Transformation Portfolio

Course	Transformative Approach	Learning Activity
Transformation to Professional Nursing I	Critical/self-reflection (questioning beliefs, values, assumptions) Critical dialogue Identification and validation of alternative points of view	Professional values Image of nursing Critical practice appraisals Disorienting dilemmas Caring
Leading and Managing in Health Care Microenvironments	Examination of alternative points of view Critical/self-reflection	Community volunteer experience Leadership moment analysis Disorienting dilemmas Book analysis
Transformation to Professional Practice II	Critical/self-reflection (questioning beliefs, values, assumptions)	Evolving nursing philosophy Evolving professional values Professional self-concept Personal career trajectory

BOX 12.1   Directions for Perspective Transformation Portfolio Activities

1. **Professional Values: A Self-Reflection for Philosophy of Nursing Development**

   In this activity, students are asked to self-reflect on professional values, identifying how prior beliefs and values impact thinking related to current values. They then rank these values and begin to develop a personal philosophy of nursing using the nursing metaparadigm.

2. **Image of Nursing**

   Students watch a list of YouTube video clips, critically reflecting on how the image of nursing is projected, identify underlying assumptions about how the image is portrayed, and state how thinking can be changed or transformed related to these images. Additionally, students identify what this means to a self-concept of professionalism. Students are also asked to identify which images conflict with current points of view and to state why.

3. **Critical Practice Appraisals**

   The purpose of this appraisal is to help students understand more about individual nursing practice and to identify and reflect upon assumptions that undergird how situations are analyzed, how decisions are made, and how actions are initiated.

   Students are asked to think back over clinical practice during the past 2 weeks and to reflect upon any "critical incidents" that occurred. A *critical incident* can be any event or patient situation that can be called to mind vividly, easily, and quickly as it is remembered. After identifying the critical incident, students complete the following:

   a. Briefly describe the incident in no more than two to three paragraphs that include details of what happened, who was involved, where and when it took place, and what it was that made the incident *critical*.

   b. Identify *assumptions* that were confirmed by this incident. What happened that led to thinking that the assumptions were accurate and valid?

   c. Identify assumptions that were challenged by the incident. What happened that led to thinking that assumptions uncovered might be inaccurate or invalid?

   d. Relate if the accuracy of assumptions were challenged. If not considered at the time, how could any assumptions be considered in the future if faced with this same situation?

   e. What sources of evidence should have been obtained?

   f. What different perspectives could be taken regarding the incident?

   g. Imagine the incident through the eyes of other people who were involved. Are there different ways the situation could be seen or the behaviors interpreted? In retrospect, are there different responses that could have been made to the incident? If so, what would these responses be, and why would they be made?

   (continued)

BOX 12.1 *(continued)*

4. **Disorienting Dilemma Identification**
   a. Identify disorienting dilemmas (any experience this term that failed to meet expectations or anything encountered that could not be understood using existing thinking) that resulted in cognitive dissonance (conflict of values).
   b. Critically reflect on the dilemma/dissonance and identify ways in which present habit of the minds might have been transformed/emancipated/liberated into a new way of thinking about the situation.

Adapted from *The Power of Critical Theory: Liberating Adult Learning and Teaching* by S. D. Brookfield. Copyright 2004 by Jossey-Bass.

5. **Caring Activity**
   a. Write a personal definition of caring. After writing the definition and reflecting, identify specific examples (at least two) of behaviors in which actions reflected the definition.
   b. Share the definition and examples with a peer in your current work setting. Through dialogue with the peer, ask them to identify assumptions that provide the foundation for the definition. Discuss with the peer how your definition impacts nursing and professional actions.
6. **Community Volunteer Experience**
   Volunteer for 4 hours in a community of choice. The student is encouraged to seek volunteer opportunities that involve cultural diversity. Submit a one-page synopsis of the experience including the purpose of the project, how and why you selected the project, and what professional values were enhanced or developed as a result of the experience.
7. **Professional Self-Concept**
   Describe your current professional self-concept. Reflect upon the description you wrote in the initial nursing concepts course and state how the two compare/contrast. How has the *Perspective Transformation Journey* changed prior habits of the mind related to thinking or describing you as a professional nurse?

OUTCOMES OF TRANSFORMATIVE LEARNING IN AN ONLINE ENVIRONMENT

Cranton (2010) believes that transformative learning can occur in an online environment and suggests a number of strategies and practices for fostering transformative learning in the virtual classroom. These include:

- Teacher presence is critical
- Learner choice in course process and content
- Ask thought-provoking questions in online discussions
- Teacher modeling of critical reflection and self-reflection by questioning points of view and providing explicit comments related to topics for discussion
- Create communities of knowers and inquirers through informal conversation
- Use learning activities that force students to view issues and content from an alternative perspective

Modeling critical reflection and enhancing learning community through informal conversation is demonstrated in an email a faculty member sent to a student in an online leadership and management course. The student posted a comment related to a "hot button" public policy issue—taking a point of view in opposition to the faculty:

Faculty member: Why do you insist on causing me to have cognitive dissonance?

Student: Did I really? Well, shoot, it's the least I can do . . . considering you've caused me to have about one hundred of them.

A learning activity is used in an online course to force students to view beliefs or preconceived ideas of what it means to be a professional nurse in a first semester transformation to professional practice course. During the first class, returning RN students are told that they are not "really professionals." Students then identify their professional self-concept, posting comments to share with peers. Cognitive dissonance is the initial outcome. However, many students begin to disagree with their initial postings midpoint in the program, and by the end of the program, almost all reflect on their inaccurate or incomplete understanding of professionalism.

Evidence to support transformative learning outcomes in online environments is limited. At the present time, anecdotal findings and practice suggestions from adult educators who use transformative approaches and strategies in traditional and online classrooms provide guidelines for nurse educators. If we are effective teachers in the traditional classroom, then we will be effective in a virtual environment. Cranton's (2010) point, "as educators, we bring our teaching styles and strengths into the online environment" (p. 8) is noteworthy.

Doering's (2006) research on adventure learning as a hybrid distance education approach can be used to determine anticipated outcomes for transformational learning online. Such outcomes could include:

- Providing an opportunity for student-to-student, student-to-expert, and student-to-teacher collaboration and interaction
- Providing students with easy access to the curriculum regardless of their location
- Providing students with easy access to both current print media in traditional format as well as up-to-the-minute knowledge from the field that may have just been released to the public
- Providing students with the opportunity to experience the advantages of transformational learning in a comfortable environment with the outcome of an increased level of motivation

Transformative principles and approaches may be used to develop learning activities that foster meaningful interactions among learners. By creating, challenging, and supporting communal knowing, the faculty can instill the trust that is needed to express opposing points of view, with a goal of change in perspectives and behaviors.

CONCLUSIONS

Stokowski (2011) noted that "as a profession, nursing is moving beyond the objective of simply increasing its numbers, to positioning itself in a healthcare environment that is being transformed to meet the needs of accessible healthcare" (section 7, p. 1). For nursing to position itself in such an environment, transformative learning must be implemented, whether in an online or traditional classroom. Because of online learning's focus on increasing student interaction, development of technological skills, and increasing the level of engagement for both faculty and students, the process of transformative learning should accelerate rapidly and smoothly without the obstacle of learners resisting the transformation process. As an end result, online transformative learning occurs. Nursing care will be of higher quality, safer in its delivery, more accessible to the patient population, and more affordable both to the consumer receiving it and the health care facility responsible for employing the nurses delivering the care.

REFERENCES

Abel, R. (2005). *Achieving success in internet-supported learning in higher education: Case studies illuminate success factors, challenges, and future directions.* Retrieved from http://www.a-hec.org/media/files/A-HEC_IsL0205_6.pdf

Brookfield, S. (2004). *The power of critical theory: Liberating adult learning and teaching.* San Francisco, CA: Jossey-Bass.

Cranton, P. (2010). Transformative learning in an online environment. *International Journal of Adult Vocational Education and Technology, 1*(2), 1–10.

Dodge, B. (1997). *Some thoughts about WebQuests.* Retrieved from http://webquest.sdsu.edu/about_webquests.html

Doering, A. (2006). Adventure learning: Transformative hybrid online education. *Distance Education, 27*(2), 197–215.

Feeg, V. D. (2004). Campaign for nursing curriculum reform in information technology: Got IT? Part I: IT and health care. *Deans's Notes, 26*(2), 1.

Glahn, R. A., & Gen, R. M. (2002). *Teaching in the next millennium: The implications of an organization's human resource management infrastructure on the adoption of online education practices.* Retrieved from http://www.genconnection.com/Ray/dissertation.pdf

Hanlin-Rowney, A., Kuntzelman, K., Abad Lara, M. E., Quinn, D., Roffman, K., Nichols, T. T., et al. (2006). Collaborative inquiry as a framework for exploring transformative learning online. *Journal of Transformative Education, 4*, 320–334.

Hartsell, T., & Yuen, S. (2006). Video streaming in online learning. *AACE Journal, 14*(1), 31–43.

Illinois Online Network. (2010). *Instructional strategies for online courses.* Retrieved from http://www.ion.uillinois.edu/resources/tutorials/pedagogy/instructionalstrategies.asp

Jobe, H. (1999). Desktop videoconferencing: Novelty of legitimate teaching tool. *Education World.* Retrieved from http://www.educationworld.com/a_curr/curr120.shtml

King, K. (2005). *Bringing transformative learning to life.* Malabar, FL: Krieger.

Lautenbach, G. (2008). Stories of engagement with e-learning: Revisiting the taxonomy of learning. *International Journal of Information and Communication Technology Education, 4*(3), 13–19.

Moon, D., Michelich, V., & McKinnon, S. (2005). Blow away the competition: Explosive best practices for cost effective excellence in distance learning. *Community College Journal of Research and Practice, 29*, 621–622.

Office of Planning, Evaluation, and Policy Development, Policy and Program Studies Service. (2009). *U.S. Department of Education evaluation of evidence-based practices in online learning: A meta-analysis and review of online learning studies.* Washington, DC: Author.

Recchiuti, J. (2003). *College students' uses and motives for e-mail, instant messaging, and online chat rooms*. Newark, DE: University of Delaware.

Ryman, S., Burrell, L., & Richardson, B. (2010). *Creating and sustaining online learning environments*. Retrieved from http://www.atypon-link.com/EMP/doi/abs/10.5172/ijpl.5.3.46

Sherman, R. (2006). Leading a multigenerational nursing workforce: Issues, challenges and strategies. *OJIN: The Online Journal of Issues in Nursing, 11*(2). doi: 10.3912/OJIN.Vol11No02Man02

Shovein, J., Huston, C., Fox, S., & Damazo, B. (2005). Challenging traditional teaching and learning paradigms: Online learning and emancipatory teaching. *Nursing Education Perspectives, 26*(6), 340–343.

Shulman, L. (2002). Making differences: A table of learning. *Change, 34*(6), 36–44.

Southern, N. (2007). Mentoring for transformative learning: The importance of relationship in creating learning communities of care. *Journal of Transformative Education, 5*(4): 329–338.

Stokowski, L. (2011). *Overhauling nursing education*. Retrieved from http://www.medscape.com/viewarticle/736236

Wicks, D. J. (2009). Emerging theories and online learning environments for adults. In K. Rice (Ed.), *Theories of Educational Technology*. Retrieved from https://sites.google.com/a/boisestate.edu/edtechtheories/Home

Woo, M. A., & Kimmick, J. V. (2005). *Comparison of internet versus lecture instructional methods for teaching nursing research*. Retrieved from http://www.sciencedirect.com/science?_ob=ArticleURL&_udi=B6WKV-4H28M02-6&_user=10&_coverDate=06%2F30%2F2000&_rdoc=1&_fmt=high&_orig=search&_origin=search&_sort=d&_docanchor=&view=c&_searchStrId=1639341796&_rerunOrigin=google&_acct=C000050221&_version=1&_urlVersion=0&_userid=10&md5=81787239060e72ec84ce25fa22f7e636&searchtype=a

IV

Transformative Learning for Specific
Educational Issues

13

Using the Transformative Process for Student Success

Julie Freeman and Ramona Browder Lazenby

Man's mind, once stretched by a new idea, never regains its original dimensions.
—Oliver Wendell Holmes

It is anticipated that 55% of practicing nurses will consider retirement between 2011 and 2020. If this holds true, an additional 1 million nurses will be needed by 2016. The market will demand that nursing programs produce 30% more graduates (American Association of Colleges of Nursing, 2008). The conundrum is that while there are many qualified applicants eager to gain access to nursing schools, an increasing faculty shortage has forced many nursing programs to limit admission numbers (Gazza, 2009). As limited numbers of qualified students are admitted, the pressure to decrease attrition and increase retention will become a reality.

A number of methods for increasing retention in nursing programs are offered in the literature (Jeffreys, 2004; Peyrovi, Parvizy, & Haghani, 2009; Stark, Feikema, & Wyngarden, 2002; Symes, Tart, Travis, & Toombs, 2002). In this chapter, we examine retention issues and offer suggestions for student success within the context of transformative learning. Using Mezirow's phases of perspective transformation (1991) and core elements of centrality of experience, critical reflection, and rational discourse, factors impacting retention from a faculty and student perspective are discussed.

Although attrition rates may be calculated differently across institutions, no matter how the rates are calculated, it is still a loss. According to Fowler and Norrie (2009), attrition and retention is multifactorial involving three general areas: faculty, student, and society. Nurse educators need to be aware of these three dimensions when evaluating factors impacting student retention.

According to Goodtrack (2010), retention rates are directly related to the relationship that is formed between students and faculty. In a study conducted by Shelton (2003), students who perceived faculty as mentors through a caring and supportive relationship were more likely to complete the nursing program. This pivotal role of faculty requires time and commitment, which can be challenging as student-to-faculty ratios increase. Inadequate numbers of faculty impede the ability for early identification of challenges that impact retention while also jeopardizing efforts to promote the transformative learning process. Swinney and Dobal (2008) further emphasized the need for faculty to be good facilitators and to empathize with students in an effort to increase diversity in the workforce.

Students are unique individuals who do not learn the same way. Faculty must respect the individuality of each student and offer support while maintaining standards. Consistent with Tinto's theory of retention (1993), students have a need to *feel* like a part of the culture. The student needs to believe he/she is connected to other students, faculty, and administration. This connection is fostered through interaction over time, again reinforcing the idea that transformation occurs gradually. Many students have grown accustomed to a paradigm of sitting in class, listening to lecture, and then regurgitating the information for the examination. With the transition from a teaching focus to a learning focus, students must relearn how to learn, and this can be a major factor impeding the ability to transform.

The third factor impacting retention is related to societal issues. The nursing shortage creates the need for schools of nursing to increase the number of graduates while educational resources are being cut. The image of nursing is also inappropriately displayed in society, distorting the reality that nursing requires not only caring but also critical thinking at the highest level. Other societal issues include the knowledge explosion and increased cultural diversity.

Not only do these factors need to be considered in light of retention but also as key components in the transformational process. For society, the transformation may begin with the realization that a nurse is not just an "angel in white" but rather a knowledgeable health care provider who continuously monitors and adjusts the plan of care as necessary.

PHASES OF TRANSFORMATION

Mezirow identified 10 phases of perspective transformation in 1991. He further specified three core elements that occur in transformative learning: centrality of experience, critical reflection, and rational discourse. These phases and elements provide an interesting perspective from which nurse educators can examine retention issues and then design opportunities to increase student success (see Table 13.1).

Centrality of Experience

Centrality of experience refers to an individual's starting point, whether student or faculty. Actions reflect a person's frame of reference which encompasses habits of the mind and an individual's point of view. An individual's frame of reference is influenced by many factors including culture, family, past life experiences, and society to name a few. Left unchallenged, this frame of reference remains stagnant and prohibits the exploration of new ideas and meaning. This element is "central" to the first four phases of the transformative process.

TABLE 13.1   Phases of the Perspective Transformation Cycle

Phase 1   A disorienting dilemma occurs
Phase 2   Self-examination with feelings of guilt or shame, sometimes turning to religion for support
Phase 3   Critically assessing personal, professional, or cultural assumptions
Phase 4   Recognizing that the process of discontentment and transformation can be shared, acknowledging that others have negotiated similar changes
Phase 5   Searching for and committing to new roles, relationships, and behaviors
Phase 6   Planning a strategy to act on commitment
Phase 7   Acquiring knowledge and skills for implementing strategies for action
Phase 8   Trying and evaluating new roles and behaviors
Phase 9   Developing personal skill and confidence in new roles and relationships
Phase 10 Incorporating behavioral change into one's life based on the new perspectives

Adapted from *A Critical Theory of Adult Learning and Education* by Mezirow, 1991, pp. 168–169.

Disorienting Dilemma

The impetus to begin to imagine that there are other options is the result of a disorienting dilemma. For example, faculty member A has always had students arrive at every class at least 10 minutes early. Students of Generation Y tend to not only show up late, but sometimes not even show up at all— what disrespect! Well, does the student see that as disrespectful? Perhaps not—the fact that they can read the book and glean the same information may have prompted them to sleep in rather than getting up early and coming to class. If transformation is an outcome, the faculty must commit to allow, and role model, transformation in his or her own role as an educator. Other disorienting dilemmas for faculty may include generational differences, which faculty may perceive as disrespectful, differences in motivating factors for different students, and transition from a teacher-centered to a learner-centered focus.

Perhaps one of the most disorienting dilemmas for the faculty related to attrition/retention issues is the perception that struggling students are passive if they do not seek or accept help. The student may be embarrassed, or cultural issues may play a role. For example, in a classroom, the faculty announced that anyone who scored less than 75% on an examination was expected to make an individual appointment. The faculty member was extremely distressed that one student had not taken the initiative to do as instructed. When the faculty member finally approached the student, it was identified that the native culture of the student prohibited students initiating contact with the professor. Only the professor was worthy enough to approach the student.

Disorienting dilemmas for the student are numerous. During lower division course work, students become accustomed to each course being considered independent of others. Knowledge gained from a history course does not impact a mathematics course. Upon entering a nursing program, the student is now expected to consider all subjects under study in relation to each other. For example, the study of pathophysiology and the disease process is threaded throughout each area of nursing education. One cannot learn the aspects and theory behind the pathophysiology of the disease process and then leave it behind upon progression to another course. This new way of learning, thinking, and knowing for nursing students creates anxiety and may impede success.

Another disorienting dilemma occurs as students realize that previous approaches to academic success may need to be altered if previous study and test-taking skills are not as effective. The expectation that the knowledge acquired in each course be carried forward and the ability to utilize all areas of knowledge can create anxiety. The students often acknowledge experiencing diminished self-confidence upon receiving lower grades after initial examinations. As admission to nursing school is highly competitive, students are often unaccustomed to attending class with peers of equal potential and are reluctant to work in groups due to the desire to be at the top of the class. This attitude requires transformation as the student recognizes that the profession of nursing engages in collaborative practice. In addition, an inability to apply information learned to a multiple choice question format of testing utilized in nursing education produces frustration.

To facilitate students during the disorienting dilemma phase, educators first make students aware that disorienting dilemmas will occur. Preparing the student in advance will help the student recognize dilemmas when they occur as well as help the student understand that these dilemmas can be expected. Making the students aware of the massive reading assignments in multiple courses, classroom plus clinical components, and expectation for critical thinking rather than rote memorization may help ease the initial shock.

Self-Examination

The process of self-examination includes reflection, evaluation, recognition of the need to transform, and altering patterns of thinking, knowing, and learning knowledge of self. While this process can be emotional and painful, it is necessary for transformation to continue. Faculty must explore the rationale for teaching strategies and determine how those strategies can be improved. Although the tendency is to teach as one has been taught, an honest self-examination may reveal that perhaps that is not the best way for others to learn. Faculty need to be encouraged to reflect on his or her personal learning style and understand that their teaching style may need to change. Novice faculty may experience feelings of guilt when students are not successful. This can be an impetus to evaluate teaching techniques, but it does not necessarily indicate that the technique is inappropriate. Self-examination also requires separating the subjective and objective to make certain that standards are being upheld. An authentic attitude is critical, but standards have to be upheld.

Students entering nursing programs expect to perform at previous levels. These students have been successful throughout their academic careers and are often ill prepared for the first set of low or failing grades. The blow to self-confidence is often expressed through anger, resentment, and a belief that the student cannot be at fault for this lack of success. As the learners' perception of self is an important component of transformative learning, it is essential to provide support during these first disorienting dilemmas (Cranton, 2006). The student is faced with the need to alter previous patterns of thinking, knowing, and learning or to acquire different patterns to better reorient the knowledge of self in relation to the present environment (Cranton). The alteration of patterns then leads to a revised self-acceptance. Acceptance of the altered patterns and transition to the modified self-confidence must then be incorporated into the revised pattern of learning. At this point, the student realizes a need to transform previous styles of acquiring and applying knowledge. Progression toward transformation requires charting a new path to success. This path includes changes in reading styles, note-taking, study habits, application, time management, and prioritization.

Critical Assessment of Assumptions

The third phase of the transformative process is a critical assessment of assumptions. Until assumptions are identified and evaluated, transformation cannot begin. For the faculty, the critical assessment of assumptions may center on the idea that all students learn the same, when, in fact, it is known that is not the case at all. The temptation to continue what has been done for years may impair the faculty's ability to question why things should be changed. Rather than examining alternative ways to teach a variety of concepts, it may be more comfortable to stay with the known. With the technology explosion, the faculty may need to examine the worth of lengthy reading assignments as opposed to computer-assisted activities or other forms of electronic learning. Although it may be distracting to some, the faculty cannot assume that the student who is surfing the web during class is not also listening to what is being said. The challenge for faculty is to become comfortable with examining personal assumptions and be open with students about the fact that each of us has to experience transformation and move forward, or we risk becoming stagnant in our learning.

Perhaps the most important assumption that must be critically assessed is that the current patterns of knowing and learning will be sufficient to be successful in nursing school and the nursing profession. Students should seek answers regarding their current learning competencies, attitudes toward the learning process, and effort put forth. The utilization of a self-assessment tool to determine areas of strength and weakness in both academic skills and personal life can provide valuable guidance (Jeffreys, 2004; Stark et al., 2002). As the student performs a critical appraisal, areas that support the students' success and areas that require change should surface (Peyrovi et al., 2009; Symes et al., 2002). Even though the goal of fostering critical thinking skills is involved in student retention, the development of a life-long learning focus is advantageous for health care professionals (Symes et al). This is of particular importance to the profession of nursing as the provision of nursing care is a fluid and dynamic environment impacted by technology, pharmacologic advances, and changes brought about by evidence-based research (Stark et al; Yuan, Williams, & Fan, 2008).

While students believe they bring individual academic skills to the nursing program, their preparation can vary greatly. Additional factors impacting academic success include the quality of previous education, natural aptitude, and the attitude toward self-learning, organization competence, study skills, and the desire to succeed (Peyrovi et al., 2009). Faculty and students need an understanding of how both previous academic preparation and the students' innate abilities affect learning (Jeffreys, 2004; Stark et al., 2002). Students frequently assume that the previous approach to learning will continue to be effective. Yet, if the student has not been provided opportunities to develop critical thinking skills, then change must take place.

Recognition That One's Discontent and Process of Transformation Are Shared

Feelings of discontent can be expected when the student experiences diminished success. Recognition of areas of discontent through critical assessment and self-reflection requires action. Is the discontent with the reality of the professional role of nurse? Is the discontent due to the struggle to balance work, personal life, and academics? Is the discontent related to the diminished academic success or disillusionment with faculty support? Is the discontent related to the realization that there are other students as capable or perhaps even stronger than the individual? Each individual's perception plays a key role in identifying areas of discontent. The ability to identify the areas of discontent allows the student to achieve another step in the transition to success. Yet, if students are unwilling to allow perspective transformation to proceed after the initial disorienting dilemma occurs, then the opportunity to succeed in pursuit of a nursing education diminishes (Peyrovi et al., 2009).

During this phase, the transformative learner should be able to identify potential new or alternate roles for success after self-reflection and faculty input. Individual and group learning activities that can be effective in moving the student forward in the transformation process will be discussed later. Working with faculty, or specified mentors, students can identify areas of need and develop a focused approach to addressing these needs. This phase can also provide the student with the opportunity to regain control of the learning process through setting realistic attainable goals.

Critical Reflection

According to Mezirow (1991), critical reflection is the distinguishing characteristic of an adult learner. Critical reflection requires the individual to question half-truths, feelings, beliefs, and actions. The questioning of assumptions and beliefs based on prior experiences is the impetus to help individuals identify personal beliefs and the reasons for those beliefs. This questioning then propels the individual to identify new methods of thinking and knowing. This is the theme throughout the next phase: exploration of options for new roles, relationships, and actions.

Exploration of Options for New Roles, Relationships, and Actions

During this phase, the faculty will begin to try new teaching methodologies that move from teacher-centered to student-centered. When met with resistance, the faculty must critically reflect on the rationale for the change and realize that resistance is inevitable with any change.

Students must try new ways of studying, note-taking, and test-taking because the former ways have not proven productive. The student may join a study group or disassociate from a previous study group that may not have been productive. Trying out new options can be frightening and often overwhelming, especially if the first attempt at something new was not effective.

Rational Discourse

At this point, the individual is objectively seeking to create understanding. Supporting arguments are based on evidence with the primary goal of promoting mutual understanding. Rational discourse is the process whereby critical reflections are converted to actions. This transformative learning element is present in the final five phases of the transformative process.

Planning a Course of Action

Planning a course of action requires dialogue among peers. Input from experienced faculty can help novice faculty develop a plan of action. For the student, transformative learning has the potential to improve retention and decrease attrition. As students dialogue with the faculty about an alternative plan of action, the faculty can offer a different perspective and help the student identify skills that may be necessary to implement the new plan.

Acquiring Knowledge and Skills for Implementing One's Plan

After developing the plan and identifying the knowledge and skills necessary to attain the goal, the faculty is ready to implement the plan. As novice faculty try out the new role, confidence will begin to develop, and the new ways of knowing and thinking can be integrated into life. Attending teaching conferences and watching others teach can be helpful in identifying and perhaps acquiring new teaching techniques.

For the student, one of the key skills needed for success and transformation is critical thinking. Critical thinking is the ability to recognize or identify issues requiring analysis, identification of knowledge or the lack of knowledge, any preconceived ideas related to the issue, and a determination of the knowledge needed to most effectively address the issue (Elder & Paul, 2003). Adept critical thinkers realize that there is more than one approach to addressing the issue and will utilize the information provided to select the best or most appropriate steps to address the issue. The faculty can role model and stimulate critical thinking through Socratic questioning, role playing, and the use of case studies.

Provisional Trying on of New Roles

This phase will require risk-taking for faculty and students. Whether it is trying new teaching techniques for the faculty or a new way of studying for the student, the possibility exists that the changes may not work. Offering support and helping the faculty and students identify what worked, what did not work, and how things could be improved will facilitate continuation of the transformative process.

Building Competence and Self-Confidence in New Roles and Relationships

Competence and self-confidence will develop over time as successes are achieved. Feedback from students about new teaching techniques will motivate the faculty to continue developing and implementing new strategies. As the student begins to experience an increase in test scores and knowledge acquisition, confidence will increase and motivate the student to continue learning and transforming.

Reintegration Into One's Life

At this point, new techniques for the faculty and student are now considered a routine part of life. Because transformation in certain areas has occurred, the process may seem less intimidating and will hopefully motivate the faculty and students to continue self-examination in other areas.

FACULTY AND STUDENT TRANSFORMATION

Mezirow (1996) espouses that a transformation in perspective is "a more fully developed (more functional) frame of reference . . . one that is more (a) inclusive, (b) differentiating, (c) permeable, (d) critically reflective, and (e) integrative of experience" (p. 163). For transformation and effective learning to occur, the faculty must establish an environment of trust, safety, and openness (Taylor, 1998). While this may seem logical on the surface, the ability to create such an environment requires a skillful educator. Simple actions such as smiling, nodding, making eye contact when the student is talking, calling the student by name, asking students to share one interesting fact about their life, and speaking to students outside the classroom, all communicate that faculty care. Literature has consistently supported the importance of that connection with faculty (Ketola, 2009; Shelton, 2003; Swinney & Dobal, 2008; Tinto, 1993).

There are a variety of enhanced learning activities to assist students through perspective transformation with the resultant outcome of successful completion of a nursing program. For example, academic support programs can meet a variety of learning needs for students. Academic support programs reinforce classroom learning, inform students and faculty how to recognize learning styles, identify gaps in knowledge, review strategies for taking notes on faculty lectures, supplement information and textbook readings, and improve test-taking, study, and organization skills. Moreover, academic support programs incorporate efforts to identify students at risk for academic failure early in the curriculum. The student acquires ownership of the learning process through utilization of the many tools available to assist in determining and achieving goals.

The faculty is instrumental in providing guidance and feedback to students in defining the goal(s). The expertise of the faculty will also provide the feedback needed to assure that the student is able to identify realistic goals. Examples of potential goals could include developing better time management, developing effective reading comprehension, developing better note-taking, moving the grade point average up to the next level, or learning to work with others to facilitate success. The student will need to decide on the method of measurement for attainment of the goals. The method of measurement could include achieving specific grades on examinations, documenting specific amounts of time to improve studying and retention, or completing exercises such as group activities or technology-based programs that require the student to utilize multiple areas of knowledge, thus providing the opportunity to further hone critical thinking skills. The process of self-reflection can provide the student knowledge of both successful and unsuccessful current learning skills and relationships. Utilizing this knowledge, the faculty and student can identify the effective skills the student currently possesses to attain success and those that need to be refined. This is an important step in attaining the goal and requires faculty input and guidance.

The student needs a realistic plan to be able to attain the goals. When determining the goal(s), the student must identify steps that they are willing to take. The student must set goal(s) to which the student can commit the skills, time, and effort, or the exercise can be self-defeating. Identifying the actual skills, time, and effort is important so that the student maintains realistic expectations. If a student is a slow reader, planning to read an additional five chapters a day is a step to attain the goal of higher test scores, but may create an obstacle to this student's success. Can the student with slow reading skills realistically add another five chapters each day? There must be a period of time for the student to identify the goal(s), attempt to attain the goal(s), and determine if the goal(s) has been met. The set time frame requires the student to maintain ownership of the learning and change process. If the original plan does not lead to the desired success, then flexibility and review will need to take place.

The Student Success Program (SSP) at Texas Women's University Houston Center is a success example of an academic support group. The main focus of the SSP was to aid students in building the skill sets necessary to evolve into accomplished and successful learners. The SSP requires the students to be active participants in, and take ownership of, the process of learning (Symes et al., 2002). Overall, students in the SSP experienced success and found that participation in the structured formal program provided the opportunity to accept transition from previous knowledge of self to the accomplished learner knowledge of self.

The specific, measurable, attainable, realistic, and time bound (SMART) model for goal-setting has also proved to be a successful academic support program. This program works well with upper division nursing students (Top Achievement, 2010). The SMART model provides the means for the student to set one or two specific goals, decide on a method of measurement, determine the steps to attain the goal, and a time frame. The tool can be an effective individual strategy, but will benefit the student more if a faculty member guides the student through the process of utilizing the SMART tool. Students can struggle with goals that are too broad or too narrow, unattainable or unrealistic, with unmanageable time frames. The faculty have more experience with goal setting and goal attainment and can assist the student in gaining the skill set to move the transformation process forward.

Another effective goal setting tool is the Loma Linda University Exam Analysis (2006). Students and faculty review an examination and identify areas of concern related to four broad categories: lack of knowledge, English skills, examination anxiety, or examination skills. These broad topics are further broken down to allow students to identify weaknesses in reading comprehension and retention, note-taking, application of knowledge, vocabulary, anxiety, diminished focus, lack of focus on the question asked, changing answers, or not identifying answers (Loma Linda University). Upon review, the student determines the goals necessary to achieve success. The Loma Linda tool increases student self-awareness of changes that need to occur to be successful in the transformation process. The faculty using this particular tool note that, initially, students arrive for an examination analysis prepared to argue about the questions, but as the mentor and student review each missed question in a methodical process utilizing the *recognize, ask, critically evaluate, eliminate options* (RACE) model, students recognize the areas in which improvement is needed to achieve desired results. The identification of and writing of the goals is another step in self-actualization and progress toward ownership of the learning process and transformation.

The RACE model for test-taking in nursing was developed by Nugent (2008) to address issues students frequently have with multiple-choice testing formats utilized in nursing education. Problems achieving mastery on multiple-choice examinations can be related to innate ability or lack of experience with this style of testing. Several common factors are expressed by students regarding test-taking success. Some of these include rushing or misreading the question, changing answers, and confusion over what is being asked. Students are accustomed to multiple-choice questions that have only one correct answer, such as can be found in history, English, or math. In nursing education, the multiple-choice format requires the student to critically think and use their full scope of knowledge to select the best answer from several that could apply. While some students may always struggle with this style of testing, others can gain mastery through structured test-taking practice.

The RACE model is used in our baccalaureate program as a structured program for test-taking mastery and to encourage critical thinking skills. The model is modified to include recognition of key words and phrases, but the *first step also includes identifying the client.* Instead of critically analyzing the question in the second step, the student is now *asked to identify the problem or issue* in the question. The third step requires the student to critically *analyze what they know about the issue and to write down applicable knowledge.* For example, if the question requires knowledge related to chronic obstructive pulmonary disease (COPD) the student is expected to write down key pieces of knowledge related to COPD. This could include shortness of breath, history of smoking, poor capillary refill, tripod posture, or low oxygen saturation. After this step, the student should critically analyze the question in relation to the knowledge listed of the disease process. The fourth step requires the student to *eliminate as many options as possible.* Mastering these test-taking strategies takes time and practice.

Another area in which students request assistance is management of the volume of reading required in nursing (i.e., How do we organize and master the readings?). It is important to maintain an organized and consistent style of reading and note-taking in nursing as each area of knowledge builds on the others. It became apparent during academic support sessions that many students complete assigned readings but cannot recall or comprehend the material.

BOX 13.1   Stop, Slow, Go

Stop	Poor understanding of the material	Highlight in red
Slow	Moderate understanding of the material	Highlight in yellow
Go	Understanding of the material	Highlight in green

BOX 13.2   Methods for Seasoned Faculty to Facilitate Novice Faculty Transformation

Offer support by affirming words when new techniques are tried
Discuss what worked and what did not work
Encourage novice faculty to videotape themselves teaching and have a
   peer offer feedback
Celebrate successes
Be open to new ideas
Ask the novice faculty to evaluate your teaching and offer suggestions
Be a good listener

Additionally, students could not recall important information when beginning
to review material for examinations. Therefore, the authors designed a simple
program that can be used when reading or taking handwritten or computerized
notes. The students utilize a red, yellow, and green highlighting pen. The reason
for using these colors is because of a familiarity with what these colors stand
for in American culture: a red light indicates stop, a yellow light indicates slow
down and prepare to stop, and a green light indicates good to go. This program
is best used when reading before class so that the student can identify what was
and was not understood in the readings and be prepared for class.

BOX 13.3   Methods for Faculty to Facilitate Student Transformation

Foster a caring environment conducive to learning
   Eye contact as appropriate
   Smiling
   Nodding affirmation
   Offering words of affirmation for even the smallest achievement
   Be aware of nonverbal messages
   Offer your undivided attention
   Keep voice tone positive
   Avoid being defensive—explain rationales, but do not become defensive
Let students know they will encounter disorienting dilemmas
Determine if a group approach is helpful or harmful
Allow the student to grieve as they give up previous assumptions and
   methods of knowing
For the struggling student, require at least one session with the academic
   success officer (then it is up to the student to continue if it is valued)
Ask the following question, "Do grading tools and objective tests stifle
   creativity and critical thinking?"
Stimulate transformative learning through the use of learning contracts,
   case studies, simulation, metaphors, and reflective journaling
Be authentic and sincere
Be willing to admit when you are wrong
Be a good listener
Challenge the students to think and learn from each other
Be willing to learn from the students—and let them know you are
   learning from them

As the student reads, the course objectives, chapter objectives, and syllabus should be available. As the objectives are determined by the chapter author(s), the material that is significant for mastery in each chapter is identified. The objectives designed by the faculty guide the student toward expected comprehension of the material (see Box 13.1). For further methods to facilitate faculty and student transformation, see Boxes 13.2 and 13.3.

CONCLUSIONS

Mezirow's transformative learning theory (1991) is well suited to nursing education. Often individuals seeking to become nurses have never had exposure to the health care system or the role of the nurse. Nurse educators using the phases of transformation will be better equipped to address student needs during the transformative process. Assisting students in facing both the comfortable and uncomfortable aspects of transformation can reduce attrition rates and increase retention. Whether it is discussing the basis of personal beliefs about a generation or discussing the rationale for the answer to a test question, the faculty can demonstrate each phase of the transformative process while also indicating that transformation occurs over a lifetime. The nurse educator who is willing to share aspects of a personal transformative journey offers students a role model, as the faculty first transformed into a nurse and then into an educator, providing another example of lifelong learning.

Though transformation is a lifelong process that can be painful, it is more often rewarding. Questioning one's beliefs and ideas can stimulate many emotions such as grief, anger, and fear, but it can also be liberating and motivating as new ways of knowing become evident. Nursing students enter a program at any level of education expecting to perform at previous levels of success. Faculty awareness during the first disorienting dilemma can provide the student with a more positive transformative experience. Benner, Sutphen, Leonard, and Day (2011) note that the nursing profession expects nurses to continue the learning process upon entry to practice. Nursing students who have experienced a successful perspective transformation will be better prepared for continued learning such as through staff development activities. The faculty must be willing to demonstrate transformation in their own teaching to facilitate transformation in the student.

REFERENCES

American Association of Colleges of Nursing. (2008). *Nursing shortage fact sheet.* Retrieved from http://www.aacn.nche.edu/media/pdf/NrsgShortageFS.pdf

Benner, P., Sutphen, M., Leonard, V., & Day, L. (2011). *Educating nurses: A call for radical transformation.* Stanford, CA: Jossey-Bass.

Cranton, P. (2006). Supporting transformative learning. In P. Cranton (Ed.), *Understanding and promoting transformative learning* (2nd ed., pp. 159–180). San Francisco, CA: Wiley.

Cranton, P. (2006). Transformative learning theory. In P. Cranton (Ed.), *Understanding and promoting transformative learning* (2nd ed., pp. 19–56). San Francisco, CA: Wiley.

Elder, L., & Paul, R. (2003). Part I: Understanding the basic theory of analysis. In L. Elder, & R. Paul (Eds.), *The foundation of analytic thinking: How to take thinking apart and what to look for when you do* (pp. 2–9). Rohnert Park, CA: The Foundation for Critical Thinking.

Fowler, J., & Norrie, P. (2009). Development of an attrition risk prediction tool. *British Journal of Nursing, 18*(19), 1194–1200.

Gazza, E. A. (2009). The experience of being a full-time nursing faculty member in a baccalaureate nursing education program. *Journal of Professional Nursing 25*(4), 218–226. doi: 10.1016/j.profnurs.2009.01.006.

Goodtrack, R. B. (2010, Spring). Engage, challenge, nurture. *The Aboriginal Nurse,* 5.

Jeffreys, M. R. (2004). Academic factors. In M. R. Jeffreys (Ed.), *Nursing student retention: Understanding the process and making a difference* (pp. 64–77). New York, NY: Springer.

Ketola, J. (2009). An analysis of a mentoring program for baccalaureate nursing students: Does the past still influence the present? *Nursing forum 44*(4), 245–255.

Loma Linda University School of Nursing Learning Assistance Program (2006). *Summary of exam techniques for multiple choice questions.* Loma Linda, CA: Author

Mezirow, J. (1991). A critical theory of adult learning and education. *Adult Education Quarterly, 32*(3), 3–24.

Mezirow, J. (1996). Contemporary paradigms of learning. *Adult Education Quarterly, 46*(3), 158–172.

Nugent, P. M. (2008). *Test success: Test taking techniques for beginning nursing students* (5th ed.). Philadelphia, PA: F. A. Davis.

Peyrovi, H., Parvizy, S., & Haghami, H. (2009). Supportive counseling programme for nursing students experiencing academic failure: Randomized control trial. *Journal of Advanced Nursing, 65*, 1899–1906. doi: 10.1111/j.1365-2648.2009.05037.x.

Shelton, E. N. (2003). Faculty support and student retention. *Journal of Nursing Education, 42*(2), 68–76.

Stark, M. A., Feikema, B., & Wyngarden, K. (2002). Empowering students for NCLEX success: Self-assessment and planning. *Nurse Educator, 27*(3), 103–105. Retrieved from http://www.nursingcenter.com/library/index.asp

Swinney, J. E., & Dobal, M. T. (2008). Embracing the challenge: Increasing workforce diversity in nursing. *Hispanic Health Care International, 6*(4), 200–204.

Symes, L., Tart, K., Travis, L., & Toombs, M. S. (2002). Developing and retaining expert learners: The student success program. *Nurse Educator, 27*(5), 227–231. Retrieved from http://journals.lww.com/nurseeducatoronline/pages/default.aspx

Taylor, E. W. (1998). *The theory and practice of transformative learning: A critical review.* (Contract No. RR93002001). Columbus, OH: Center on Education and Training for Employment (ERIC Document Reproduction Service No. ED423422).

Tinto, V. (1993). *Leaving college: Rethinking the causes and cures of student attrition* (2nd ed.). Chicago, IL: University of Chicago Press.

Top Achievement. (2010). *Creating S.M.A.R.T. Goals.* Retrieved from http://www.top-achievement.com/smart.html

Yuan, H., Williams, B. A., & Fan, L. (2008). A systematic review of selected evidence on developing nursing students' critical thinking through problem-based learning. *Nurse Education Today, 28*, 657–663. doi: 10.1016/j.nedt.2007.12.006.

14

Self-Regulation Through Transformative Learning

Arlene H. Morris, Debbie R. Faulk, and Michelle A. Schutt

You can motivate by fear, and you can motivate by reward. Both those methods are only temporary. The only lasting thing is self-motivation.
                                                                              —Homer Rice

Threaded throughout the first 12 chapters is how transformative learning is fostered through the key approaches of critical reflection, self reflection, and dialogue. The very behavior of becoming reflective can be a transformation. In this chapter, we focus on these learning approaches to examine the issue of self-regulated learning (SRL) in nursing education. To critically reflect for transformation of perspectives, learners need to develop awareness and skill required to be self-regulated. Development of a deliberate process for self-regulation involves self-monitoring, planning, and goal setting by learners (Belles, Cihiwsky, Hall, Schindwolf, & Shober, 2008). SRL as defined by Zimmerman (2000) is "self-generated thoughts, feelings, and actions that are planned and cyclically adapted to attain personal goals" (p. 14). Successful completion of nursing programs and development of nurses' motivation and skills for lifelong learning requires development of self-regulation skills. The three main components of thinking in SRL are planning, monitoring, and evaluating. These components are used throughout the practice of nursing. Nurses must be able to plan for providing care, yet also identify personal learning needs and methods for continuing professional development. Patients must be monitored to provide quality and safe nursing care, and evaluation of patient outcomes is essential to determine if the interventions have been effective. Similarly, nurses must monitor their personal practices as nurses to assure continued competence and to determine effectiveness of interventions that are selected to continually develop personal expertise.

Several examples follow to illustrate a learner who is developing self-regulation skills and one who is not. After these examples, we briefly discuss SRL in nursing and the teaching strategies that can be used to promote development of self-regulation.

Jonathan is a second degree nursing student who is well-liked by faculty and peers. He has had a lifelong dream of becoming an emergency room nurse. In obtaining his first degree, Jonathan maintained a B average and had few difficulties planning his study habits or with motivation. However, after the middle of the first semester of nursing school, Jonathan begins to question his past methods for learning. He thinks about trying different ways to learn the vast, complex material. He partners with a senior nursing student whom he believes can help him to organize his thinking and who can serve as a mentor. This relationship works well until the senior graduates. Jonathan is actually frightened and excited at the same time. He wonders if he will be able to continue his present methods of studying by himself or should he change his plan for learning again? He even wonders if he might fail.

We see from the example that Jonathan was self-regulated to plan, organize, and monitor his learning. By seeking a partnership with a senior nursing student, his learning actually became directed by another individual. However, when the mentor was no longer available, Jonathan had to reevaluate his plan for learning. His goal of becoming an emergency room nurse and his fears and anxieties about receiving failing grades actually served as motivation to help him organize his thinking about the best methods to continue to be successful in the nursing program.

Martha on the other hand is not as outgoing as Jonathan and many of her peers do not know her last name. Martha's mother is a nurse and Martha believes she should follow in her mother's footsteps and become a nurse as well. Although she has no idea in which area of nursing she is most interested, she thinks she might like to work in Labor and Delivery once she graduates. Martha often tells classmates that she does not understand why nurses have to learn leadership and management skills. She simply does not see the value in learning this content because she never plans to be a leader or manager. During class, Martha is often seen surfing the web, trying to engage those around her in side conversations, and often distracting those sitting close to her. She rarely completes assignments on time as she has no plans, nor does she understand how to organize her thoughts around the readings and class lectures. She visits with faculty several times to talk about projects or learning assignments, but never finishes assignments as directed.

There is simply no planning, monitoring, or evaluating of learning in Martha's example.

SELF-REGULATED LEARNING

To situate SRL within transformative learning, a brief description of the concept, its components, and strategies for helping learners to develop self-regulated behaviors are offered. SRL is an elusive concept but includes the learner processes of *thinking ahead* (including task analysis with goal setting and strategic planning, and self-motivational beliefs such as self-efficacy), *performance* (including motivation, self-control/organization, and self-observation), and *self-reflection* (including self-judgment, evaluation, and self-reaction). Use of self-regulatory learning strategies can increase the perception of self-control and thereby provide motivation to continue to use self-regulation (Zimmerman, 2000).

Nursing faculty expect that students will enter a nursing program as independent, autonomous, empowered, motivated, and self-regulated learners, with an overarching goal of being successful. In fact, the faculty strive to create SRL environments whereby learners take full ownership for motivation and learning and in which new perspectives are developed and old perspectives can be transformed. However, the reality is that many learners are concurrently developing self-regulation skills, emotional intelligence, and the ability to identify personal assumptions, points of view of self or others, and self-reflection throughout nursing programs. Nurse educators must be aware that although some learners will engage and participate in critical self-reflection, others will not choose to do so at a particular time. Educators should continue to use transformative learning approaches throughout the curriculum, providing further opportunities for learners to choose to critically self-reflect.

Learners in the discipline of nursing require development of high-level thinking skills for critical thinking, clinical reasoning, and self-observation/self-reflection. Nurse educators can teach SRL behaviors, model, and dialogue regarding appropriate use of these behaviors to promote learner development of SRL skills throughout the nursing curricula. The potential outcome is development of a nurse who values and is committed to using these strategies throughout his/her career.

Self-Regulated Teaching Strategies

Learners can initially observe the use of SRL by faculty members and then apply the new SRL behaviors with faculty feedback, developing to the point of independently using SRL behaviors. Therefore, nursing faculty must incorporate modeling their own thinking and learning strategies to allow opportunity for learners to apply newly learned content with the concurrently learned SRL skills, and provide feedback, then plan for opportunities for learners to independently apply the content and SRL skills. For example, in designing content to stimulate development of SRL skills in returning nursing students, educators ask all learners in the class (online or traditional) to consider their initial thoughts about how they, in the role of nurse, would intervene with a person who comes into an emergency department expressing a distorted reality. The educator encourages each learner to *think ahead* about how they believe they would initially respond. Then, the educator asks each learner to recall any prior experiences they may have had with an individual whose reality was different from their own and to recall how they interacted with that individual (*review of personal performance*). This introduction of content is intended to help learners think ahead of situations that they may not have considered and to prime learners to engage in content as they consider how it may be used in their nursing practice. Additionally, the thinking ahead *self-reflection* can help learners to provisionally try out the new role of caregiver for a person with cognitive issues. The intentional discussion prompt that asks learners to recall past performance is designed to achieve at least two outcomes: comparing past role behavior before nursing (family member, another employment setting, etc.) to behaviors that the learners may believe a nurse would perform in this situation and to identify any assumptions as the learners self-reflect. In threaded online discussion or class dialogue, learners are exposed to perceptions of others and may identify assumptions that had not been realized and subsequently can develop a deeper appreciation of possible client needs. From this introduction, nurse educators can then continue presentation of course content to include possible etiologies of cognitive changes such as reaction to a medication or illicit substance, fluid or electrolyte imbalance, infection, oxygenation, dementia, delirium, developmental issues, etc. The intention of this component of content presentation is to stimulate *motivation* to become engaged in the learning opportunity and to help learners consider what may not have been considered independently. In this way, learners can become motivated to engage and to seek information or methods of clustering information that will be retrievable to them at a later time.

In another example, a nurse educator plans class content to enable development of SRL skills. The nurse educator structures discussion about wound prevention by asking learners to think about what is involved in wound development and how wounds could be prevented in those who experience immobility. After listening to student responses, the educator provides additional information, encouraging the learners to think further about the relationships of concepts, the impact of other concepts such as protein and oxygenation, and the relevance of the content to their own transition to becoming a nurse and how this content potentially affects the patient's outcome.

The educator then asks learners to further think about what they currently know about wound prevention and related concepts and what is desired to be known. Next, learners are asked to complete a case study or view a clinical vignette in which some of the concepts can be applied, followed by discussion among group members to gain additional points of view. Then, learners apply the content in the clinical or simulated setting by providing actual care for a person who is immobile. At the next class meeting, the educator asks learners "What was your thinking about wound prevention while you were caring for those who are immobile?" The educator praises learners for improved thinking about various factors that contribute to wound formation and various interventions to prevent development, adding content that was not included by the learners. With each subsequent faculty–learner interaction, the educator input decreases, and learner thinking and awareness increases. Eventually, the educator is not needed, as the learner has developed SRL skills to use or obtain information that is needed for the practice of nursing.

A number of factors can inhibit learners from developing or maintaining SRL skills. Accurate learner perceptions of motivation, self-efficacy, and self-control are most significant in the development of SRL and must be considered by the learner and educator to develop SRL skills. If a learner enters a nursing program with a background in which self-regulated skills have not been developed in prior learning or other environments, the learning and personal application of SRL skills will be more difficult. Learners who have been told either that they possess skills and abilities that, in fact, are not possessed or have been told that they cannot perform at adequate levels may find SRL difficult.

The delicate balance for nurse educators is between structuring learning situations and allowing independence for SRL. Furthermore, educators must understand the necessity of emotional intelligence and control of personal emotions needed for concentration in learning nursing content and processing the feedback that is required for continued development. Therefore, self-discipline in goal setting and strategic progression to attain personal goals is crucial. To help learners, nurse educators must create an environment of trust through authenticity and opportunities for teacher and learner reflection and dialogue. In the structuring of this learning environment, transformative learning can be fostered.

TRANSFORMATIVE LEARNING FOR SELF-REGULATION

In Part IV, transformative learning as it applies to specific nursing education issues, beginning with student retention and empowerment, is discussed. In this chapter, transformative learning approaches are considered as effective methods in promoting SRL in nursing for lifelong learning. Use of critical self-reflection to identify prior assumptions, values, and beliefs can enable learners to realize the power or impact that prior beliefs have on points of view and resultant behaviors. Outcomes from this critical self-reflection and identification of personal factors can assist learners to consider their own perceptions of self, the education process, and personal motivation for engaging in learning required in nursing education.

Examples best illustrate changes in learners' perspectives. In the first example, one nursing student experienced difficulty in initial nursing courses. She was trying to memorize isolated facts, without considering how these facts would interact or be used. In a discussion with a faculty member, she self-reflected about her prior experiences with the health care delivery system, which included accompanying her mother to seek care for her physically challenged younger brother. She recounted how some of the experiences were more negative than positive. She then expressed her difficulty in imagining herself in the role of a nurse if she would be expected to make decisions like the nurses she had observed. After this brief, but powerful, self-reflection and dialogue, she identified that her difficulty in learning the content might actually be that she did not want to act like some of the nurses had acted toward her family. As the faculty guided her to identify her personal values, beliefs, and motivation for becoming a nurse, the student's thinking and approach to her courses changed as her ownership of her own learning increased with identification of her personal goals.

A second example of personal transformation was shared during a final seminar in an RN to BSN program. The student gave permission for the story to be told in this book:

> I attended a small high school in a small town in Alabama. I made average to above average grades in high school because I was a good memorizer. When I began the 9th grade and had to take algebra, I panicked as I found that I could not use memorization to learn algebra. I had developed the mindset that I would never be able to learn math and received reinforcement of this mind set from my mother and classmates who often stated that most girls were weak in math. This mindset followed me throughout most of my adult life. The math that I had to take when I went to LPN and ADN school was basic, so I managed to get through. However, when I decided I wanted to return to school to obtain my BSN, I let my assumptions that I could never learn algebra because I did not have the cognitive abilities and that I could not use behaviors (memorization) that had always gotten me through, delay that dream or goal for many, many years. Finally, I decided that I would give it a try, going into the algebra class knowing

that I would fail. This was my mindset. The disorienting dilemma that caused me to critically reflect on my assumptions and mindset was the first exam. For some reason, the fact that I knew I was going to fail the exam, made me realize that I could transform my thinking about not being able to learn. I actually wanted to learn algebra at that time. I finished the exam to the best of my ability, handed in my paper to the teacher, and told him I would be back, but I would be back after receiving tutoring. I hired a tutor, slowly began to see that my prior assumptions about not being able to learn algebra were wrong. I could learn. . . . I never made below a 90 on the rest of the exams in the class. From this experience, I was empowered to transform my way of not only thinking about math, but thinking about my overall ability to learn and to succeed in furthering my education. I realized that it was not so much about my cognitive abilities, but about my willingness and desire to learn, and to critically examine prior frames of references and to realize the power of these points of view on my decisions and behaviors. Thus I learned to take charge of my own learning and when I could not use personal resources, to ask for help.

This true account provides an example of a transformative learning activity in which learners are asked to write their personal transformation stories. In online and in-class venues, students, who are comfortable, with their personal transformation stories can share in small- or large-group dialogue. Through the creation of an authentic, caring learning environment, students can be encouraged to offer alternative points of view to help each other to further identify personal assumptions or habits of mind and to consider alternative ways of thinking. These examples reveal the overlap and interaction among transformative learning teaching approaches, progression through phases of perspective transformation (Mezirow, 1991), and principles for self-regulation.

A number of transformative learning activities have been provided in Parts II and III for use in teaching particular nursing courses. To describe the interaction between using transformative learning approaches and development of SRL, we continue with the example of using SRL teaching strategies for wound prevention to demonstrate how the transformative learning approaches of critical self-reflection and dialogue can promote SRL.

When implementing transformative learning approaches, nurse educators become facilitators or encouragers for learners to consider questions regarding personal confidence, autonomy, and motivation. Questions can be structured for pre-nursing interviews or courses early in the curriculum to help learners begin to self-reflect about their own assumptions (see Box 14.1). Various learner style inventories can assist learners, as can different value clarification exercises.

Nurse educators can intentionally incorporate questions to promote learner reflection and dialogue by asking students to *put on their thinking caps* to consider, for example, wound prevention and immobility. Questions to prompt self-reflection related to immobility or wounds may include:

1. What do you know about the concepts of immobility and/or wounds?
2. Do you have any past experiences with either of these? If so, what does that experience add to your knowledge, or what assumptions do you have about either immobility or wounds because of your personal experience?

3. Do you have any ideas regarding the prevalence or contributing factors for either of these or any related concepts?
4. What do you think will be your role as a nurse in providing care for those who experience immobility, wounds, or both?
5. Why does this content matter?
6. How do you assume that content about immobility or wounds will be taught?
7. What are your expectations for your own learning about immobility or wounds?
8. How do you anticipate that you will demonstrate that you have learned how to apply new information about immobility or wounds?

Learners may record and monitor their thoughts about any or all of these questions in a self-reflection journal or may discuss in pairs or small groups. Dialogue regarding reflections to these questions can allow learners to share their points of view and to organize and transform information while considering the points of view of classmates. Motivation for engaging in this content may occur from past experience, dialogue with others, or from thinking ahead about how the information will likely be used in nursing practice.

Educators can present additional information, with examples of how the content has been used in personal nursing care, or integrate a case study or clinical video clip as a basis from which the educator can model application of content to the depicted situation. Learners can then apply the content to answer class response system questions, apply to a further unfolding of the

---

BOX 14.1   Questions to Identify Personal Motivation and Assumptions

I. Why am I in nursing school?
   a. Is this my desire, or am I doing this to please someone else?
   b. What is my personal motivation for pursuing a nursing education?
   c. What do I hope to gain from this education or from future employment as a nurse?
II. What are my expectations (or assumptions) regarding how nursing courses should be taught?
   a. In what type of situations or courses have I performed well in my past?
   b. In what way do I prefer to learn?
   c. How would I describe my usual method of studying?
      1. Do I plan ahead for how I will learn relevant content?
      2. Am I actively engaged in my own learning? If so, how?
      3. Do I prefer to have educators to present facts or show how I will use those facts?
III. What level of commitment do I have for my own learning?
   a. What personal behaviors demonstrate this level of commitment?
   b. Are there other behaviors that I would like to develop?
IV. How would I describe my level of confidence in gaining new knowledge?
V. How would I describe my confidence in applying new knowledge in situations?

case study, or create additional questions to be considered. Learners are then asked to consider what content areas remain unclear and to identify and plan learning strategies to address the unclear areas.

A disorienting dilemma may occur for some learners who have anticipated that content related to immobility and wound prevention will be provided by the teacher, rather than actively engaging in learning that can be applied to various situations to achieve a sense of salience for critical thinking and clinical judgment ability. These learners may experience difficulty in application activities in which overlapping of the content areas requires interpretative judgment for identifying possible contributing factors or priority interventions. Learners may choose not to engage or may be motivated to engage by self-reflection and dialogue activities. Group dialogue can then progress to teaching others in the group or by enabling group members to rehearse information for providing nursing care. Mental imagery can be used to visualize the pathophysiology of the concepts, or concepts maps can be created if desired.

Learners must be able to check their own progress in understanding wound development and immobility and the relationship of these concepts to each other and to other concepts. If learners have been unable to dialogue within the group activity, unclear points may be self-identified. Courage is needed to admit personal accountability for seeking environmental resources (i.e., library, internet, textbooks, faculty, peers, etc.) that can be helpful for individual needs and learning preferences (Common self-regulation strategies, 2011). Further self-evaluation occurs in clinical or simulated settings through seeking opportunities to apply the concepts and determining if additional information is needed. Feedback from faculty members occurs through clinical discussions, formative and summative evaluations, or exam scores.

Nurse educators must intentionally plan methods to achieve the goal of creating transformative and SRL environments. Teaching strategies may include development of intentional questions that allow time for faculty and learner reflection and dialogue in which other points of view may be considered. Opportunities should also allow learners to develop a valuing of the content for use in practice. Modeling and discussing SRL behaviors can help learners develop effectiveness in planning, organizing, monitoring, and self-evaluating their own learning.

CONCLUSIONS

Nursing education is ripe for changes in teaching approaches. Learners need not memorize isolated facts, but to be able to determine what knowledge is needed and how to access the needed knowledge, how to use the knowledge by relating understanding of nursing concepts to other concepts and situations, while using interprofessional relationship skills. Change in teaching approaches includes planning activities that encourage transformative learning and the development of self-regulated behaviors. Graduates of nursing programs who develop SRL skills are positioned to impact the health care delivery system culture. However, without transformative learning, the commitment to do so may not be present.

REFERENCES

Belles, A., Cihiwsky, J., Hall, T., Schindwolf, M., & Shober, C. (2008). Self-regulated learning. Retrieved from http://www.unco.edu/cebs/psychology/kevinpugh/motivation_project/349_spring08/final4/psy/selfregulation.htm

Common self-regulation strategies. (2011). Retrieved from http://www.gifted.uconn.edu/siegle/selfregulation/section7.html

Mezirow, J. (1991). *Transformative dimensions of adult learning.* San Francisco, CA: Jossey-Bass.

Zimmerman, B. J. (2000). Attaining self-regulation: A social-cognitive perspective. In M. Boekaerts, P. R. Pintrich, & M. Zeidner (Eds.), *Handbook of self-regulation* (pp. 451–502). San Diego, CA: Academic Press.

15

Being an Educator: Bringing Ourselves Into Teaching Practice Using Transformative Learning

Debbie R. Faulk and Arlene H. Morris

When we achieve new growth in our personal development, we also spontaneously achieve increased self-awareness, which we bring into our professional development.

—Patricia Cranton

In this chapter, we will discuss how Mezirow's (2000) six habits of mind can be used by educators to self-reflect on what they bring individually to their teaching practice. Novice and experienced educators can benefit from using transformative learning approaches to examine how habits of mind influence teaching behaviors. This self-examination can increase awareness of personal authentic transformation. As faculty transform personally and professionally, the process is modeled for students and colleagues.

Educators in the discipline of nursing are not unique in that they have identities of self in a practice and an academic role. Each of these roles informs the other, yet expertise in practice does not necessarily lead to expertise in teaching. Educators may teach in the manner that they have been taught or in a manner that highlights areas in which they are expert, yet ignore innovative options for teaching approaches. Educators can become focused on tasks required by the faculty role, rather than considering their personal and professional strengths and areas in which improvement is needed. In the fast-paced world of academia, educators can project competence by completing the tasks, while actually hiding behind a cloud screen of busyness. Fear of self-reflection and a focus on the mechanics of teaching can lead to hesitancy to focus on self-development or personal/professional transformation. Strength originating from commitment to self and the professions of nursing and education can motivate novice and experienced educators to self-reflect and continue development and transformation. If a teacher can be self-reflective, there is a greater likelihood that the teacher will be authentic.

Several assumptions drive the discussions within this chapter:

1. Most educators never think about the "self" as an educator.
2. Self-awareness is an essential component for good teaching.
3. Self-awareness establishes the foundation for transformative learning in teaching.
4. Subjecting personal teaching practice perspectives to critical questioning/examination increases self-awareness.
5. Subjecting personal teaching practice perspectives to critical questioning/examination sets the stage for comprehensive assumption hunting and identification of beliefs about being a nurse educator.
6. Teacher authenticity is a critical foundation for developing a trusting relationship with learners and other faculty colleagues.

SELF-REFLECTION

Self-reflection has been shown to be valuable for improving both nursing practice and teaching (Asselin & Cullen, 2011; Brookfield, 1991; Cranton, 2006). Asselin and Cullen's definition of reflection was discussed in Chapter 6 but warrants repeating as it relates to educator self-awareness: "Reflection is a conscious, dynamic process of thinking about, analyzing, and learning from an experience that gives you insights into self and practice" (p. 45). In clinical, administrative, and academic practice settings, major outcomes from reflection may include awareness of personal strengths and need for development, enhancement of critical thinking skills and clinical reasoning that allow for changes in approaches to care delivery or teaching, and greater skill in communication.

The concept of reflection is elusive, often not considered in workload, nor is it evident to others unless discussed or a behavior change occurs. Motivation for self-reflection must come from the self as a desire to further develop personally or professionally. Motivation can also occur if reflection is shared among trusted colleagues or valued by administration as a planned component of development. Evidence indicates that using some type of structure to initiate and guide the process of self-reflection is important (Forneris & Peden-McAlpine, 2009; Peterson, Bergstrom, Sumuelsson, Asgerg, & Nygren, 2008). Key to the process of transformative learning is questioning habits of mind that influence personal points of view. Mezirow's (2000) six habits of mind can provide a structure for self-reflection.

HABITS OF MIND

According to Cranton (2006), "habits of mind are ways of seeing the world based on background, culture, and personality" (p. 24). Mezirow (2000) identified six habits of mind (epistemic, sociolinguistic, psychological, moral–ethical, philosophical, aesthetic) that explain how individuals develop points of view that result in behaviors. Who we are as a person, how we think, and how we act—in other words, our personal story, is influenced by these six interrelated habits of mind. Within these six habits of mind, we offer suggestions for how novice and expert nurse educators teaching at vocational, associate, baccalaureate, and graduate levels, or in professional staff development can engage in meaningful self-reflection for the outcome of teacher authenticity, or the "bringing of one's sense of self into teaching practice" (Cranton, 2006, p. 183). Reflecting on habits of mind involves a realization of assumptions, and questioning assumptions and how these assumptions influence teaching in either a positive or negative manner. Examples of ways in which educators can engage in self-reflection in the six habits of mind are included in Table 15.1.

Epistemic

Epistemic habits of mind are those related to how an individual acquires and uses knowledge. This includes how we learn using preferred learning styles, how we know what we know, and finally how this can lead to knowing what we do not know. When reflecting about this habit of mind, educators first determine personal learning style or personality strengths from a variety of different views (e.g., Myers-Briggs, Kolb, VARK, etc.) because learning style influences how teaching is approached. For example, if a teacher is a strong visual learner, PowerPoint slides may be the selected approach. However, as an educator develops greater awareness and values others' learning styles, the educator will consider and incorporate multiple teaching strategies. Self-reflection can be prompted when learners ask, "How is it that you know that?" Reflection may reveal that repeated experience is the source of the knowledge, rather than empirical facts. Often this reflection progresses to an awareness of what is actually not known when learners then ask for the evidence to support a practice. Additionally, educators can design instruction to promote learner awareness that much may remain unknown regarding those for whom care is provided.

Sociolinguistic

Sociolinguistic habits of mind involve an individual's developmental background and choices to conform (or not) to social norms, cultural expectations, and how language is used.

Ways of thinking based on these factors may be subconscious, yet powerfully influence behavior. Intentional consideration of the origin of personal points of view may help identify some sociolinguistic habits of mind and allow an individual to reconsider or recommit to one or more of their points of view based on self-reflection.

Examination of sociolinguistic habits of mind is involved in the socialization process to the profession of nursing and, again, when taking on a faculty role. Considering the origin of personal motivation in entering nursing practice, further education and role development, and expectations of others' response to the role of educator may be included in sociolinguistic self-reflection.

Psychological

The psychological habit of mind involves identification of perception of self: who we are, what our personality traits are, what our source for approval is, what our strengths and needs are, and what our perceptions of self-efficacy or areas in which we lack self-efficacy are. For example, an educator may be reticent to teach an online course due to performance anxiety if the educator has limited experience in using online technology. Various methods can be used to identify personal strengths and needs. However, an intentional, deep self-reflection may include a potentially uncomfortable reality check to determine if the self is perceived as authenticated by the perceptions of others.

The metaphor of a journey may help educators to identify their personal life story to reveal psychological habits of mind. Pondering psychological habits of mind may overlap consideration of sociolinguistic and/or philosophical habits of mind as a personal story unfolds. An educator can build on a life journey by including motivation and expectations for professional choices, any associated anxieties or inhibitions, and discovery of expected end points for the journey.

Moral–Ethical

Moral–ethical habits of mind involve perceptions of what is inherently right or wrong, rationales for these perceptions, and the level of commitment to a particular belief that a person demonstrates through behaviors. Everyday choices and behaviors in nursing practice and education are influenced by points of view based on habits of mind within the moral–ethical area. Individuals may not be aware or able to readily articulate foundational moral–ethical habits of mind, yet be passionate about an issue or cause. People may be reluctant to ponder personal habits of mind in the moral–ethical area, preferring to discuss or argue about issues without realizing their personal foundational habits of mind. Moral–ethical habits of mind may overlap reflecting about sociolinguistic habits and may continue to develop over time. Reflecting on why we believe what we believe and how our actions reflect our beliefs requires courage.

Ethical comportment is critical in the current health care arena. Ethical comportment is the demonstration of behaviors based on ethical–moral values. To help nursing students develop and commit to ethical comportment, educators must first reflect on the development of their own moral–ethical values. Reflecting on one's personal story may reveal contributing factors for the development of moral–ethical habits of mind, or an educator may use case studies of moral–ethical dilemmas to identify preferred outcomes and basis for the preference. See Table 15.1 for further examples of reflective activities in the ethical–moral habit of mind.

Philosophical

Philosophical habits of mind are complex and form a foundation for personal world views (a representation of points of view). Systems, such as family or culture, influence development of religious or philosophical beliefs. Religious or philosophical beliefs are also influenced by other intrapersonal or interpersonal experiences occurring throughout an individual's life span. For example, the relationship a child has with parents or other family members influences development of religious or philosophical beliefs. However, during adulthood, the person may interact with others through discussions that result in the person reconsidering their prior beliefs, leading to transformation by either revising or recommitting to the original world view. Another example would be the nursing student who believes that people with mental illnesses are contriving the illness or are resistant to care until the student experiences a personal depression.

TABLE 15.1 Reflection Within Six Habits of Mind

Habit of Mind	Reflective Activity	Intended Outcome
Epistemic	1. Use unfolding case studies in content areas not in area of expertise.	1. Personally recognize what is known and what is not known.
	2. Review an exam in an area not in expertise.	2. Consider what is and is not known.
	3. Create case studies related to nursing students who are experiencing difficulty with specific content.	3. Consider possible learner situations and pedagogical options that may affect learning specific content.
	4. Journal regarding experiences with learners in classroom, clinical, or simulated environments.	4. Determine personal learning and teaching approaches.
	5. Review a recorded teaching session. Compare to a colleague's review of the same teaching session.	5. Reflect on teaching style, choice of pedagogy, and identify assumptions.
	6. Use the scenario of Mary, the novice nurse educator who questions what is good teaching presented in Chapter 2 to imagine that you are Mary's mentor. The following questions might guide reflection: a. What knowledge as a nurse educator do I have to mentor Mary? b. What would I tell Mary that is the most important thing a teacher needs to know?	6. Explore personal knowledge of teaching, content, and mentoring abilities.
Sociolinguistic	1. Create a blog with educators from other schools of nursing to identify and contrast institutional norms and how these influence teaching behaviors.	1. Consider if these setting-based norms match what is important to me in my role as a teacher. Become a change agent if norms need revising.
	2. Observe faculty member interactions during a curriculum meeting. Journal observations related to the following questions: a. What words were used that have specific meaning in nursing education? b. Would a novice nurse educator attendee have understood the implications of these words?	2. Clarify if nurse educators actually share a meaning for terms used in curricular planning. Determine if a lack of shared meaning is a barrier for curricular planning.
	3. Create a metaphor that would describe the nursing education culture.	3. Identify assumptions related to the power that cultural expectations have on behaviors of nurse educators.

(continued)

TABLE 15.1 *(continued)*

Habit of Mind	Reflective Activity	Intended Outcome

Psychological	1. Reflect on these questions:
	  a. What criteria do I use to determine if I am a good teacher?
	  b. How do I get approval from self, administration, and/or students?
	  c. Why is this approval important to my perception of what a good teacher is?
	  d. How do I identify personal strengths and areas in which improvement is needed?
	  e. How would I describe myself as a teacher?
	  f. How would students and/or colleagues describe me as a teacher?
	  g. Do I need to reconsider my answers to any of these questions? If so, why?
		1. Awareness of how one's self-concept impacts self-efficacy and teaching effectiveness.

Moral–ethical	1. Complete one or more values clarification activities of choice. 2. Reflect on factors that have contributed to my choice of personal values. 3. Journal over a period of time to determine if values are seen in choice of behaviors. 4. Dialogue the issues surrounding cheating on nursing exams and possible implications. 5. Imagine that you believe cheating is unethical and that the implications go beyond the classroom setting and have serious potential consequences. Your colleague, however, believes that cheating indicates a deeper need or desperation. Identify personal moral–ethical habits of mind and how you might be able to view this issue through your colleague's point of view.	1. Prioritization of values to identify bases for personal ethical decisions in the educator role. 2. Awareness of influence during formative years and the power of assumptions. 3. Understanding that values impact behaviors and that behaviors may be based on stated values (or not). Determine if changes in behavior are indicated. 4. Determine the foundation for moral–ethical point of views. 5. Understand how assumptions and habits of mind of another person influence points of view and behaviors.

(continued)

TABLE 15.1 (*continued*)

Habit of Mind	Reflective Activity	Intended Outcome
Philosophical	1. Construct a narrative to describe personal worldview and how it developed.	1. Understand basis for beliefs.
	2. Develop a personal teaching philosophy or evaluate current teaching philosophy.	2. Compare teaching philosophy with teaching behaviors.
Aesthetic	1. Observe various classrooms to determine ways in which learners appear to respond to certain environmental conditions (i.e., lighting, arrangement of seats, temperature, colors, wall décor, etc.)	1. Determine which environmental conditions engage learners.
	2. Interview colleagues of different ages and backgrounds regarding characteristics desired in learning environments.	2. Understand how perceptions of a good learning environment vary.
	3. Reflect on the following questions:	
	a. In what way do the physical appearances of students affect my teaching?	a. Determine subconscious response to personal perceptions of beauty.
	b. How do group dynamics or interactions with students, colleagues, or administration impact my personal attitude?	b. Awareness of basis for attitude and response.
	c. Do I make judgments from a rational or emotional basis?	c. Awareness of basis for making judgments.

Reflecting on philosophical habits of mind can enable a nurse educator to develop and write a personal teaching philosophy. Further reflection on the teaching philosophy may reveal preferences for particular teaching strategies and may help educators to understand why other activities may be avoided, such as seminars or debates in which power is shared or controlled by the learners rather than the educator. Sharing a personal teaching philosophy with learners allows learners to understand what is important to an educator to provide a basis for learning interactions.

A nurse educator, when reflecting on philosophical habits of mind, may imagine a teaching situation in which the strategy of debate is used for the first time. During the debate, students with opposing world views argue aggressively regarding the economics of health care reform. If the educator has a psychological habit of mind that includes fear of conflict, he or she may refrain from again using debate as a teaching strategy. Reflecting on philosophical habits of mind, however, the educator may have a greater awareness that the students' opposing worldviews, rather than the selected teaching strategy, contributed to the argument.

Questions that might be considered in this reflective activity include:

1. Would adding a learning activity in which learners identify methods to present personal views while showing respect for those whose views may differ decrease the aggression?
2. What is the basis for the educator's personal political ideology?
3. How could the educator's personal political ideology impact his or her response to the conflict?
4. In what way could the educator's personal political ideology be threatened by the students who express an opposing view? If threatened, how does the educator interact with the students in further encounters?
5. How could the educator avoid swaying the argument to the educator's personal point of view?
6. Is the grade influenced if a student has an opposing or a similar point of view as the educator?

Honest self-reflection about personal philosophical habits of mind is challenging. However, reflection can lead to change or recommitment to a point of view with an outcome of a more authentic, transformed educator. Awareness of the difficulty of reflecting on philosophical habits of mind can enable the authentic educator to design instruction that encourages learner reflection regarding philosophical habits of mind, which can then lead to transformative learning.

Aesthetic

Personal values, attitudes, judgments, determination of what is considered beautiful, personal tastes or preferences such as regarding choice of style are all components of aesthetic habits of mind. Aesthetic habits of mind are influenced by sociolinguistic and/or philosophical habits of mind. For example, a person's social and cultural background influences perception of what is beautiful in personal appearance, art, music, arrangement of the environment, etc. A person's worldview influences attitudes and judgment regarding what is valued as priority importance. The practice of nursing is influenced primarily by personal values, attitudes, and judgments, and therefore, these components of aesthetic habits of mind should be the focus of self-reflection for educators. An educator's awareness of personal aesthetic habits of mind can potentially motivate the educator to design instruction that will help learners to consider different points of view and to help learners develop awareness that those for whom nursing care will be provided have personal, and likely different, aesthetic habits of mind.

Educator reflection regarding personal aesthetic habits of mind can lead to value clarification and reveal how personal attitudes and biases impact interactions with students and colleagues in the educational setting. Further reflection on personal aesthetic habits of mind can enable awareness of how judgments are made regarding a variety of issues or situations. For example, some educators may devalue learners who take limited responsibilities for their own learning and may ignore or be reluctant to address contributing factors (i.e., learners' life demands). Another example may be an educator limiting interactions with learners that the educator suspects of cheating. Questions to consider for reflection regarding aesthetic habits of mind are presented in Box 15.1.

Self-reflection is a component of deeper learning as discussed in recent research regarding mind/brain/education (Tokuhama-Espinosa, 2011). Reflective behaviors are now encouraged in nursing literature, and the development of reflective skills is incorporated into essential educational standards. The use of the six habits of mind as previously discussed and awareness of how these habits of mind interact to determine one's point of view and resultant behavior

---

BOX 15.1   Reflection Questions Regarding Aesthetic Habits of Mind

Reflecting on personal values:

1. What do I value about the educator role?
2. How do my personal values influence my ability to be an educator?
3. How do my personal values impact my personal interactions with colleagues and students?
4. How do I perceive my personal affirmation of being valued?
5. What do I consider to be my most valuable skill as an educator?
6. In what way do I value theories of education?
7. In what way do my values influence my perception of what occurs in the educational process?
8. Do I value an individual who looks or acts differently than I look and act?

Reflecting on personal attitudes:

1. What are my attitudes toward those who are similar to me? Those who differ from me?
2. What are my attitudes regarding my role as a member of a faculty or health care organization?
3. What are my attitudes regarding learner responsibility or accountability?

Reflecting on personal judgment:

1. What do I consider when forming a judgment regarding a controversial issue?
2. What do I consider when forming a judgment regarding prioritization of how I spend my time?
3. Are my judgments rational or emotional?
4. Do I use a systematic process to make judgments to solve a problem?

can serve as a starting point for reflection. The following example illustrates how this can occur. An educator reflecting on philosophical habits of mind realizes the assumption that a strong personal value for individual accountability formed a foundation for personal political views. The educator then acknowledged avoidance of learners who did not demonstrate individual accountability for their learning, thus showing the interaction between philosophical and aesthetic habits of mind. Greater self-awareness leads to teacher authenticity.

TEACHER AUTHENTICITY

As stated in the beginning of this chapter, we believe the ultimate outcome from self-reflection is a transformed, authentic teacher. We believe that teacher authenticity is knowing oneself and using that knowledge to develop a personal teaching approach in which the teacher is genuine in interaction and connection with learners. Learners are more likely to trust an authentic teacher and the content presented by this teacher, and then to develop courage to engage in personal reflection for transformation.

Cranton and Carusetta (2004) developed a guide for teachers to reflect on a personal transformative journey for an outcome of authenticity. Questions for self-reflection are presented in the areas of self-awareness, awareness of others, relationship building, awareness of context, and development of reflective skills. Through this self-reflection, teachers,

> are finding their place, learning the expectations of their profession and their institution. They are trying to fit in, and during that process, they adopt the persona of teacher, the role of teacher that society expects of them. With experience and making meaning of that experience, teachers find their own way that is sometimes different from and sometimes the same as the teacher persona. (Cranton, 2006, p. 196)

We strongly believe that building a trusting relationship with learners is at the heart of being an authentic teacher. However, today's educators may be challenged to find their place in teaching settings or in developing ethically appropriate relationships with students. Issues have arisen from misuse of social media as a method for communicating and interacting with students, risk for development of codependency if the faculty create a relationship that meets their own needs, or other inappropriate personal relationships in which either the faculty member or student goes beyond acceptable boundaries. Awareness of these potential issues informs authentic faculty relationships with learners, with the goal of assisting learners to develop their potential.

Although the faculty do not form synergistic relationships with all learners, when synergy does occur, it is often transformative for the learner and faculty, enhancing the authenticity and development of both. Synergy is a term that refers to two or more functioning together, using the strengths and energy of each, thus leading to an end result that is greater than what would have been possible by either of the independent parts. The term *synergy* comes from a *Greek* word that means working together.

As nurse educators, we continue to be amazed when we witness learners developing teamwork skills that lead to a group product that exceeds what any of the group members had anticipated. Working together is a synergistic process that includes (a) identifying what each does best, (b) respecting different points of view, ideas, and approaches, (c) having flexibility to evaluate progress, (d) readjusting as needed, and (e) incorporating new findings that become available. Additionally, often the most powerful end result is an increased awareness of how to work with others more effectively than alone. Striving for synergy in group processes is critical in nursing.

Learners may connect with a teacher in such a way that synergy occurs. We have been more familiar with this occurring in graduate-level education when a learner and faculty advisor develop a shared interest that deepens with progressive work and relationship building. This synergy can also develop at the LPN, ADN, or BSN level. Teacher authenticity, a true passion for content, and openness to learning with and from students is often the precursor to students approaching faculty with ideas that they desire to share or develop.

For example, one student in an RN to BSN program admitted that she came "only to get the piece of paper" [BSN diploma] to get a promotion. She believed that she was skilled in her nursing practice, effective in her unit manager role, and really had nothing more to learn. However, after [required] participation in critical reflection and critical self-reflection for some assignments in courses that used transformative learning principles and approaches, she wrote in her course journal that she was realizing that her development was just beginning. Subsequently, she sought opportunities for further development in the areas she identified as personal goals, identifying strengths of which she was previously unaware. Relationships with faculty members deepened when she brought new thoughts and ideas, variations of applications that energized her to further thinking, reflection, dialogue, and which shaped some of the direction of the class and group projects. In further courses, she deepened her working relationships with class peers and with additional faculty, again leading to more personal and professional transformation than she had ever anticipated. She stated, "It is as if the volcano has erupted, and I am so much more productive in my classes and at my work. I did not anticipate that I would be able to grow as much personally." Furthermore, the faculty discussed the impact that this student had on them, how they were energized by her enthusiasm, and how witnessing her transformation actually had transformed them. After the student graduated, she and one faculty member continued to collaborate for nursing presentations at local and state levels. The student developed a mentor–mentee relationship with the faculty member when she pursued graduate study and became a faculty member at another school of nursing.

Another example illustrates unanticipated personal transformation in foundational points of view. After two semesters, one student from a different cultural background shared an article that she had read about mentors with a class peer. The author of the article had suggested that the best mentors would be someone from the same cultural background, from which a shared understanding of cultural values would promote trust and mutual development. During a brief planned dialogue period in the face-to-face course, the student shared with the peer that she did not agree with the article's thesis, explaining that she believed it was actually a racist point of view. The pair of students then shared this discussion with other class members, asking their points of view, and discussing that the shared cultural background was not as important to them as faculty trustworthiness and authenticity in all actions, or "walking the walk, not just talking the talk." Student discussion and consensus revealed that the faculty characteristic most desired was a perception that the faculty had the best interest of the learners in mind in all learning activities, seeking actual development of learners and modeling their own development.

At times, working through difficult situations creates an opportunity for development of synergy between faculty members and students. One student had an extremely difficult preceptorship experience in which the nurse preceptor created obstacles for student attainment of course outcomes. The faculty member encouraged the student to critically reflect on the situation, to critically self-reflect and identify what was being learned through the difficult preceptorship, and to dialogue with the faculty through weekly clinical journaling. The student developed an awareness of her own strengths and areas of control, setting boundaries with the preceptor and seeking alternate opportunities to fulfill course requirements. Faculty support of the student's efforts with pertinent feedback eventually led to some revisions in the course structure through sincere collaboration with students.

Faculty members can be surprised by the development of synergy. One beginning student had extreme difficulty mastering sterile technique and requested one faculty member's assistance and feedback before the final evaluation. The faculty weighed the time required for remediation after regular teaching hours with the expressed need of the student, deciding that the student's request should be honored because it likely was an expression of trust and openness at a vulnerable time. The student did learn sterile technique in a calmer environment in which she trusted the faculty member. In subsequent semesters, the student volunteered to assist other students who had difficulty with sterile technique. The student continued to seek feedback from the trusted faculty member, including requesting collaboration when seeking her first job—as a surgical nurse. This student later pursued graduate education to become a nurse faculty member.

Final examples illustrate that synergy may develop between students and faculty when the faculty consider the holistic needs of the learners. Students who are responsible for financial support of family members, whether local or remote, who experience acute or chronic health issues, or who are caregivers for others may seek counsel from authentic faculty members that are perceived as trustworthy. When faculty members observe the heroic efforts of learners to pursue and excel, the faculty can be transformed.

CONCLUSIONS

Just as nursing students' professional development leads toward a level of commitment to actions, educators' development of reflective skills can lead to a commitment to authentic behaviors. According to Fishman and Davis (2006), teacher development occurs along a continuum from preparatory education for teaching, induction into teaching, and continues through mastery within the profession of teaching. They suggest that "the most effective professional development also requires teachers to examine their own practice, reflect, [and have] opportunity for social supports" (p. 526).

An educator who demonstrates authenticity will reflect on knowledge of content, method of teaching, and its effectiveness. Shulman (1986) suggests that educators must not only know the content and know about pedagogy, but must be able to integrate content knowledge with pedagogy in such a manner that the pedagogy effectively supports the teaching of the particular content. The authentic educator with courage and awareness can identify from their own behaviors some of their underlying assumptions, habits of mind, and points of view from which behaviors arise. Reflection regarding personal and professional behaviors over time provides opportunity for educators to consider or reconsider points of view, dialogue with others, further reflect, and then choose to commit to particular actions, possibly integrating transformative learning principles and approaches into their educational practices.

REFERENCES

Asselin, M. E., & Cullen, H. A. (2011). Improving practice through reflection. *Nursing 2011, 4*(4), 44–47.

Brookfield, S. D. (1991). The development of critical reflection in adulthood. *New Education, 13*(1), 39–48.

Cranton, P. (2006). *Understanding and promoting transformative learning: A guide for educators of adults* (2nd ed.). San Francisco, CA: Jossey-Bass.

Cranton, P., & Carusetta, E. (2004). Perspectives on authenticity in teaching. *Adult Education Quarterly, 55*(1), 5–22.

Fishman, B. J., & Davis, E. A. (2006). Teacher learning research and the learning sciences. In R. K. Sawyer (Ed.), *The Cambridge handbook of the learning sciences*. New York, NY: Cambridge University Press.

Forneris, S. G., & Peden-McAlpine, C. (2009). Creating context for critical thinking in practice: The role of the preceptor. *Journal of Advanced Nursing, 65*(8), 1715–1724.

Mezirow, J., & Associates. (2000). *Learning as transformation: Critical perspectives on a theory in progress* (pp. 35–69). San Francisco, CA: Jossey Bass.

Peterson, U., Bergstrom, G., Sumuelsson, M., Asberg, M., & Nygren, A. (2008). Reflecting peer-support groups in the prevention of stress and burnout: Randomized controlled trial. *Journal of Advanced Nursing, 63*(5), 506–516.

Shulman, L. S. (1986). Those who understand: Knowledge growth in teaching. *Educational Researcher, 15*(2), 4–14.

Tokuhama-Espinosa, T. (2011). *What mind, brain, and education (MBE) can do for teaching.* Retrieved from http://education.jhu.edu/newhorizons/Journals/Winter2011/Tokuhama2

16

Transformative Learning for Change

Arlene H. Morris and Debbie R. Faulk

> *Transformative learning involves reflectively transforming the beliefs, attitudes, opinions, and emotional reactions that constitute our meaning schemes or transforming our meaning perspectives.*
>
> —Jack Mezirow

In this final chapter, we would like to focus on the ethical issues related to transformative learning and provide a few concluding thoughts as to why we believe principles and approaches of transformative learning theory offer a signature pedagogy for nursing and for consideration by nursing staff educators. Transformative learning provides practical innovative methods for designing nursing curricula and for creating learning activities. The call for reformed or transformed ways of teaching in nursing presents the perfect thinking environment for change. However, we agree with Benner, Sutphen, Leonard, and Day (2010) that changes in pedagogy and curricular design are not the only areas in nursing education where change is needed. Change in educational policies must also come from unified efforts of all stakeholders (Benner et al., 2010).

ETHICAL ISSUES RELATED TO TRANSFORMATIVE LEARNING

Our personal teaching philosophies include the value that we, as educators, give voice to our students through authentic teaching and learning. We believe that an authentic teacher encourages and motivates students to be lifelong learners. While we are passionate about teaching and learning, we do realize that there may be unintended outcomes of learning, especially in transformative learning. Two questions are pertinent for critical self-reflection when considering ethical issues related to transformative learning: How do we as educators ethically create an environment for transformative thinking without indoctrination? How do we ethically support and foster learner accountability for transformative learning?

Transformative learning outcomes may come with a high price for the learner. An educator cannot force changes in perspectives, and therefore, the transformative educator must be critically aware of the risks that the learner may experience within all learning situations. When we ask future nurses to critically question long-held assumptions, we must realize that this can be very uncomfortable and could result in extreme anxiety for the learner. As King (2005) points out, "if we facilitate and encourage critical examination of values, beliefs, and assumptions, must we not be ready to support such questioning?" (p. 110). Transformative learning is powerful learning and has the potential for impacting an individual's worldview and resultant choices for behaviors. According to Mezirow (1991), "encouraging learners to challenge and transform meaning perspectives raises serious ethical questions" (p. 201). Mezirow encourages educators to critically reflect on possible ethical questions related to transformative learning. For example, should the transformative educator:

- attempt to manipulate a learner's thinking without the learner being aware of what transformative learning means?
- foster transformative learning when the outcome(s) may result in conflict or extreme anxieties for the learner, which may lead to feelings of hopelessness/insecurity?
- selectively dictate which particular belief or point of view learners should question?
- influence learners by stating personal perspectives?
- refuse to assist learners when the educator's personal values are in conflict with the learners' values?
- become involved in a therapist-type relationship with learners who experience psychological distress in response to cognitive dissonance?

Baumgartner (2001) poses a more basic question by asking if educators have the right to encourage transformational learning. Although ethical issues regarding transformative learning have been articulated in different ways by different authors, the issues must be addressed.

ETHICAL LEARNING ENVIRONMENTS

In light of the fact that there are ethical considerations inherent in most pedagogical approaches, we believe that educators can create ethical transformative learning environments. This requires informing learners at the beginning of courses, curricular orientations, or continuing education offerings that transformative learning principles and approaches will be used to stimulate critical reflection, critical self-reflection, and dialogue. For example, in a transformative learning curriculum, students are presented with written and verbal descriptions of the transformative learning process, environment, phases, and approaches during orientation. This initial discussion assists learners to determine expectations for faculty and learner roles. Dialogue in traditional and online classrooms allows learners to question transformative principles and approaches and develop a level of comfort with faculty and peers.

In addition to the orientation information about transformative learning theory, a metaphor of a perspective transformation journey is used to describe learning as a process that may involve starts, stops, side trips, individual or group participation, and helps students to visualize the anticipated educational process. In one situation, students became so engaged with the metaphor that it now serves as a guide for linking perspective transformation adult learning theory to the development of renewal or changes in professionalism (Faulk & Morris, 2010).

Encouraging learners to initially identify personal values, assumptions, and points of view related to learning and personal goals for learning can foster identification of potential areas of discomfort. Offering a choice of learning activities allows learners to select those not anticipated to be overwhelming or to create undue psychological anxiety. However, unanticipated anxiety may arise in either planned or happenstance learning situations. Providing opportunities for learners to express concerns through dialogue or journaling can assist them to identify and clarify underlying issues. Although the faculty role includes responding to learner needs, delineating the role of faculty to promote learning rather than to provide psychological counseling is necessary, and referrals may be needed.

In Chapter 2, we discussed transformative learning through the lens of the educator and emphasized the need for educators to create a trusting, open, and caring learning environment to foster transformative learning. Awareness that transformative learning may spark emotional responses from both learner and teacher requires that educators carefully consider timing and opportunities for reflection and dialogue, within trusting environments for faculty to learner or learner to learner interactions. For example, one nursing class included the learning activity of a debate regarding health care policy issues. Learners were beginning to become polarized and emotional as individual political and philosophical ideologies were revealed. The faculty reminded learners that the outcome was to consider others' points of view and suggested taking a week for critical reflection regarding the values that were assumed during the critical discourse. De-escalating the situation allowed interpersonal respect to continue within the learning situation. A follow-up journal assignment encouraged learners to critically self-reflect and identify how both assumptions and personal self-concept/identity were involved in the values revealed during the debate and then to consider opposing points of view in a less emotional manner.

Education for adults rests on the premise that adults desire to create meaning, solve problems, and enhance decision making. Education for nursing necessitates consideration of potential dissonance in beliefs when nursing concepts and interventions are taught and within interactions during clinical experiences. Learners are encouraged through transformative learning approaches to identify their assumptions and points of view, consider those of others, and then are allowed freedom to uphold, renew, or revise their personal convictions. For example, in one learning activity in an RN to BSN program in which learners deconstructed a leadership experience, one learner identified a personal assumption that colleagues would be honest which had resulted in her resigning from an administrative nursing position after being lied to by an associate. As she identified the assumptions and realized the impact these had on her behaviors, she became tearful and fearful of the possible impact of her tears on her group's grade for the activity. The faculty member demonstrated caring, assuring all learners that, at times, learning and realizations can be very emotional and powerful, thus providing a profound opportunity for all of the learners to experience personal and professional growth.

In further consideration of ethical transformative learning environments, educators must be aware and plan for potential conflicts that may arise between faculty and learners. Mezirow (1991) emphasizes that there is no such thing as a value-free educational environment. Thus, the faculty must critically self-reflect to identify personal values, assumptions, points of view, and honestly evaluate if any hidden agendas are involved in choice of content or methods of teaching. Educators need to be transparent and open regarding personal values for learners to consider points of view that may be the same or different than their own. Transparency, in effect, prevents indoctrination or "selling" of the point of view. Creating an environment of freedom to agree or disagree can limit the risk of manipulating learners through grade assignment or other methods of approval only if they agree with the faculty. Designing activities in which issues can be evaluated and personal assumptions and values honestly discussed can lead to critical reflection without coercion.

Emancipatory learning occurs in ethical learning environments whereby learners critically self-reflect to identify personal assumptions, values, and points of view. As these are then compared to informational and experiential knowledge gained in nursing curricula, learners are motivated to not just memorize isolated facts to pass courses, but rather to critically analyze concepts within the context of personal assumptions, values, or points of view and are provided the freedom to retain, renew, or revise points of view. Subsequently, the points of view form the basis for choices and behaviors. Use of these approaches of critical reflection, critical self-reflection, and dialogue can become a lifelong process for transformative thinking.

CONCLUDING THOUGHTS

Is it possible for nurse educators to use transformative learning as pedagogy in nursing education? Our answer is yes! We offer the caveat, however, that transformative learning can be complex and difficult for both learners and educators and that more research is needed to support this pedagogy. However, from our extensive experience in using transformative learning principles and approaches, we have seen the outcomes and believe that the benefits far outweigh the difficulties. These benefits involve transformative thinking in individual nurses, and lead to improved health outcomes from a commitment to quality and lifelong learning, and ultimately to strengthening nursing as a profession.

Similar to the feedback and interaction between research, education, and clinical practice in nursing, the outcome of transformative thinking transcends one environment. Motivation for quality nursing practice requires a commitment to the valuing of others, the valuing of personal contributions to health care, and a commitment to continually seek personal improvement.

In thinking about how to end this book, we believe that transformative learning can best be illustrated through the words of former nursing students. The following excerpts have been taken from completion of course learning activities and course evaluation comments:

> This experience made me realize how important volunteer work and community outreach is and how many people it helps and gives chances to that would otherwise not be attainable. In undergoing self-examination, I did not realize how

many assumptions I had about different topics or issues. Analyzing work experiences and identifying assumptions and alternate ways of thinking really was a "wake up call" for me personally.

Through the entire perspective transformation process I was urged to look into myself and see what I wanted, where I was going and how I was going to achieve it. I have made three big turns in this program, 1) No CRNA School for me, 2) I am on a lifelong journey to becoming a professional and 3) There is a big difference between leaders and managers.

The perspective transformational journey has led me to new ways of caring for myself as a nurse and an individual. Everyone has different ways of speaking, writing and managing, just because I may not agree with it, does not mean that it is wrong. My new experiences have taught me to be open minded so that I may open myself up to new learning activities and ways of thinking.

Reflection on my future career trajectory and on my nursing philosophy, values and personal self concept has reminded me of why I wanted to continue my education. The career trajectory has given me a plan with dates that I now need to hold myself accountable towards achieving those stated goals. When I reflect on the 10th phase of perspective transformation, I believe that I am now armed with the knowledge and skills needed to succeed in successfully reintegrating into society as a professional. I am empowered to continue to use these new skills. I plan on joining nursing organizations, continuing my education and seeking new employment where my full potential as a nurse and a leader can be recognized and utilized.

I really had to wake up and smell the coffee when I realized that I too have a responsibility not only to the nursing profession, but to my community as well. I was one of those nurses who was "so busy" and always assumed someone else would do it. Then one day I realized, what if every nurse thought like me? Who would "someone else" be? When I completed my volunteer hours for this semester, I was so excited when the school nurse asked me back. Not only did I have fun teaching the class, I felt like I had been a safe sounding board for misinformed teenagers. I guess I had never seen the value in participating in community service because I had yet to find something I believed I needed to be doing or was interested in doing.

I truly am integrating back into society with a transformed perspective. A year ago, I would have said that I was on a transformation journey through hell. I had bitten off way more than I could chew with work, school, and kids. I mean, how much busy work can one program give you in a semester?!? And how in the world can any of this junk help me in "the real world of nursing?" Oh my! Stamp idiot on my forehead! As I look back, I can almost visualize myself changing. How stupid I was not to see it as I was first going through it. It was not until the end of last semester when I really noticed the difference in how I would advocate for my patients, or a policy that was much needed. It was then that my co-workers started commenting on the difference in how I handled adverse situations and how the relationship between my co-worker and me had changed for the better. I am so grateful to have experienced what this program has offered.

Many times as nurses we run into situations that make us question the decisions we make in patient care. Our attitudes and personal beliefs sometimes influence the direction of care that we provide as nurses. Sometimes, I have to redirect my own personal feelings. I am especially biased when it comes to gender. I was raised by a woman, never meeting my biological father for the first time until I had almost reached the age of thirty. So, I have a soft spot in my brain and heart for female patients, especially in mental health where some of the patients may remind me of a motherly image. I tend to be more lenient when it comes to certain forms of treatment and more restrictive with male clients. I have to step back many times and say to myself to refrain from treating one patient differently from the next. What really brought this home for me is when I saw a frail, one hundred and fifteen pound woman hurl a chair across the room when she got frustrated, and I thought that she was physically incapable of lifting such a heavy object, nor did I think she was aggressive in nature. In mental health nursing, it is very easy for staff to get injured by patients in the blink of an eye. Through a self-examination, I can say that I have begun to rethink my approach to ANY patient regardless of age, size, and gender. I try to treat my patients in the way I would like for my mother to be treated by the nurse, but at the same time, this process is carried out with better precautionary measures.

What's the next milestone? A question I have asked myself. The way that I plan to introduce the things that I have learned into society is patient-driven teaching and the encouragement of others to pursue lifelong learning. My new perspective is still based upon the elements of humbleness and willingness to learn and improve my nursing skills, but moreover, I hope to further kindle the flame of learning through better patient teaching and education so that my nursing will not only be direct, but also preventative care.

Personal growth is something that never dies unless the learner becomes unreceptive to change, new perceptions, and ideas. I focused on the notion of growing and learning as a precursor of the path into the professional role of nursing. My mind has been transformed in the sense that I have developed alternate methods of nursing implementation and thinking outside of the box from a managerial and leading standpoint; however, I feel that I have remained grounded with the same initial declaration to be committed and open to the continuance of learning. That's how a professional nurse strives to become more professional. For example, one year ago, I probably would have just collected a lot of text book knowledge and leave that information to rest, but my current, more professional approach would be to know why I have the information, research its effectiveness for the patient, or study how others in leadership roles have applied this information to different types of settings. My "habits of the mind" could almost be considered complacent as I reflect upon my professional self-concept one year ago. It's as if I would retain information for the sake of doing so, but not really exploring how I could fully put that knowledge into productive use. I believe that my self-concept has been transformed for the better, a professional nurse now, and still aspiring to learn.

From a professional standpoint, I see myself as an ever-evolving person. I believe that because of my capacity to possess an open mind and learn new things, even at the expense of my current ways of thinking, I have the capacity to change and create change in my immediate surroundings as well as my world. I have become an effective agent for change in my facility as well as my profession, and I plan to exercise my voice as well as my rights. I believe in empowerment; empowering coworkers, clients, and families helps to shape the health care world as we see it and help it progress to new heights.

The most profound assumption I had about nursing philosophy was evident because I never sat down to actually decide what MY philosophy was. Just the word PHILOSOPHY sounded lofty and felt much like it was over my head and nothing for me to be concerned about. Perhaps I assumed that only advanced degree nurses needed a philosophy, and that I as an Associate Degree Nurse (ADN) just needed to focus on getting my job done and carrying out safe, competent care. Obviously, my point of view changed as soon as I sat down to examine my personal nursing philosophy. Suddenly, I felt as though my work had a purpose, a focus, and a foundation on which to firmly stand. This is very important for a professional nurse . . . a philosophy is everything a nurse stands for, as well as why the nurse stands for it. The philosophy serves as the vision for the nurse's professional journey. Nothing that anyone does should be done without a definite purpose, and a philosophy gives the action its said purpose. My personal philosophy will forever be engrained in my professional career. It seems that after sitting down and determining what my philosophy was, I searched for that philosophy in everything I did. Simply having brought it to life has given my work a focus, and it will continue to provide that focus. I will heavily rely on my philosophy when getting involved in the legislative realm of nursing. As my father would say . . . "If you stand for nothing, you may as well just sit down."

It is our sincere hope that you, our colleagues as nurse educators, will become convinced through these students' words that transformative thinking can actually happen. We also hope you will use our experiences with transformative learning theory that we have shared to develop further applications of the principles and approaches, thus promoting your own transformative thinking as you plan and integrate transformative learning activities into your courses.

REFERENCES

Baumgartner, L. M. (2001). An update on transformational learning theory. In S. B. Merriam (Ed.), The new update on adult learning theory (pp. 15–24). *New Directions for Adult and Continuing Education*, No. 89. San Francisco, CA: Jossey-Bass.

Benner, P., Sutphen, M., Leonard, B., & Day, L. (2010). *Educating nurses: A call for radical transformation.* San Francisco, CA: Jossey-Bass.

Cranton, P. (2006). *Understanding and promoting transformative learning: A guide for educators of adults* (2nd ed.). San Francisco, CA: Jossey-Bass.

Faulk, D. & Morris, A. H. (2010). The perspective transformation journey: Using a metaphor to structure progression of thinking and exploration of attitudes in the RN to BSN student. *Nurse Educator, 35*(3), 103–104.

King, K. P. (2005). *Bringing transformative learning to life.* Malabar, FL: Krieger.

Mezirow, J. (1991). *Transformative dimensions of adult learning.* San Francisco, CA: Jossey-Bass.

Appendix A: Additional Transformative Learning Activities

The learning activities listed in this appendix have been used in various levels of nursing education and in traditional and online classes to engage students in transformative learning. Although this is certainly not a comprehensive list, the learning activities are offered for novice and expert educators of nursing students and for professional staff development educators as an impetus for thinking about transformative learning and as a resource for developing transformative learning activities.

NAME OF ACTIVITY/SOURCE

BaFa BaFa: A Cross Culture Simulation© by R. Garry Shirts (2008). Available from Simulation Training Systems, P.O. 910, Del Mar, CA 92014 (1-800-942-2900). www.SimulationTrainingSystems.com

Instruction/Description

A role-play activity in which learners divide into the Alpha culture and the Beta culture to behave according to directed cultural norms for each of these contrived cultures. After participation, critical reflection of questions included in the BaFa BaFa kit using in-class or online dialogue is followed by critical self-reflection and a two-page writing assignment or journal entry.

Anticipated Learning Outcomes

1. Development of cultural awareness and humility.
2. Critical reflection of other points of view when trying to navigate within a different culture.

3. Critical self-reflection regarding personal assumptions about behaviors of those from another culture.
4. Critical self-reflection about personal adaptation to behaviors of another culture and how this could relate to socialization or resocialization to the health care delivery system culture.

Level of Education and/or Suggested Courses

- All levels of nursing education in face-to-face learning environments
- Beginning-level nursing concepts courses
- Ethics courses
- Leadership/management courses
- In-service for health care delivery settings

NAME OF ACTIVITY/SOURCE

Interprofessional Healthcare Delivery Communication Exercise. *Team STEPPS™: Strategies and Tools to Enhance Performance and Patient Safety* (2008). Agency for Healthcare Research and Quality (AHRQ) Pub. No. 06-0020-2. www.ahrq.gov

Instruction/Description

This role-play includes interprofessional health care delivery team members' communication about a newly admitted hospital patient. Learners in pairs assume the role of different health care team members to practice communication using each technique.

Anticipated Learning Outcomes

1. Awareness and valuing of roles of health care delivery team members.
2. Awareness and valuing of interprofessional communication techniques such as *SBAR, Call-Out, Check Back,* and *I Pass the Baton.*
3. Awareness of health care delivery team members' decreased effectiveness from incomplete communication.

Level of Education and/or Suggested Courses

- All levels of nursing education in face-to-face or virtual learning environments
- Beginning-level nursing concepts courses

- Leadership/management courses
- In-service for health care delivery settings

NAME OF ACTIVITY/SOURCE

Personal Values Card Sort by W. R. Miller, J. C'de Baca, D. B. Mattherws, & P. L. Wilbourne (2001). University of New Mexico. http://casaa.unm.edu/inst/Personal%20Values%20Card%20Sort.pdf

Instruction/Description

Learners download cards labeled with various value terms and self-reflect to place into the following categories: Very important to me, Important to me, Not important to me. Within each category, values are then placed in rank order. Learners record their placement of the values within each category. Four to six weeks later, the activity is repeated, and results are compared with the initial results. Learners further self-reflect to consider if decisions and behaviors that have transpired during the intervening weeks were based on the values identified as very important, and if not, why not. Dialogue with a self-selected individual who knows the learner (not necessarily a classmate) provides opportunity for another view of the learner's usual patterns of behavior.

Anticipated Learning Outcomes

1. Awareness of personal values and/or beliefs.
2. Self-reflection to determine if decisions/behaviors are actually based on stated values/beliefs.
3. Dialogue with a trusted other person to provide an alternate point of view regarding congruity between actions and stated values.
4. Awareness of hidden assumptions or frames of reference on which values are based.

Level of Education and/or Suggested Courses

- All levels of nursing education in face-to-face or virtual learning environments
- Beginning-level nursing concepts courses
- Ethics courses
- Leadership/management courses
- Public policy courses
- In-service for health care delivery settings

NAME OF ACTIVITY/SOURCE

Interpersonal Process Recording

Instruction/Description

Learners divide into dyads to assume role of nurse and client in scenarios provided by faculty (scenarios include settings across the health care delivery system and various levels of acuity). Learners in the role of nurse practice therapeutic communication techniques during a 5-minute interaction. Following the interaction, both learners complete an interpersonal process recording form in which therapeutic communication techniques and barriers to communication are identified.

Anticipated Learning Outcomes

1. Awareness of vulnerability of the client seeking health care in the various scenarios.
2. Identification of verbal and nonverbal therapeutic communication techniques.
3. Self-reflection to identify personal discomfort triggers (sensitive issues, periods of silence, etc.).
4. Interaction with co-learner regarding perceptions of what unintentional component was perceived as a barrier to the communication process.

Level of Education and/or Suggested Courses

- All levels of nursing education in face-to-face or virtual learning environments
- Beginning-level nursing concept courses
- In-service for health care delivery settings

NAME OF ACTIVITY/SOURCE

Cultural Assessment PowerPoint Presentation

Instruction/Description

Each learner identifies a person from another culture to be interviewed for approximately 30 minutes using a cultural interview/assessment tool that includes health promotion behaviors. Learners may select classmates, older family members who are not well known, or ask individuals from ethnic restaurants or other settings to participate. Confidentiality of the interviewee is maintained. After the interview, learners create a PowerPoint presentation that summarizes information obtained. Learners present in face-to-face or virtual classrooms. Learners compare interview findings to personal cultural assumptions or stereotypes, personal experience, depictions in health care texts, and other learners' presentations. Patterns and individual differences are discussed. Individuals then self-reflect to compare personal cultural competence to levels discussed by Campinha-Bacote.

Source for self-reflection to identify current personal level of cultural competence: Josepha Campinha-Bacote's (2005) *Transcultural C.A.R.E. Associates* www.transculturalcare.net

Anticipated Learning Outcomes

1. Awareness of personal cultural assumptions or stereotypes.
2. Self-reflection to determine if decisions/behaviors for nursing care have been based on accurate information.
3. Dialogue with others to consider alternate points of view regarding possible motivators for health promotion or health management decisions for individuals from various ethnicities, socioeconomic levels, or age groups.
4. Awareness of hidden assumptions or frames of reference on which nursing behaviors are based.

Level of Education and/or Suggested Courses

- All levels of nursing education in face-to-face or virtual learning environments
- Beginning level nursing concept courses
- Ethics courses
- Population-based courses
- Public policy courses
- In-service for health care delivery settings

NAME OF ACTIVITY/SOURCE

Personal Health Lifestyle Review

Instruction/Description

Learners identify personal lifestyle strengths and risk factors using an age-appropriate heath behavior screening tool, complete a family genogram that includes illnesses of at least three generations of family members, and use a literature search to identify appropriate health-promotion activities based on lifestyle and genetic risks. Learners then select health-promotion activities in which they desire to participate, then determine realistic, specific, and timed goals for behaviors. Learners self-reflect to determine which level of health promotion (according to Pender's levels) they most identify with and identify potential barriers and driving forces for the health-promotion behavior. After 1 month, learners self-reflect to evaluate personal progress toward achieving the health behavior changes.

Anticipated Learning Outcomes

1. Awareness of how personal health is influenced by genetic factors and lifestyle choices.
2. Awareness of personal valuing of health-promotion behaviors.
3. Self-reflection to determine if decisions/behaviors have been based on accurate information.
4. Awareness of hidden assumptions or frames of reference in which personal behaviors are based.
5. Consider alternate points of view regarding motivators for health promotion or health management decisions.

Level of Education and/or Suggested Courses

- All levels of nursing education in face-to-face or virtual learning environments
- Beginning-level nursing concept courses
- Population-based courses
- In-service for health care delivery settings

NAME OF ACTIVITY/SOURCE

Think-Pair-Share. First developed by Frank Lyman at the University of Maryland (1981). http://www.eazhull.org.uk/nlc/think,_pair,_share.htm

Instruction/Description

Learners have 2 minutes to write what they consider to be the most pertinent class content from the last 15 minutes of discussion. In dyads, learners compare what each believes is the most important. Then, learners discuss their thinking and rationale for ranking the content as important. Volunteers from each dyad share their thinking with a larger class group. At the end of the class, learners self-reflect about their responses to each content area and identify areas in which further learning is needed.

Anticipated Learning Outcomes

1. Recall and prioritization of facts.
2. Awareness of thinking processes used for prioritization.
3. Identification of personal assumptions.
4. Awareness of powerful influence of individual points of view.

5. Review chunks of content within the content presented during the entire class.

Level of Education and/or Suggested Courses

- All levels of nursing education in face-to-face learning environments
- Beginning- or advanced-level nursing courses

NAME OF ACTIVITY/SOURCE

The Jig-Saw Puzzle

Instruction/Description

After presenting a problem-based learning scenario, place students in small groups to discuss the following:

Group 1—students will identify symptoms
Group 2—students will identify outcomes
Group 3—students will identify potential interventions
Group 4—students will identify potential nursing responsibilities

During discussions in each group, students are encouraged to review their thinking and to reflect on alternative ways of thinking.

Anticipated Learning Outcomes

1. Perspective transformation related to how the pattern of empirical knowledge relates to the aesthetic knowing pattern necessary for holistic practice.
2. Perspective transformation related to how the sociolinguistic knowledge pattern influences valuing for decisions or behaviors.

Level of Education and/or Suggested Courses

- All levels of nursing education in face-to-face learning environments
- Beginning- or advanced-level nursing courses

NAME OF ACTIVITY/SOURCE

Audience Response Systems

Instruction/Description

After a segment of content is discussed, students use digital handheld devices to anonymously respond to questions related to class content. Once the questions have been answered, learners dialogue with co-learners to determine alternate points of view and then the faculty about rationales for correct answers.

Anticipated Learning Outcomes

1. Allows learners to answer questions regarding content without risk of embarrassment.
2. Allows learners to validate use of new knowledge.
3. Allows learners to identify missing information or misperceptions.
4. Allows learners to identify personal assumptions.
5. Allows learners to consider alternative ways of thinking.

Level of Education and/or Suggested Courses

- All levels of nursing education in face-to-face or virtual learning environments (using WIMBA Live classroom)
- Beginning- or advanced-level nursing courses

NAME OF ACTIVITY/SOURCE

The Perspective Transformation Portfolio. Selected examples of learning activities that can be included are provided below.

Instruction/Description

1. Using Huber's (2005) *Leadership Moment* model, critically analyze a situation in which you were the leader. Identify hidden assumptions you might have had related to this particular leadership role. How did these assumptions impact your behaviors? From what you know now about leadership and followership, what would you do differently?
2. In one paragraph, describe the best decision making you have seen by a nurse in a client situation. In one paragraph, describe the worst decision making you have seen by a nurse in a client situation. Compare these two situations in terms of the following:
   - The thought process(es) used
   - The underlying assumptions of the nurse(s)
   - The accuracy of available information
   - The interpretation of information
   - The soundness of the decision reached

Huber, D. (2005). Leadership and nursing care management. St. Louis: Elsevier Health Sciences

Anticipated Learning Outcomes

1. Enhanced critical thinking, perspective transformation, reflections, and learning over the course of the nursing program.

2. Monitoring of personal and professional growth over the course of a nursing program.
3. Creation of a document that will demonstrate knowledge and creative abilities to future employers and/or graduate admission committees.

Level of Education and/or Suggested Courses

- All levels of nursing education in face-to-face and virtual learning environments
- Leadership/management courses
- Personal and professional self-reflection of novice/expert educator

NAME OF ACTIVITY/SOURCE

Leadership Literature Circles

Instruction/Description

Students are assigned to faculty-selected literature circles. Each member of the group must read two research articles related to leadership from referred journals published within the last 3–5 years. Each group member will write a synopsis (no more than two paragraphs) of each article (articles within groups cannot be repetitive). The synopsis must include identification of the author's primary thesis and how the information is useful to a nursing manager/leader at the microsystem/macrosystem level. Post the synopsis in the appropriate group room by assigned due dates. The groups will decide on a date and time to "meet" in a WIMBA Live classroom for critical dialogue. Notify the professor of the date and time for the discussion. Select a leader for the group. This individual will lead the dialogue and ensure that the session is archived. Before the discussion begins, state how and why the leader of the group was chosen. There are no specific guidelines for the dialogue but it should include identification of assumptions, beliefs, values, and alternative ways of thinking about the information.

Anticipated Learning Outcomes

1. Enhanced critical thinking, perspective transformation, reflections, and learning related to leadership.
2. Examine and critique evidence related to leadership for use in practice settings.
3. Enhanced group/team dynamics.
4. Broadened perspectives by dialoguing to learn others' points of view.
5. Development or enhancement of technology skills.
6. Consideration of possible use of WIMBA Live classroom as a client teaching medium.

Level of Education and/or Suggested Courses

- All levels of nursing education in face-to-face and virtual learning environments
- Leadership/management courses
- Professional development within health care delivery settings

NAME OF ACTIVITY/SOURCE

Reflective Management Journal

Instruction/Description

Interact with an identified preceptor in a leadership/management position in a health care delivery setting (microlevel only) for a minimum of 40 hours. The relationship should be one of *mentorship* to assist learning the managerial role. No direct patient care will be performed. The student will participate with the preceptor in a variety of management/leadership activities to include, but not limited to:

- Management activities such as planning, organizing, staffing, leading, and controlling
- Interactions with others in the organizational structure
- Use of motivation, communication, authority, power and politics, and conflict engagement/resolution processes
- Decision-making/problem-solving activities
- Use of evaluation for personnel, client, and agency needs
- Financial planning and implementation
- Discussion of evidence-based practice (EBP) clinical question and related findings.

Collaborate with the preceptor to develop individual learner outcomes for the preceptor experience. The outcomes must be approved by the course faculty before beginning the preceptorship. The outcomes must address the following aspects of the preceptor/student interactive learning experience:

- Analysis of management activities observed at the microhealth delivery system, including management functions, principles, processes, roles, and leadership style of the preceptor.
- Other learning outcomes that reflect individual learner areas of interest.
- Development of a reflective management journal of all related preceptor activities.

During each clinical encounter, students reflect on their strength and weaknesses when working with the preceptor. Identify assumptions related to the leadership/management role, the consequences of those assumptions, and alternative ways of thinking about the role of manager.

At the end of the preceptorship:

1. Provide an analysis of your personal beliefs, opinions, assumptions, values, and current meaning perspectives. Explain how these may impact your role as a manager.

2. Provide an analysis of your thinking related to your preceptor's style of leadership and use of the management process (planning, organizing, controlling, directing).
3. Compare the preceptor's leadership, management activities, and functions (i.e., use of management processes) with those learned through literature review and class discussions. Give specific examples to illustrate theoretical application to practice.
4. Evaluate achievement of learner outcomes by providing at least two examples that illustrate how you met the outcomes.

Anticipated Learning Outcomes

1. Application of theory to practice.
2. Enhanced critical thinking, perspective transformation, reflections, and learning related to the management/leader role.

Level of Education and/or Suggested Courses

- All levels of nursing education in face-to-face and virtual learning environments
- Leadership/management courses

NAME OF ACTIVITY/SOURCE

Cinema Critical Thinking Exercise

Instruction/Description

Motion pictures can provide unique learning experiences for students in a variety of educational settings. The movie, *My Life*, was selected as it addresses numerous life issues that are concepts for this class. As you will see, the movie is a topic for dialogue regarding dysfunctional communication, sexuality, motivating clients for lifestyle changes, family systems, life transition, spirituality, complementary health care, and grief and loss. The film's characters portray behaviors of individuals facing the aforementioned issues. Media reflects life and as such, *My Life* brings to "life" the subtleties of human behavior in a poignant and moving way.

During and after viewing the movie, reflect upon the following questions:
1. Early in the movie, how would you describe Gail's behavior? Bob's?
2. What can you tell about Bob's social life? Professional life?
3. Describe Bob's relationship with his family of origin.
4. Recognize and discuss examples of dysfunctional communication. Provide literature-supported rationales for your response.

5. Why do you think Bob does not want to disclose his diagnosis to his parents or friends?
6. What are your thoughts and feelings about the professional behavior of Bob's primary doctor?
7. How is complementary health care portrayed in the movie? Using current literature, briefly discuss complementary health care. What are your thoughts and feelings about the role of this health care delivery alternative?

Parker, F. M. & Faulk, D. R. (2004). Lights, camera, action: Using feature films to stimulate emancipatory learning in the RN to BSN student. Nurse Educator, 29(4), 144–146.

Anticipated Learning Outcomes

1. Self-awareness about personal points of view related to each of the concepts.
2. Evaluation of the effectiveness of personal thinking.
3. Propose alternate ways of thinking.

Level of Education and/or Suggested Courses

- All levels of nursing education in face-to-face or virtual learning environments
- Beginning-level nursing concept courses
- RN to BSN or RN to MSN family system courses
- Life span courses

NAME OF ACTIVITY/SOURCE

Senior Prom

Instruction/Description

Learners volunteer 3 hours to assist with the Area Agency on Aging senior resource center annual banquet and prom. During the activity, learners assess physical functioning or adaptation, cognition, psychosocial interactions, and developmental levels of the participants.

Anticipated Learning Outcomes

1. Self-awareness about personal assumptions or points of view about aging related to each of the assessment dimension concepts.
2. Critical reflection to compare personal assumptions with observed behaviors during interactions.
3. Valuing of older adults' efforts to maintain independence/normalcy.

4. Dialogue with other learners in online or face-to-face settings to discuss how a personal awareness of independence of older adults or community resources could affect discharge teaching.

Level of Education and/or Suggested Courses

- All levels of nursing education in face to face or virtual learning environments
- Beginning-level nursing concept courses
- RN to BSN or RN to MSN family systems or community courses
- Life span courses

NAME OF ACTIVITY/SOURCE

Teaching About Coping Strategies at Mental Health Group Homes

Instruction/Description

Learners research current evidence regarding coping strategies that can be used for assigned topics (grief/bereavement, time management, goal setting, anger management, medication adherence, health promotion behaviors, etc). A six-slide PowerPoint presentation is created by student triads and presented to participants in a mental health group home.

Anticipated Learning Outcomes

1. Self-awareness about personal assumptions or points of view about individuals coping with mental health issues.
2. Critical reflection to compare personal assumptions with observed behaviors during interactions.
3. Valuing of individuals experiencing mental health issues and their efforts to maintain independence/normalcy.
4. Dialogue with other learners in online or face-to-face settings to discuss how a personal awareness of independence of those experiencing mental health issues or community resources could affect discharge teaching.

Level of Education and/or Suggested Courses

- All levels of nursing education in face-to-face or virtual learning environments
- Special population nursing courses
- RN to BSN or RN to MSN family system or community courses
- Life span courses
- Public policy courses

NAME OF ACTIVITY/SOURCE

Vulnerable Family Assessment

Instruction/Description

Learners research current evidence regarding coping strategies that can be used for assigned topics (abuse, homelessness, grief/bereavement, posttraumatic stress disorder, anger management, etc.). Learners sign a confidentiality agreement when volunteering to interact with children in a community shelter for abused family members. During an initial observation, children are assessed for developmental and psychosocial needs. Learners return 1 week later to use appropriate play techniques for developmental and psychosocial needs.

Anticipated Learning Outcomes

1. Self-awareness about personal assumptions or points of view about families coping with abuse.
2. Critical reflection to compare personal assumptions with observed behaviors during interactions with children.
3. Valuing of children who have experienced abusive or other situations that contribute to increased vulnerability and their efforts to maintain independence/normalcy.
4. Dialogue with other learners in online or face-to-face settings to discuss how a personal awareness of independence of those who have experienced traumatic events or community resources could affect discharge teaching.

Level of Education and/or Suggested Courses

- All levels of nursing education in face-to-face or virtual learning environments
- Pediatric nursing courses
- Special population nursing courses
- RN to BSN or RN to MSN family system or community courses
- Life span courses
- Public policy courses

NAME OF ACTIVITY/SOURCE

Ethical Case Study Analysis/Asynchronous Discussions

Instruction/Description

Each student is required to participate in two out of four ethical case studies by
- Responding to questions posed for each case study analysis
- Supporting answers with sound rationales using resources

- Reading two other student's postings (responses to case questions) and offering support and/or refute of responses in one to two paragraphs
- Posting responses in the appropriate online discussion room by due dates and times

Responses to questions and to peers will be evaluated for quality, substance, and utility.

CASE ANALYSES

CASE ANALYSIS 1: *The Bill That Was for Sale*

Senator Pond from the great state of Zeno is a proud liberal Democrat. He has been in the U.S. Congress for 25 years. He knows that the time is right for health care reform and is exhilarated that he will be a part of this historical event. Health care costs are too high, there are too many uninsured Americans, too many insurance companies charging too high premiums and making too much money, etc. The current bill being debated in the Senate appears to be one that will be the greatest good for the greatest number. However, Senator Pond is against using federal funds to pay for abortions and has decided to vote NO. If he votes NO, the bill will not pass. He believes, however, that he must vote his conscious and not for the greatest good. Two days before the bill is to be voted on, Senator Pond gets a call from the Senate Majority Leader, Senator Whipp. He asks to meet with Senator Pond. The meeting takes place at noon at a very expensive restaurant that is Mr. Pond's favorite. Senator Whipp asks Senator Pond, "What will it take for you to vote YES?" Senator Pond replies, "remove the part about federal funds paying for abortions." Mr. Whipp says, "We cannot do that George. What will it take for you to vote YES? If we do not pass this bill, our window of opportunity will pass and the administration will have failed on a very critical piece of legislation. Many Americans will blame our party for not passing healthcare reform and we (you and me) may lose our senate seat in the next election. Do you want this on your shoulders?" Senator Pond turns pale and suddenly no longer feels hungry. He is experiencing cognitive dissonance (conflict of values). Senator Whipp lets him ponder for a few moments and then he says, "What if we give your great state of Zeno 10 million dollars in federal funds to build a new bridge. Would you vote yes then?" Senator Pond looks horrified—Did Senator Whipp just try to buy his vote with a bribe?

1. Define this dilemma.
2. What values are at stake in the dilemma?
3. What principles are at stake in the dilemma?
4. Pretend that you are Senator Pond. What ethical framework would you use to arrive at a decision, why this framework, and what would be your answer?

CASE ANALYSIS 2: *The Governor Wants Me*

The governor of XYZ asks you to serve on a panel that will provide expert testimony to the state legislature on physician-assisted suicide. The governor wants the legislature to pass a Death with Dignity Bill and believes that your nursing leadership and clinical expertise is what is needed to "sway" the legislators to vote for such a bill. This is a very prestigious honor and one that you have been waiting for a long time. It is considered to be the pinnacle in your career as a nurse leader. As you hang up the phone, you look out the window as many questions race through your mind: "What must I do? I am opposed to assisted suicide for religious and moral reasons. How can I turn the Governor down? What would my friends and colleagues think? What would my family or members of my church think? How can I make this decision?

1. Define this dilemma.
2. What values are at stake in the dilemma?
3. What principles are at stake in the dilemma?
4. What personal issues are at stake in the dilemma?
5. Imagine that you are this nurse. What ethical framework would you use to arrive at a decision, why this framework, and what would be your answer?

CASE ANALYSIS 3: *Nurse Candidate*

You have been a nurse for 25 years and recently decided to toss your hat in the ring for a seat in the state senate. Your opponent is also a nurse whom you know personally. However, you believe that his election would be a disaster. This is because you disapprove of your opponent's character and you think that if elected, he will try to implement bad policies. Here is what you believe that you know about your opponent, but voters do not have this information:

• He has had numerous extramarital affairs;
• He used cocaine while in nursing school;
• His sister is a member of a racist political party;
• His wife has been involved in illegal financial dealings in the past.

During the campaign, your opponent has said many harsh and untrue things about you. His campaign attacks have been brutal, and you have thought many times about quitting the race. One week before election, the polls show that the race is even.

1. Define this dilemma.
2. What values are at stake in the dilemma?
3. What principles are at stake in the dilemma?
4. What personal issues are at stake in the dilemma?
5. Would you reveal any of this information to the public before election day? Why or why not?
6. What ethical framework would you use to arrive at a decision, why this framework, and what would be your answer?

CASE ANALYSIS 4: *Terrorism or Health Care*

You live in an urban city that is home to a large military base. Six months ago, two terrorists tried to get on base to kill as many soldiers as possible. The public clinic that is located at the entrance to the base was full that day, and when the terrorists could not get onto base, they opened fire in the clinic, killing 100 people. Because of major budget deficits, the state legislature must decide how to use tax revenues in response to the terrorism. Specifically, they are debating whether to use tax monies to build a new emergency hospital or to pay more security officers. They lack the money to do both. There are many people who support building the new hospital and many who support funding more security officers.

1. Define this dilemma.
2. What values are at stake in the dilemma?
3. What principles are at stake in the dilemma?
4. Imagine that you are a legislator. What ethical framework would you use to arrive at a decision, why this framework, and what would be your decision?

CASE ANALYSIS 5: *The Lobbyist and the Senator*
One evening, you and your significant other are enjoying dinner in a posh restaurant in DC. After a long day on Capitol Hill in which you were racing back and forth from Senator Pond's office to the senate chamber to bring information about the health care reform bill, you want nothing more than to relax, enjoy the meal, and forget about politics. As you are on your second glass of wine, in walks Senator Pond with a lobbyist who represents a large health insurance company. They do not see you and sit down close enough for you to overhear the conversation. After you observe them sharing many drinks and talking intimately, you hear the lobbyist tell Senator Pond that she can secure a large donation for his reelection campaign if he votes NO on the bill.

1. Define this dilemma.
2. What values are at stake in the dilemma?
3. What principles are at stake in the dilemma?
4. What personal issues are at stake in the dilemma?
5. Pretend that you are Senator Pond's legislative assistant. What ethical framework would you use to arrive at a decision, why this framework, and what would be your decision?

Anticipated Learning Outcomes

1. Development of analytical skills.
2. Awareness of various ethical decision-making models.
3. Concise articulation of points of view related to ethics.

Level of Education and/or Suggested Courses

- BSN and MSN levels in face-to-face or virtual learning environments
- Ethics courses
- Leadership/management courses
- Public policy courses
- In-service for health care delivery settings

NAME OF ACTIVITY/SOURCE

Assumption Busting

Instruction/Description

Students are given 30 minutes to find a statement from assigned readings that "grabs" them. Directed dialogue then includes the following questions:
- What about this statement "grabbed" you?
- What assumption(s) are made in the statement?
- Are the assumption(s) valid? If so, why? If not, identify an alternate point of view.

Anticipated Learning Outcomes

1. Development of analytical skills.
2. Awareness of information presented by authors of nursing texts.
3. Awareness of various assumption(s) made by authors of nursing texts.
4. Concise articulation of points of view.
5. Consideration of alternate points of view.

Level of Education and/or Suggested Courses

- All levels of nursing education in face-to-face or virtual learning environments
- All levels of nursing courses
- In-service in health care delivery settings

NAME OF ACTIVITY/SOURCE

Health Care Issue/Problem Resolution

Instruction/Description

Learners complete the following:
- Identify a health issue/problem
- Investigate underlying problems/causes of the issue problem and the current and/or future effects on community
- Identify all stakeholders including individuals, communities, organizations, and official and unofficial policymakers. Why do you believe these stakeholders are important to the issue/problem
- Examine the issue from a socioeconomic, ethical, legal, and political aspect
- Develop a resolution related to the issue for presentation to the Executive Director of the XYZ State Nurses Association. Request that the resolution be considered by the Annual House of Delegates

Anticipated Learning Outcomes

1. Awareness of political activism and policy advocacy.
2. Critical self-reflection to identify a personal level of commitment to policy advocacy.

Level of Education and/or Suggested Courses

- BSN and MSN level public policy courses

NAME OF ACTIVITY/SOURCE

Nursing Process Activity

Instruction/Description

Select a client from your current work situation. Maintaining anonymity of the client, provide the following: date(s) and time(s) of your assessment, care planning, and implementation of the teaching plan. Provide a brief description of the client's condition, priority diagnoses, priority problems, treatments and a brief physical assessment. Using subjective and objective data:

1. Identify one priority nursing diagnosis in each of the physical, psychosocial, spiritual, and educational domains.
2. Identify one priority desired client outcome.
3. What issues need to be addressed to achieve the priority outcome?
4. Who, what, when, where, and why will need to be involved in helping the client achieve the outcome?
5. How does the client define health, and how will this influence the achievement of the priority outcome?
6. What client values, beliefs, and/or cultural influences are pertinent to achievement of the priority outcome?
7. What resources are needed to help the client achieve the outcome?
8. What personal or professional assumptions/beliefs may influence your thinking related to the client, the situation, and the outcome?

Prepare and implement a teaching plan to address the identified educational needs. You may utilize any format for the teaching plan, but it must include an assessment of the learner (learner readiness), learner-focused objectives, teaching-learning strategies, and an evaluation of both the learner and teacher.

Anticipated Learning Outcomes

1. Prioritization of client data to plan and implement care.
2. Communication and collaboration between nurse–client/family and nurse–health care team

3. Awareness of thinking processes used for prioritization.
4. Awareness of client values, beliefs, and cultural influences on achievement of outcomes.
5. Awareness of how a client's definition of health influences achievement of outcomes.
6. Collaboration with client/family to increase motivating factors and decrease barriers to health behaviors.
7. Enhanced competency in teaching role, with linkages between priority outcome, client preferences, teaching content and methods, and evaluation methods.
8. Identification of evidence-based rationales for content to be taught and method(s) selected for teaching/learning.
9. Awareness of powerful influence of individual points of view.

Level of Education and/or Suggested Courses

- ADN, BSN, or MSN nursing education in face-to-face or virtual learning environments
- All levels of nursing courses
- In-service in health care delivery settings

NAME OF ACTIVITY/SOURCE

Nursing Process Interviews

Instruction/Description

Interview two LPNs, two ADNs, two BSNs, and two advanced practice nurses (MSN or higher) and ask the following questions:
1. How do you use the nursing process in your practice?
2. What are your assumptions, beliefs, values related to, and the use of the nursing process?
3. How does use of the nursing process impact client care?
4. Analyze the responses as an aggregate (one written page) and be prepared to discuss in class (this becomes part of your professional portfolio).
5. Plan an in-service for staff of this unit to explore how the various points of view influence decisions and actions of the staff and client outcomes.

Anticipated Learning Outcomes

1. Increased collaboration with other nursing staff.
2. Enhanced understanding of various applications of the nursing process.

3. Awareness of various points of view in using the nursing process.
4. Analysis of strengths and needs of the various points of view that are identified for both client outcomes and nursing staff workload.

Level of Education and/or Suggested Courses

- All levels of nursing education in face-to-face or virtual learning environments
- All levels of nursing courses
- In-service in health care delivery settings

NAME OF ACTIVITY/SOURCE

Cultural Awareness Diary

Instruction/Description

Throughout this semester, record interactions that you have with people from different cultures. In your diary entry, critically reflect on the possible influences on the process and outcome of your interaction from:

1. Influence of your assumptions, beliefs, values, or points of view about the particular culture.
2. Identify any stereotyping that you may have about the particular culture.
3. Identify any cultural preferences from nursing or cultural literature.
4. Identify differences in verbal and nonverbal communications.
5. Analyze 1–4 for accuracy or individual differences.
6. Review your feelings about the process of the interactions.
7. Review your feelings about the outcome of the interactions.
8. Identify strategies for improving communication.
9. Read about cultural leverage as a communication strategy, and state your thoughts about this concept based on your personal interactions.
10. Reflect on the outcomes from using these strategies.
11. Analyze your level of cultural humility, awareness, competence, etc.
12. Reflect on any change that occurred either in your communication or cultural thinking during the semester to identify why the change occurred.

Anticipated Learning Outcomes

1. Cultural humility, awareness, and competency.
2. Enhanced communication.
3. Awareness of thinking processes when communicating with others from a different culture.
4. Awareness of cultural influences on communication.

Level of Education and/or Suggested Courses

- All levels of nursing education in face-to-face or virtual learning environments
- All levels of nursing courses
- In-service in health care delivery settings

NAME OF ACTIVITY/SOURCE

Group Dynamics Reflection

Instruction/Description

Reflect about a group in your work setting where you were the leader. If you have not been a leader of a group in your work setting, think about a personal situation in which you were a leader. Record your answers to the following questions. Be prepared to dialogue related to your responses to these questions in the virtual class.

1. Do you believe you were an effective group leader? Why or why not?
2. What thoughts, assumptions, and beliefs do you have about being a group leader?
3. What are the consequences to these assumptions/beliefs, and what alternatives would be appropriate?
4. What changes do you need to make for future leadership roles in groups?

Anticipated Learning Outcomes

1. Enhanced understanding related to group dynamics.
2. Awareness of leadership competencies needed to lead followers.
3. Awareness of the power of influence of individual points of view.
4. Awareness of the importance of critical self-reflection/dialogue for changing perspectives.

Level of Education and/or Suggested Courses

- RN to BSN/MSN courses
- In-service in health care delivery settings

NAME OF ACTIVITY/SOURCE

Developing Competence in the Roles of the Nurse

Instruction/Description

This activity can be used in a voice-over PowerPoint in an online environment or as a short response application activity in a face-to-face classroom or in-service setting to promote dialogue. Although the role of teacher is presented in this activity, other nurse roles can be added in subsequent activities.

Answer the following questions as you critically self-reflect on your nurse role of teacher:

1. What assumptions do you have about the nurse as teacher?
2. On what beliefs, values, and past experiences are your assumptions based?
3. What are the consequences of your thinking related to the teacher role?
4. Are there alternative ways of thinking related to the nurse role of teacher?
5. Identify your strengths and areas which need improvement to fulfill the teacher role.
6. In your current work or education setting, what resources are available for you in the role of teacher?
7. Are there factors or issues in your current work or educational environment that limit your role as teacher? How can you overcome these obstacles or barriers?

Anticipated Learning Outcomes

1. Enhanced understanding related to nurse roles.
2. Awareness of competencies needed for different nurse roles.
3. Identification of resources for personal development in various nurse roles.
4. Awareness of the powerful influence of individual assumptions or points of view.
5. Awareness of the importance of critical self-reflection/dialogue for changing perspectives.

Level of Education and/or Suggested Courses

- RN, BSN, or MSN courses
- In-service in health care delivery settings

NAME OF ACTIVITY/SOURCE

"It's Not About Me" Journal

Instruction/Description

Over the next 10 days, self-reflect and record your thoughts in your perspective transformation journal about the following questions:

Day 1
What aspects, if any, in your professional career are just "not working" right now?

Day 2
When your colleagues/patients *look* at you as a nurse, they see *something*. How do your choices and values influence what they see or reflect that "it's not all about you?"

Day 3
As you move toward a more person-centered practice, what *part* do you think you might play? How does a focus on the patient/family influence your desires and goals?

Day 4
What do your goals in your roles as nurse reveal about you? Describe how you strive to achieve these goals. What do your behaviors reveal about your view of colleagues on the interprofessional team? What do your behaviors reveal about your view of those for whom you provide nursing care?

Day 5
What are some steps you can take to resist focusing on self?

Day 6
How can you begin to appreciate points of view of other members of the health care team or patients/families and view situations as they may view them? Can you enjoy this way of looking at situations?

Day 7
We often think of health care as something complicated and unknowable at times. What actions and attitudes are evident in your attempts to provide person-centered care?

What other purposes, events, or ideas do you spend most of your nursing time and energy promoting? What are some practical ways you can purposefully "declare a person-centered approach?"

Day 8
Person-centered care is a rather abstract concept. How would you explain it in more concrete terms? What does it mean to *be* person-centered versus *acting* person-centered?

Day 9
As we begin to more fully understand person-centered care, more of our true motivators and points of view about ourselves as a nurse become apparent. In what way does this approach to health care delivery influence human boasting? In what way does this approach to health care delivery influence your sources for personal or professional approval?

Day 10
Reflect on what you have learned about yourself as a person-centered nurse over the past 10 days. Why is it important to recognize that your *life* as a nurse can be viewed as encapsulated during a moment in time in a patient's *life*?

Anticipated Learning Outcomes

1. Awareness of personal assumptions and expectations regarding personal identity as a nurse.

2. Awareness of personal valuing of others' points of view.
3. Identification of personal needs and motivators for behaviors.
4. Identification of sources of personal approval.
5. Increased skill in critical self-reflection.
6. Increased skill in critical reflection required to express abstract concepts or awareness of self in a journal entry.
7. Increased sense of the unknowing pattern of knowing in relation to health care team colleagues and clients/families.

Level of Education and/or Suggested Courses

- Nursing fundamental courses at all levels of education
- In-service in health care delivery settings

NAME OF ACTIVITY/SOURCE

Reflective Cyberspace Journal

Instruction/Description

The student will select and address one question from either of the topic areas within the assigned week. These questions are intended to help you identify and evaluate the processes you use for thinking in clinical situations. Your descriptions should be about your thinking, not about actual activities you do in clinical settings. In each answer, provide information about what happened in only enough detail to put the situation in context. The writing is intended to be about your thinking and your evaluation of the processes you use in your thinking.

Topics

Ethical Considerations
1. Over the assigned time period, did I consciously think about my personal and professional values, and if so, what impact did this thinking have on my behaviors/actions while delivering care?
2. Did an ethical dilemma(s) occur during the assigned time period? If so, put the dilemma into words, including the statement: "I resolved or addressed the dilemma by using_____." (Focus reflecting here on thinking processes and not so much on the actual dilemma.)
3. Did I experience any cognitive dissonance during the assigned time period? If yes, how did I become aware of my conflict in values?
4. As I analyze my thinking, can I identify a preferred ethical framework in my thinking processes? Am I comfortable with being drawn to that

ethical framework? Are there other frameworks that I desire to become more comfortable using?

Legal Considerations
1. Describe any situation(s) where there was a threat to patient confidentiality. (Focus on the thinking process and not the actual situation.) How did I handle the situation(s)?
2. I was a client advocate when I _____.
3. I was concerned with patient safety/errors when _____. I prevented this safety issue/error from happening by_____. In the future, I will prevent this safety issue/error from occurring by _____. (Reflect on your thinking about the safety issue/error and your thinking process(es) that lead to correction of the issue/error).

Professional Growth
1. I incorporate evidence into my practice when I _____ (identify how you become aware that more information was needed). I evaluate the evidence as valid and reliable because _____. I considered the client/family's values in this situation by _____.
2. I need to improve my nursing practice by _____. In my particular practice setting, the following barriers prevent incorporating evidence into my clinical practice. (Provide specific examples.)
3. During the assigned time period, did I consider all dimensions of care while planning care for my assigned patients? (Describe your thinking about these dimensions.)
4. As I analyze my thinking, are there dimensions of care that I tend to omit in my planning? If so, why?
5. During the assigned time period, was I completely accountable for my actions and judgments related to patient care? What variables affected this accountability and my judgments? What methods did I use to evaluate the effectiveness of my clinical judgments?
6. My behaviors reflected those of a professional when I _____.

Clinical Judgment/Reasoning
1. I was open-minded and aware of how my personal assumptions impact my thinking related to clinical actions when I _____.
2. I used problem solving when I _____. An evaluation of my decision making in the problem-solving example includes _____. (Identify examples of alternative solutions and describe why you chose the solutions.)
3. I considered another's point of view when I _____. Was I cognizant and sensitive to the feelings of others when I _____?
4. How did I relate content from NURS _____ to my work setting and experience? (Give examples of your thinking in terms of course content.)

5. As I analyze my thinking and clinical reasoning, how do I evaluate the outcomes from the care I have provided? Are there areas I need further development? If so, where can I obtain resources for further growth?

Anticipated Learning Outcomes

1. Increased self-awareness about personal view of the world of nursing.
2. Evaluation of the effectiveness of the thinking processes.
3. Consideration of alternative ways of thinking.
4. Increased competency in clinical reasoning.
5. Increased competency in critical and self-reflection.

Level of Education and/or Suggested Courses

- All levels of nursing education in face-to-face or virtual learning environments
- All levels of nursing clinical courses
- In-service in health care delivery settings

NAME OF ACTIVITY/SOURCE

Group-Directed Online Chat Session

Instruction/Description

Each student will participate in one group online synchronous chat session by the date specified. Groups can decide among themselves when to do the chat, but they must be completed by the date specified. The chat session will include a discussion of thoughts related to the following:

1. Miller's (1984) Wheel of Professionalism includes eight *spokes* or characteristics for a profession. At the center of the *wheel* is education at the university level and the scientific basis for nursing. Discuss the significance of each of the *spokes* to the nursing profession as a whole. What other indicators/characteristics do you believe makes a nurse professional?
2. Discuss the characteristics as they apply to you as an individual nurse. What other indicators/characteristics do you believe that you possess or specific behaviors that you routinely do that make you a professional?
3. Dialogue about your thoughts about Miller's Wheel as a particular model for professionalism.

Anticipated Learning Outcomes

1. Increased awareness of models that identify characteristics of professions.
2. Increased self-awareness about personal points of view about self as a professional.
3. Evaluation of the accuracy of any assumptions about nurses as health care professionals.
4. Consideration of alternative ways of thinking.
5. Awareness of areas for personal professional growth or development.
6. Identification of resources that can facilitate personal professional development.
7. Increased competency in critical and self-reflection.

Level of Education and/or Suggested Courses

- All levels of nursing education in face-to-face or virtual learning environments
- Professional concepts courses
- In-service in health care delivery settings

NAME OF ACTIVITY/SOURCE

Perspective Transformation Leadership Portfolio

Instruction/Description

Your portfolio will include areas in which you seek to develop or transform. These will include areas such as how you will be or are a leader in clinical settings, in the profession of nursing, in one or more health care systems, and in one or more personal areas in which you have influence. Initially:
1. Identify any assumptions that you have about leaders in each of these areas.
2. What values, beliefs, or past experiences could be influencing your assumptions or points of view?
3. Then identify one or more personal professional goals that you have in each of these leadership spheres of influence (clinical, professional, systems, other).
4. Critically self-reflect to identify your personal characteristics that can be strengths or weaknesses in each of the leadership spheres of influence.

From an *LPN* perspective, consider how you are or will be a leader in the clinical setting.
1. My spheres of influence include_____.
2. I believe that I have this influence because _____.

3. My scope of practice related to leadership according to my state nurse practice act is _____.
4. One specific example of my scope of practice related to leadership is___ _____.
5. My scope of practice influences my leadership or sphere of influence in the following manner: _____.
6. Clinical leaders engage in mentorship. Specific situations in which I can mentor others include:_____.
7. To mentor others, I need knowledge and skills such as _____ _____.
8. As I critically self-reflect, I have determined that I do or do not _____ desire to be a mentor because _____.
9. I can further develop my mentorship abilities by _____.
10. I was a clinical leader when I _____.
11. The outcome from the situation in which I was a clinical leader was_____ _____.
12. To be a clinical leader, I need to know the following about being a follower: _____.
13. Clinical leaders empower others. I do _____ or do not _____ desire to empower others because _____.
14. Specific situations in which I have empowered others include _____.
15. The outcome from the situation in which I empowered others was_____ _____.

From an *LPN* perspective, consider how you are or will be a leader in the professional sphere.
1. I do _____ or do not _____ desire to be a leader in the professional sphere because _____.
2. I can be aware of issues that influence nursing/ health care delivery systems/patient outcomes by _____.
3. I demonstrated activism related to health policy when I _____ _____.
4. My scope of influence in the professional sphere includes _____ _____.

From an *LPN* perspective, consider how you are or will be a systems leader (micro or macro).
1. I do _____ or do not _____ desire to be a systems leader because _____ _____.
2. System leaders are change agents. I do _____ or do not _____ desire to be a change agent because _____.
3. To be a change agent, I need knowledge and skills such as _____ _____.
4. System leaders are innovative. I do _____ or do not _____ desire to be innovative because _____.
5. To be innovative, I need knowledge and skills such as _____ _____.
6. I was an innovative agent for change when I _____ _____.

7. The outcome from the situation in which I was an innovative agent for change was _____.
8. As I critically self-reflect, I have determined that I can further develop my ability to be an innovative agent for change by _____
_____.
9. My scope of influence in the systems sphere includes _____
_____.

From an *LPN* perspective, consider how you are or will be a leader in other spheres of influence (family, community, other civic or religious groups, etc.).

Revisions for other levels of nursing education:
From an *ADN* perspective, consider all of the questions above that prompt critical reflection and critical self-reflection. Answer according to the ADN roles and responsibilities/scope of practice.
-or-
From a *BSN* perspective, consider all of the questions above that prompt critical reflection and critical self-reflection. Answer according to the BSN roles and responsibilities/scope of practice.
-or-
From a *MSN* perspective, consider all of the questions above that prompt critical reflection and critical self-reflection. Answer according to the MSN roles and responsibilities/scope of practice.

Anticipated Learning Outcomes

1. Increased awareness of spheres of influence for leadership in nursing.
2. Increased awareness of the need for leadership in nursing.
3. Identification of characteristics of effective leaders.
4. Critical reflection about past experiences with leaders.
5. Critical self-reflection to identify hidden assumptions or points of view about leaders or personal desire to take on leader roles/responsibilities as appropriate for level of education and scope of practice.
6. Increased awareness of personal characteristics, including identification of strengths and areas in which improvement is desired.
7. Critical self-reflection about how personal leadership in areas outside of nursing can help or hinder development as a leader in nursing.
8. Identification of resources for personal development.
9. Critical self-reflection to intentionally commit or choose to not commit to leadership thinking and behaviors.

Level of Education and/or Suggested Courses

- All levels of nursing education in face-to-face or virtual learning environments

- Leadership and management courses
- Health care delivery system courses
- Health care administration courses
- In-service in health care delivery settings

NAME OF ACTIVITY/SOURCE

Perspective Transformation Political Environment Scan

Instruction/Description

Conduct a political environment scan in your home state to identify improvements or changes that may be needed for the good of patients and health care. Answer the following questions:

1. What are your assumptions about the political environment in your state?
2. Why would nurses be involved in conducting a political environment scan?
3. What knowledge and skills are needed to conduct a political environment scan?
4. Critically self-reflect about your personal and professional values and goals. Identify if these would influence your involvement in a political environment scan.
5. Are the identified needed improvements or changes in the health care-related issues, relevant during the past 2 years, currently being discussed in your state?
6. Do these issues continue to be priority? Why or why not?
7. Do you personally care about these issues? Why or why not?
8. Critically reflect about potential effects of various solutions for the needed changes.

Anticipated Learning Outcomes

1. Increased awareness of knowledge and skills needed for political advocacy.
2. Critical reflection regarding roles and the power of unofficial and official players in political decision making.
3. Increased awareness of the relationship between the advocacy process and policy change.
4. Enhanced knowledge related to the criteria and methods for conducting a political environmental scan.
5. Development of strategies for enacting and continuing policy changes.
6. Critical self-reflection regarding personal desire to be involved in political activism.

Level of Education and/or Suggested Courses

- All levels of nursing education in face-to-face or virtual learning environments
- Leadership and management courses
- Public policy courses
- In-service in health care delivery settings

NAME OF ACTIVITY/SOURCE

Analysis of a State Legislative Agenda

Instruction/Description

Research then select one current State Legislative Agenda Initiative in a state of your choice. Use this information to create a presentation for a group of health care consumers and/or practicing nurses in a practice setting of choice. The presentation should include the following:

1. Situate the issue within the health care delivery system.
2. State how the issue will impact health care in the state.
3. Identify the stakeholders and why you believe they have power regarding this issue.
4. Critically reflect on the legislators who have supported or blocked any prior efforts within committees and the possible reasons/agendas. From this reflection, identify if there are invisible stakeholders and why they have power regarding this issue.
5. Critically reflect on possible effects, using effect-based reasoning. From this reflection, identify what first-, second-, or third-order outcomes can be anticipated.

Anticipated Learning Outcomes

1. Increased awareness of knowledge and skills needed for political advocacy.
2. Critical reflection regarding roles and the power of unofficial and official players in political decision making.
3. Increased awareness of the relationship between the advocacy process and policy change.
4. Critical self-reflection regarding personal desire to be involved in political activism.
5. Increased role modeling for others in the health care delivery system or consumers of nurses' role in the political process.

Level of Education and/or Suggested Courses

- ADN, BSN, MSN levels of nursing education in face-to-face learning environments
- Public policy courses
- Community courses
- In-service in health care delivery settings

NAME OF ACTIVITY/SOURCE

Professional Nursing Issues—Scenarios 1–8

Instruction/Description

The following brief scenarios (1–8) can be used in fundamental courses across all levels of nursing education or for staff development in either a seminar format or as individual 30- to 60-minute discussion groups.

Scenario 1

During nursing school, a student was observed by other students to be cheating during both online and classroom exams. This student stated, "I am proud that I only do what is absolutely necessary to get by." This student had "taken short cuts" with other work, such as copying and pasting areas from online resources for paper assignments and had complained to other students when the teacher asked to meet regarding this issue. This student was known to drink heavily on nights before clinical experiences, stating to classmates that it was necessary to reduce stress. After graduation, several students from that nursing program were working on the same unit as this graduate. A pattern in client outcomes was discovered on that unit: clients experienced sudden significant changes in vital signs during the shift after care provided by the nurse who had taken shortcuts in school. The unit manager asked all employees to verify accuracy of charted information such as assessments including vital signs, medication administration, position changes, etc. The unit manager also requested further information that would help identify and/or prevent the pattern of significant clinical events and asked former classmates of the nurse in question for specific information.

1. What are your assumptions or expectations about the graduate who had cheated on exams, plagiarized, and used excess alcohol as a coping strategy?
2. How would you identify if your assumptions or expectations are valid and accurate?
3. What issues are involved in the unit manager's request for background information from former classmates?

4. What do patterns of behavior have to do with trust among the interprofessional team?
5. Imagine that you were one of the former classmates. If you could return to the point when you were classmates during nursing school, would you do anything differently? If so, what? If not, why not?
6. What are potential effects of the patterns of past behaviors on client outcomes? What would be your point of view if this graduate was providing care for one of your family members?

Anticipated Learning Outcomes

1. Enhanced understanding of how the ANA Code of Ethics can be used for ethical decision making.
2. Awareness of student integrity and reporting issues.
3. Increased awareness of legal issues.
4. Incorporation of principles of integrity and accuracy in documentation.
5. Value clarification and identification of any value conflict.
6. Personal commitment to professional behaviors.
7. Analysis of factors that influence health care team collaboration and trust.
8. Critical reflection and self-reflection about effective versus ineffective coping strategies.

Level of Education and/or Suggested Courses

- All levels of nursing education in face-to-face or virtual learning environments
- All levels of nursing courses
- In-service in health care delivery settings

Scenario 2

During a clinical experience, a student nurse approaches the nurses' station and witnesses two staff nurses having a disagreement regarding housekeeping services and discussing what the nurses "should not have to do." The same nurses were disagreeing during morning report regarding who had the greater patient workload for the shift. During the discussion about housekeeping, a family member approaches the nurses' station to ask a question regarding a patient. The two nurses continue their discussion, ignoring the family member.
1. What are your assumptions or expectations about health care delivery team communication?

2. How would you identify if your assumptions or expectations are valid and accurate?
3. What issues are involved in the staff nurses' definition of nurse and housekeeping responsibilities?
4. What do patterns of behavior have to do with trust among the interprofessional team?
5. What would you do if you were one of the nurses at the nurses' station?
6. What are potential effects on the organizational image? What would be your point of view if you were the family member who approached the nurses' station during this disagreement?
7. What impact might these nurses' behavior have on the work environment for staff and patients?

Anticipated Learning Outcomes

1. Value clarification and identification of any value conflict.
2. Personal commitment to professional behaviors.
3. Analysis of factors that influence health care team collaboration and trust.
4. Critical reflection and self-reflection about effective versus ineffective communication strategies.
5. Increased awareness related to conflict resolution.

Level of Education and/or Suggested Courses

- All levels of nursing education in face-to-face or virtual learning environments
- All levels of nursing courses
- In-service in health care delivery settings

Scenario 3

A student has a strong personal connection to the information contained in a research article related to family presence during resuscitation efforts. The student decides to write a letter to the editor of the nursing journal about personal assumptions and points of view about family presence during codes. In this letter, the student relates a personal situation that the student witnessed, using actually names of the family member and the patient. The student also recounts a situation observed during a clinical rotation in a critical care setting in which the nurses conducting the cardiopulmonary resuscitation were shouting profane language throughout the code. After the person was resuscitated, he asked the student what had happened and what had he done to cause all of the profanity. The editor responded back to the student that the tone of the letter was not professional and that it would not be published.

1. What issues are involved in this scenario?
2. What are your personal assumptions and points of view regarding each of these issues?
3. What is professional communication?
4. Where should professional communication take place?
5. How can the student respond back to the editor in a professional manner?
6. Critically self-reflect about your level of commitment to professional communication in verbal or written format.

Anticipated Learning Outcomes

1. Awareness of ethical issues regarding communication.
2. Critical self-reflection regarding personal points of view about family presence during resuscitation efforts.
3. Value clarification and identification of any value conflict.
4. Personal commitment to professional behaviors.
5. Critical reflection and self-reflection about effective versus ineffective communication strategies.

Level of Education and/or Suggested Courses

- All levels of nursing education in face–to–face or virtual learning environments
- All levels of nursing courses
- In-service in health care delivery settings (revise the scenario to be a nurse rather than a student)

Scenario 4

You and a group of friends decide to spend one Saturday volunteering at a homeless shelter. While there, you meet a single mother with AIDS. After several conversations during the day, this mother shares that she does not know how to provide health care for her five children and is very worried.

1. What can you, as a student or nurse, do in this situation?
2. Describe the role of patient advocate and how it differs (or does not differ) in a workplace setting versus a community service setting.
3. How does community service impact the profession of nursing? How does it impact you personally?

Anticipated Learning Outcomes

1. Awareness of ethical issues regarding communication.
2. Critical self-reflection regarding personal points of view regarding those in a homeless shelter.
3. Critical self-reflection regarding personal points of view about those who have AIDS.
4. Value clarification and identification of any value conflict.
5. Personal commitment to professional behaviors.
6. Critical reflection and self-reflection about settings for nursing care.
7. Critical reflection and self-reflection about service learning opportunities.

Level of Education and/or Suggested Courses

- All levels of nursing education in face-to-face or virtual learning environments
- All levels of nursing courses
- In-service in health care delivery settings

Scenario 5

A senior student has been working with a staff nurse during a preceptorship experience for 3 weeks. The student has an opportunity to start an IV for a patient being cared for by another nurse. However, the preceptor and the other nurse are too busy to supervise the student and tell the student to go ahead and start the IV. The student had validated on starting IVs in the school of nursing skills lab and had tried to start an IV twice in other clinical rotations. The student decides to "go for it." The student is told the name and room number of the patient, collects the supplies, and enters the patient's room to start the IV alone. The student does not get the IV started on the first attempt, although there is flashback, but it will not thread up the vein. The student is very worried about telling the preceptor and other nurse that the IV is not inserted, so the student tries five more times until the IV is started and working properly. However, the student had brought only two IV catheters into the patient's room. The student decided it was better to keep using the same two IV catheters rather than leave the room to get new ones because that is what they did during practice in the skills lab. After an hour, the student comes out of the room and documents the successful insertion of the IV in the left forearm. While documenting, the student notices that the patient had a left mastectomy last year. When the nurse asked how everything went, the student replies, "It was just fine."

1. What are the issues here?
2. How would a more professional nursing student have handled the situation?
3. What does it mean to attain and maintain competence?

Anticipated Learning Outcomes

1. Awareness of ethical and legal issues regarding nursing skill performance.
2. Critical self-reflection regarding personal points of view about sources of approval in clinical settings.
3. Critical self-reflection regarding personal points of view about maintaining client safety.
4. Value clarification and identification of any value conflict.
5. Critical self-reflection to identify level of personal commitment to professional behaviors.

Level of Education and/or Suggested Courses

- All levels of nursing education in face-to-face or virtual learning environments
- All levels of nursing courses
- In-service in health care delivery settings

Scenario 6

A new graduate started his first nursing job 3 days ago. Today, he was instructed by the charge nurse to administer a medication intravenously that is classified as a chemotherapeutic agent. The new graduate is very concerned because he is unfamiliar with this drug classification apart from the information that he received during the basic nursing program. However, the graduate RN remembers learning how caustic these drugs can be when administered. The new graduate wants to make a good impression in his first job and also does not want to be seen as a "troublemaker" by his unit manager.

1. What is the graduate RN's scope of practice in your state regarding this procedure?
2. How can the new graduate determine if he is able to perform the procedure?
3. How can the new graduate deal with the situation if similar instructions are given by the charge nurse regarding another procedure?

Anticipated Learning Outcomes

1. Awareness of ethical and legal issues regarding nursing skill performance.
2. Critical self-reflection regarding personal points of view about sources of approval in clinical settings.
3. Critical self-reflection regarding personal points of view about maintaining client safety.
4. Value clarification and identification of any value conflict.
5. Critical self-reflection to identify level of personal commitment to professional behaviors.

Level of Education and/or Suggested Courses

- All levels of nursing education in face-to-face or virtual learning environments
- All levels of nursing courses
- In-service in health care delivery settings

Scenario 7

Imagine that in your state during the past legislative session, 2.5 million dollars was transferred from the Board of Nursing (BON) budget to the General Fund Budget. BON operating cost predictions are such that in 3 months, the BON will no longer have the funds to operate and will be mandated by the state legislature to be subsumed under the Board of Medicine. In other words, nursing will no longer have a separate BON and will be governed by the medical board. It is anticipated that the Board of Medicine will require mandatory overtime by every nurse working in a hospital and that the Board of Medicine will require a nurse licensing fee increase to $350.00 every 2 years.

1. What are your assumptions or expectations for state Boards of Nursing?
2. What would you expect the State Nurses Association to do about the problem?
3. Critically reflect to identify what/anything you could do to prevent this scenario from happening.
4. Critically self-reflect to identify skills and knowledge you will need to prevent this from happening.
5. Critically self-reflect to identify a personal level of commitment to pursuing questions 3 and 4.

Anticipated Learning Outcomes

1. Awareness of ethical and legal issues regarding nursing regulation.
2. Critical self-reflection regarding personal assumptions or expectations about autonomy of the nursing profession.
3. Critical self-reflection regarding personal points of view about becoming involved in efforts to maintain nursing's autonomy.
4. Critical reflection about the possible effects of various possible actions.
5. Critical self-reflection to identify the level of personal commitment to behaviors that support the autonomy of nursing as a profession.

Level of Education and/or Suggested Courses

- All levels of nursing education in face-to-face or virtual learning environments

- All levels of nursing courses
- In-service in health care delivery settings

Scenario 8

A recent graduate nurse begins work at a local hospital. The graduate nurse is preparing an intramuscular injection with her mentor and states that she will administer the 3 ml injection in the ventrogluteal injection site. The mentor states, "Well, I always give it in the buttocks. You can just give it there." The graduate nurse declines, stating that evidence has shown a greater risk of sacral nerve damage when injections are given in the dorsogluteal muscle. The mentor states "Well, our protocol states either injection site is acceptable."
1. What immediate action is most appropriate for the graduate nurse?
2. What can the graduate nurse do to promote evidence-based practice on this unit?

Anticipated Learning Outcomes

1. Awareness of ethical and legal issues regarding evidence for practice of nursing skills.
2. Critical self-reflection regarding personal points of view about translation of evidence findings into practice settings.
3. Critical reflection about the possible effects of various possible actions.
4. Critical self-reflection to identify the level of personal commitment to behaviors that support quality and safe nursing practices as shown by findings of well-designed research studies/systematic reviews.

Level of Education and/or Suggested Courses

- All levels of nursing education in face-to-face or virtual learning environments
- All levels of nursing courses
- In-service in health care delivery settings

Appendix B: Case Studies for Transformative Learning

In Appendix B, we offer examples of case studies that can be used as a basis for learning activities within a variety of courses or in teaching specific content/concepts. A number of these case studies have been used in traditional and/or online venues to engage students in transformative learning. Other cases have been developed specifically for this work to illustrate either a "stand alone" case to engage learners in a specific concept or to show how an unfolding case could be used by multiple faculty members in various courses simultaneously or across semesters. These cases are presented for consideration by novice and expert nurse educators to modify or revise, or to spark creativity for developing other cases that could be the impetus for engaging learners in transformative thinking, thus leading to a commitment for decisions and behaviors throughout a nursing career.

CASE STUDY 1

Mary Parker is a registered nurse on a 50-bed medical/surgical unit in an urban not-for-profit hospital. Mary has been the charge nurse on the 7 a.m. to 7 p.m. shift for over 5 years now. For the past 3 years, due to the nursing shortage, Mary has had to take a patient assignment, as well as fulfill her management responsibilities. She prides herself on completing thorough nursing assessments of her assigned group of patients and feels stressed if her management duties keep her from accomplishing this goal. Most patients admitted to Mary's unit are indigent and are usually extremely ill by the time they are hospitalized. Mary experiences firsthand the health outcomes of people who are uninsured or underinsured and thinks often about what she can do to help her patients.

Suggested Courses/Content/Concepts

- Macro-leadership/management
- Public policy
- Health care disparities

- Policymaking process
- Ethical principles
- Foundational concepts of delegation

Suggested Questions to Guide Critical Reflection/ Self-Reflection/Dialogue

1. What does Mary need to know about herself to determine how she will make decisions about providing care for indigent persons? (This presents an opportunity to add in a values clarification activity if not yet done within the curriculum.)
2. What competencies does Mary need to address health care issues related to the uninsured and underinsured patients?
3. In what phase of the policymaking process would Mary enter to initiate changes?
4. How would Mary's personal and political ideology/values impact her actions in advocating for her patients?
5. How does Mary use a decision-making framework to determine which patients will be delegated?
6. What information would need to be included in admission reports for Mary to know how to make appropriate assignments?

CASE STUDY 2

A visitor enters a client's room at 9:00 a.m. The first thing observed is the urinary catheter bag that is ¾ full of bright yellow urine hanging on the side of the bed nearest the door. A blood-stained 2 × 2 is lying on the floor below the urine bag. The client has a white residue surrounding her lips that are obviously dry and stick together when she responds to the visitor's hello. The client's blanket has large drops of Betadine, and the pillow is under the client's shoulders, not her head. The phone is dangling off the bedside table out of the client's reach, as is the call bell, and the water pitcher and cup is on a bedside table on the other side of the bed, also out of the client's reach.

Suggested Courses/Content/Concepts

- Foundational nursing concepts
- Value clarification for motivation to become committed to quality and safety
- Professionalism

Suggested Questions to Guide Critical Reflection/ Self-Reflection/Dialogue

1. What are your thoughts as you read this?
2. Identify and list any concerns that you have about the quality of care or safety of this person in the situation described.
3. If you were the nurse in this setting, list in order of priority what you would do after you entered the room.

4. What value(s) does this prompt you to consider?
5. What are your assumptions about the dignity of the client or the nursing care?
6. Does this situation in any way reflect the assigned nurse's values? If so, describe how.
7. What other assumptions do you need to consider?
8. Do you believe there would be any situation in which the described situation would be "appropriate"?

CASE STUDY 3

For many years, you have identified yourself as a professional nurse. Today, during a discussion on professionalism, you learned an alternative way of thinking about what it means to be a professional nurse. Your prior assumptions related to being a professional nurse included being organized, having integrity in your interactions with clients and coworkers, dressing professionally, and completing your tasks on time and in an efficient manner. The alternative way of thinking about professionalism that was described in nursing literature does not *fit* into your current world view. You now experience a disorienting dilemma because you still believe you are a professional, yet your actions do not reflect professional characteristics. You have identified that you value a personal identity of being a professional in fulfilling your roles of nurse.

Suggested Courses/Content/Concepts

- RN to BSN transition to professional nursing courses
- Professionalism/professionalization
- Values as identified by American Association of Colleges of Nursing (AACN), National League for Nursing (NLN), American Nurses Association (ANA) Code of Ethics
- Self-reflection as a skill for identifying values, beliefs, and assumptions

Suggested Questions to Guide Critical Reflection/ Self-Reflection/Dialogue

1. Identify how your self-concept relates to your personal identity and professional identity.
2. Ponder how encountering a disorienting dilemma feels to you. Label the emotions that you feel.
3. Evaluate if you agree with the definition of professional as stated by various nursing organizations or other literature sources. Why do you agree or disagree? How strongly do you feel about your agreement or disagreement? Why?
4. On what foundational beliefs do you base your answer to case number 3?
5. On what assumptions do you base your answer to case number 3?
6. Identify past experiences that have led to your answer to case number 3.

7. If you identify that you want to make any changes in your own professional behaviors, what would help or hinder those changes?
8. How can your current thinking about professionalism become emancipated?

CASE STUDY 4

After completing your preceptorship at a local hospital, you are hired to work on a busy orthopedic unit. During your preceptorship, you noticed that the unlicensed assistive personnel (UAPs) on the unit would often hide from the nurses when total lift patients needed to be turned or assisted out of the bed. You asked your preceptor if this happened often and she said, "Yes, many of them are just plain lazy and do not care about the patients." Although this concerned you as a student, you believed that if hired to work on this unit, you could work with the UAPs and might even be able to effect change. Within 2 weeks of working on the unit, you are frustrated and feel stressed when the UAPs will not help you move total care patients. They seem to disappear when they are needed most. You ask your nurse manager if you could develop team-building sessions to address the issue. She smiles and says, "Sure go ahead. It will not work, however." During the first meeting with the UAPs, you ask them these questions: "What do you need from the nurses to make your day go better? What is important for you to have the best working relationships on this nursing unit?" The UAPs almost in unison say they need to feel welcomed, appreciated, valued, and respected for what they contribute to the care of patients on the unit. You tell them you will meet with the nursing staff to relay this information and that you will get back with them. In the staff meeting, you ask the nurses these questions: "What do you need from the UAPs to make your day go better? What is important for you to have the best working relationships on this nursing unit?" Almost in unison, the nurses state, "We need to feel competent as managers and to have UAPs comply with requests and give feedback about assigned activities. We are embarrassed when the UAPs fail to comply with our requests." You share the UAPs answers to these questions. A week later you are allowed to meet with the nursing staff and UAPs together. During this meeting, the UAPs state they did not realize that the RNs were expected to plan, supervise, and evaluate their work, nor did they realize that the nurses felt embarrassed when they did not do their work. They also stated they did not realize that it was actually the patients who suffered when they hide from the nurses. The nurses stated they did not realize all the work that the UAPs were required to do. Both groups voiced their commitment to working together to meet the patients' needs.

Suggested Courses/Content/Concepts

- Micro-leadership/management
- Civility
- Team building

- Collaboration
- Communication
- Delegation

Suggested Questions to Guide Critical Reflection/ Self-Reflection/Dialogue

1. What values do the responses of the UAPs reveal?
2. What values do the responses of the nurses reveal?
3. Is there any value conflict?
4. Is the term "have the UAPs comply" value laden? If so, in what way?
5. Identify three lessons learned from this case.
6. What point(s) does this case make related to assumptions?

CASE STUDY 5

Y. Jones, an African American woman in her 50s has come for her yearly physical examination. Her regular doctor is not available so she will be seen by Dr. Smith, a nurse practitioner, whom she has never met. Dr. Smith, a Caucasian woman approximately the same age as Ms. Jones, enters the exam room and introduces herself, saying, "Hello Y, I'm Dr. Smith, It is nice to meet you." Dr. Smith continues with the examination, noticing that Ms. Y is quiet and unresponsive to many of her questions, although she had been smiling and friendly when she first walked into the room. Dr. Smith is concerned that she might have missed important information about Ms. Y's health history because of her reticence to talk, but no matter how friendly she tries to be, Ms. Y remains reluctant, even refusing to talk.

Suggested Courses/Content/Concepts

- Basic communication (verbal versus nonverbal)
- Assessment
- Cultural awareness
- Community nursing

Suggested Questions to Guide Critical Reflection/ Self-Reflection/Dialogue

1. What assumptions come to your mind that might have influenced the communication or interaction (verbal or nonverbal)
2. What do you know about the cultures of each of the people described?
3. What else would you like to know about the individuals that may not be based on cultural influences?
4. What type of miscommunication happened between Ms. Y and Dr. Smith?
5. Is it an assumption that most people prefer to be on a first name basis? How do you decide whether to address your patients by their first or last name?

CASE STUDY 6

You are the nurse assigned to care for a 68-year-old lady for the evening shift. She is 2 days post-op after hip fracture surgery. No problems were noted at nursing sign-out (change of shift) other than c/o pain, for which she was receiving pain medication. When you perform your initial assessment on this patient, you find her to be confused.

Suggested Courses/Content/Concepts

- Communication
- Assessment skills
- Pain management safety principles
- Assertiveness
- Collaboration
- Clinical reasoning

Suggested Questions to Guide Critical Reflection/ Self-Reflection/Dialogue

1. What additional information do you need to gather before contacting the physician?
2. How would you state your concerns and question to the physician?
3. Turn to the person sitting next to you and give a brief summary (no more than 60 seconds). Have that person give you feedback on:
   - What was effective about your communication?
   - What could have been clearer?

The resident physician asks that you obtain the following tests: chest x-ray (CXR), arterial blood gas (ABG), electrocardiogram (EKG), and routine blood work (chemistry studies and complete blood count).

Suggested Questions to Guide Critical Reflection/ Self-Reflection/Dialogue

1. Is there any additional information you need to know at this time? If so, what? If so, where would be your best resource for obtaining the additional information?

The CXR suggests pneumonia, and the resident orders an IV antibiotic. Two hours later, as you start the antibiotic, you note that the patient is more short of breath. You request that the physician reevaluate the patient. The patient's O_2 sat is now 88% on 50% face mask, and her respiratory rate is 30/minute. You believe she needs almost 1:1 nursing and is worried about how you will provide the care she needs and care for your other three patients. You ask if the physician will move the patient to the ICU, but he states he wants to first see how she responds to the antibiotic.

Suggested Questions to Guide Critical Dialogue

1. Practice assertive communication to the person sitting next to you:
   - State your concern
   - State information that supports your concerns
   - Suggest a course of action
   - Recap why you believe this action is the best option

Suggested Questions to Guide Critical Reflection/ Self-Reflection/Dialogue

1. Identify how you feel about yourself at this point in your nursing education related to being able to communicate with physicians or other health care team members who are involved in planning or directing client care.
2. What assumptions do you have about your role as a nurse and the role of other health care team members? On what foundation are these assumptions based? Are they accurate and valid? Do you think that these assumptions hold validity throughout health care settings?
3. What is your personal motivation for assuming the nursing role of advocate?
4. Identify what would help you personally in your skill interacting with other health care team members.
5. If your effort at assertive communication does not have the desired effect, what other options are available to you?
6. How would using standardized communication tools such as SBAR or Call-Out for the communication changed or not changed your dialogue? If so, what were its strengths or weaknesses?
7. Do you believe that using a standardized communication tool would have led to a change in the response by the physician? Why or why not?
8. What changes would need to be made on this unit to empower members of the health care team who identify that client needs are not being met?

CASE STUDY 7

The client is a 32-year-old divorced woman with adenocarcinoma of the lung that has metastasized to her brain and liver. She is the single parent of a 5-year-old daughter. Her husband died 4 years ago while serving in the Iraq War. She has expended her military benefits and now has no health insurance and no immediate family. She continues to smoke one to two packs of cigarettes a day (she has been smoking since she was 12). *Past Medical History (PMH)*: Appendectomy 2 years ago from which she developed infection postsurgery and had an extended hospital stay. In May of last year, she developed scapular and arm pain on her left side and was diagnosed at your hospital with adenocarcinoma of the lung. She underwent a wedge resection of the upper left lobe of the lung. No insurance resulted in no follow-up care (no radiation, no chemo). She tells you that she knows she will die soon and that she welcomes death. She denies belief in a higher being and states "I do not attend church regularly." When asked her definition of health, she states, "dying as quickly as I can." Her daughter is living with her aunt and uncle (father's sister). They try to take care of their niece as best as they can while she attends high school. The client states, "my only regret is leaving her behind with no one I trust to take care of her." The current admission began with pain in her left temple, which started 48 hours ago. She was seen in the emergency department (ED) and received Velosef. She had a seizure and was diagnosed as allergic to Velosef. She has lost 22 pounds over the past year and is receiving Loritab for bone pain. She states she takes one or two 5-mg tabs every 2 hours. However, this is not the way the medication is ordered. A CT scan revealed a large mass in the left frontal area. Her treatment plan includes Decadron IV, seizure precautions, Hydrocodone, one to two 5 mg every 3–4 hours. Vital signs: B/P 160/98, 100, 24, 100.2 (orally).

Suggested Courses/Content/Concepts

- Clinical reasoning
- Assessment
- Communication
- Pharmacology
- Life span courses
- Death and dying
- Health care policy

Suggested Questions to Guide Critical Reflection/ Self-Reflection/Dialogue

1. Identify what initial personal feelings you have in response to this case study.
2. Can you identify any personal assumptions that you make in response to this case study?
3. What process would you use to begin assessing the needs of this person?
4. What process would you use to begin planning care for this person?
5. How would you respond to this person's definition of health?
6. What would be your role as a nurse in response to her statements about leaving her daughter to be cared for by the father's family?
7. In what way does the lack of insurance impact your thinking about this client and the care to be provided?
8. In what way do past or current behaviors impact your thinking about this client and the care to be provided?
9. What is your role as a policy advocate, and what skills do you need for this role?
10. Discuss your answers with one classmate. In what way do your answers differ? Why?

CASE STUDY 8

Patient: Ms. N
Case Manager: Mr. C

Ms. N, a 78-year-old former long-term care patient was found unresponsive, placed on ventilator support, and transferred to the hospital. Ms. N has stage four lung cancer with little hope of being weaned from the vent. Because of her poor prognosis and the fact that she has a terminal illness, she is close to exhausting her lifetime Medicare reserve days. As the case manager assigned to Ms. N, Mr. C has had difficulty finding a long-term care facility that will accept transfer. To complicate matters, Ms. N does not meet the criteria to be admitted to another acute care facility, she does not qualify for a long-term acute-care hospital, and she has no family that will take her home on a ventilator. Today, Ms. N is awake and alert. Her doctors have expressed that the most humane plan of care is to take her off of the vent and let her die of natural causes. The plan is to make her as comfortable as possible during the dying process when she is extubated. Once the ventilator support is discontinued, she will most likely die. It may not be right away, but she will not last long without the vent. Her only family is a stepdaughter and stepson who live in Texas. The stepchildren's initial wish was to place the patient in a ventilator facility. To reiterate, there is no ventilator facility that will accept her as a patient. Right now Mr. C believes he has two options: Option one is to extubate, and option two is to keep the patient on the ventilator until she dies, which could be several months. Hospital administration and the doctors want to extubate Ms. N. Ms. N's stepdaughter is listed as the responsible person. The stepdaughter has had minimal involvement and has only visited the patient a couple of times. The stepson has never visited. Mr. C knows through prior conversations with the stepdaughter that she is extremely uncomfortable with the thought of extubating Ms. N. Surprisingly, she came from Texas last weekend and met with Mr. C's supervisor (the director of case management) who happened to be on call. The director told the stepdaughter that the patient has no quality of life and that she was basically in a "prison cell" left to die. The stepdaughter returned to Texas without giving consent to extubate. The director has asked Mr. C to call the stepdaughter to follow up. After calling the stepdaughter, Mr. C told the director that she (the stepdaughter) wanted to wait until the 26th of December to extubate. Mr. C stated, "She kept repeating something about the Christmas holiday." The director said, "Why wait and prolong her suffering? Get the Department of Human Resources (DHR) involved so they can appoint someone to make the decision." The director then asked Mr. C to call the stepdaughter back and tell her that DHR was going to get involved. The thinking is that DHR will appoint a legal guardian who will make decisions with guidance from the doctors. Mr. C was also told to instruct the stepdaughter that she would not be allowed to make funeral preparations if DHR was involved. Mr. C was totally perplexed by these instructions as he has never heard of this before. The stepdaughter said she would call back later in the day, which she did and gave consent over the phone to withdraw life support. Her one request was to, "let me know when it is to be done." As this was somewhat of a unique situation, the hospital decided that a consent form needed to be created for this case. The form basically read: "I know that if the hospital removes the ventilator, the patient will die, but it is the best thing for the patient." The consent form was faxed to the stepdaughter and she signed for the patient to be extubated. The director then asked Mr. C to sign as a witness to the step-daughter's signature. Mr. C refused, stating that he did not actually witness the stepdaughter signing the consent form. In fact, Mr. C had inquired if a notary should witness signing of the consent form and have it mailed instead of faxed. The director told Mr. C that this was not necessary. Mr. C further expressed to his supervisor that he did not feel comfortable signing the consent, as he believes that there are legal implications of signing as a witness to a signature obtained via phone call and faxed. The director stated, "They do it all of the time and it is part of the nursing world. We get phone consents all the time as long as two people are there." Mr. C stood his ground as he believes the consent basically gives the MD the okay to remove life support. The MD had stated that consent from the family is all he required to order removal from life support. That afternoon, the consent was "witnessed" by another case manager and the nursing supervisor. Mr. C overheard a group of nurses caring for Ms. N talking about the ethical and legal implications of this case. Several of the nurses have grown close to the patient. As stated above, Ms. N is aware and alert and the nurses stated they view the removal of the vent as murder.

Suggested Courses/Content/Concepts

- Ethical principles/ANA Code of Ethics
- Legal principles of health care
- Death and dying
- Clinical reasoning
- Communication
- Values clarification
- Advocacy
- Health care policies and procedures
- Public policy

Suggested Questions to Guide Critical Reflection/ Self-Reflection/Dialogue

1. What is your initial response to this case?
2. In what way would you, as a nurse, begin to unravel the issues involved?
3. What assumptions and expectations for behaviors do you have regarding the client, the family, and the various members of the health care team?
4. If you were Mr. C, the case manager, what would you determine to be the priority issue?
5. How would your personal values influence your decisions and actions?
6. How would what you know at this point in time about professional nursing values influence your decisions and actions?

7. Identify if and why your level of commitment to any decisions and actions that you believe you would take would change if you knew that this case was based on an actual occurrence versus composed for the class activity.
8. Identify components from the ANA Code of Ethics that would apply to this situation and why.
9. How would your actions or decisions be influenced by legal implications? What else do you want to know about this case?
10. What is your role as a policy advocate, and what skills do you need for this role?

CASE STUDY 9

Imagine that you are the licensed practical nurse (LPN) first line manager on Hall B at XYZ long term care facility. You have agreed to work on your weekend off. On Friday March 8th, Mr. J.G., an 80-year-old male, was admitted to your hall. His admission diagnoses include: diabetes type I, hypertension (HTN), dementia, and end-stage renal disease. He has been being cared for at home by his long-time companion, Sally Patriot. Admission assessment determines that Mr. J.G. requires total assistance with his activities of daily living (ADLs). The doctor has discussed Mr. J.G.'s condition with Sally and his 15 children. However, the 15 children cannot agree that he should be classified as "do not resuscitate (DNR)" or "allow natural death." On Saturday, you find Sally sitting by Mr. J.G.'s bed cross stitching and singing softly to him. It is 3:45 p.m., and you do a quick assessment, finding that his lungs sounds are clear, his vital signs are: B/P 180/110, 90, 28, 100.1. His color is ashen, but skin is warm to touch. You note severe swelling of his ankles. He is alert to person but not to time and place. You leave the room and return to the nurses' station to begin you medication pass for the shift. While you are passing medications, the supper trays come on the hall. You see Joan, the certified nursing assistant (CNA) assigned to Mr. J.G. take his tray in the room. She comes out and you ask her if she is going to feed Mr. J.G. She states that his companion said that she would. An hour later, you are sitting at the nurse's station talking to a group of CNAs. Sally screams, "come quick I think J.G. is dead." When you get to the room, Mr. J.G. is blue, unresponsive, and has a large piece of meat hanging from his mouth. Mr. J.G. is pulseless and appears to have expired, having no vital signs, and is not breathing. As you leave to call the doctor and the RN supervisor, you hear Sally say, "good, it worked. Now he will not have to suffer anymore." Mr. J.G.'s next of kin as listed on the admission sheet (Mr. G) is notified and tells you to call the Funeral Home. At 9:45 p.m., Mr. J.G.'s body is released to the funeral home.

Suggested Courses/Content/Concepts

- Values clarification
- Communication
- Ethical principles/ANA Code of Ethics
- Legal principles

- Death and dying
- Clinical reasoning
- Advocacy
- Leadership/management
- Health care management and financing
- Public policy

Suggested Questions to Guide Critical Reflection/ Self-Reflection/Dialogue

1. What is your initial response to this case?
2. Identify what initial personal feelings you have in response to this case study.
3. In what way would you, as a nurse, begin to unravel the issues involved?
4. What assumptions and expectations for behaviors do you have regarding the family, the significant other, and various members of the health care team?
5. If you were the nurse, what would you determine to be the priority issue?
6. How would your personal values influence your decisions and actions?
7. How would what you know about professional nursing values at this point in time influence your decisions and actions?
8. Identify if and why your level of commitment to any decisions and actions that you believe you would take would change if you knew that this case was based on an actual occurrence versus composed for the class activity.
9. Identify components from the ANA Code of Ethics that would apply to this situation and why.
10. How would your actions or decisions be influenced by legal implications? What else do you want to know about this case?
11. What is your role as a policy advocate, and what skills do you need for this role?
12. Can you identify any personal assumptions that you make in response to this case study? For example, would it matter to you that Sally was the patient's lifetime companion unbeknownst to his wife?
13. Would your thinking about this case be any different if the nurse had done what is implied in the case? If the CNA had done what is implied?
14. What is your role as a policy advocate, and what skills do you need for this role?
15. Discuss your answers with one classmate. In what way do your answers differ? Why?

CASE STUDY 10

Imagine that you are the charge nurse on a unit in XYZ facility. You receive a letter from a staff member describing an incident that took place during your weekend off. A nursing assistant left the building, took a 2-hour lunch break and did not clock out. Upon returning, the nursing assistant did minimal work, hid in a resident's room, and did not volunteer to help others. Reflect on the following examples and decide which one you would prefer to use to address the issues as the leader of the unit, or state how you would respond to the situation:

1. Confront the CNA immediately as there is no need to verify the facts by speaking with the writer of the letter. A witness should be present.
2. Verify the facts by speaking with the writer of the letter. Then, confront the CNA with the information and ask for her resignation. A witness should be present.
3. Speak with the writer of the letter to verify the facts and to obtain more detail. Then, speak with the CNA to ascertain problems he/she is having and ask for suggestions on how the facility can meet the needs of the CNA. There is no need to document the incident or have a witness present.
4. Speak with the writer to verify facts and to obtain more details related to the incident. Give the CNA an opportunity to explain the situation. Ask if the CNA has any problems working on the unit and invite suggestions. Document the incident in the employee's record and follow up with a meeting. A witness should be present in all interactions with the CNA.

Suggested Courses/Content/Concepts

- Health care team roles/responsibility
- Leadership/management
- Communication
- Decision making
- Civility/conflict management

Suggested Questions to Guide Critical Reflection/ Self-Reflection/Dialogue

1. Identify assumptions or expectations that you have about the role of charge nurse.
2. Write a short paragraph that expresses how your answer to number 1 could have influenced your selection for how you desired to respond.
3. Identify your current strengths that would be useful as a charge nurse.
4. Reflect individually about what the goal(s) for care are in various facilities and if these would influence your selected response. If so, why?
5. Pretend that all possible responses stated above are correct. Provide sound rationale that would support each of the responses.
6. Dialogue with one peer to identify why you and your peer selected the responses.

CASE STUDY 11

An 80-year-old female with a history of dementia, congestive heart failure, diabetes mellitus, and peripheral vascular disease is recovering from a fractured ankle sustained in a fall. There is a 4-cm laceration over the fracture site. A right ankle splint was applied in the emergency department on 1/08/2012. Documentation in the nurses' progress notes included:

1/09/2012: The resident complained of throbbing pain. CNA reported to LPN. Two Tylenol given as ordered.

1/10/2012: 1600: Odor noted upon entering room. Complaining of pain. Tylenol given as ordered. Splint in place.

1/11/2012: Strong odor noted during bed bath. Crusty drainage noted between toes. Resident screamed and cried when turned. Turned on right side.

1/12/2012: CNA reported foul odor and pain in the foot to LPN charge nurse. Tylenol given. Pillow placed under ankle. Splint in place.

1/13/2012: 2300: Odor worse. Temperature 104. MD called. Orders received to transport resident to the emergency department. Admitting diagnosis: Septicemia.

The resident expired 4 hours later.

Suggested Courses/Content/Concepts

- Fundamental nursing courses at all levels of education
- Wound care principles
- Assessment
- Clinical reasoning
- Documentation
- Standards and scope of practice
- Ethical/legal principles
- Decision making

Suggested Questions to Guide Critical Reflection/ Self-Reflection/Dialogue

1. What are your assumptions and expectations for the responsibilities and role performance standards of each member of the health care delivery team?
2. What ethical principles apply to this case study?
3. What legal principles apply to this case study?
4. If you had been the LPN charge nurse in this situation, what, if anything would you have done?
5. What information do you know at this point about wound healing, infection, immunology, cognitive changes, etc.?
6. What other information would you need to make decisions related to this situation? Why?

7. List all missing elements from the above documentation. Why would this be important information to document?
8. Does the fact that the person died 4 hours after arrival at the emergency department influence your level of commitment to actions or decisions in any way? If so, why? If not, why?

CASE STUDY 12

A 75-year-old male has been living in XYZ LTC for 2 years. His medical diagnoses include diabetes mellitus, peripheral vascular disease, arthritis, cardiovascular accident, and emphysema. He is totally dependent for full assistance in all ADLs. On 2/6/2012, the doctor orders a urinary catheter to genitourinary (GU) bag. Further orders include irrigate catheter with 30 cc normal saline as needed (PRN). On 2/15/2012 at 11:00 p.m., the night shift CNAs are making rounds, and the resident is moaning. He states that his groin area is hurting. This is reported to the night shift LPN. From 1:00 a.m. until 5:00 a.m., the CNAs report to the LPN that the resident complains of pain each time they make rounds. At 5:00 a.m., the LPN goes into the resident's room and finds that he has pulled his catheter out with the bulb inflated. The catheter is reinserted with a return of cloudy urine. Documentation in the nurses' progress notes include:
2/15/2012: 10–6 shift: Resident pulled catheter out with bulb inflated. New catheter 16 French Foley inserted per protocol and connected to drainage bag with yellow cloudy urine noted.
2/16/2012: 10–6 shift: Resident complaining of lower abdominal pain throughout the shift.
2/17/2012: 6–2 shift: Resident sent to the ED for continued complaint of severe lower midline abdomen pain.

The resident was admitted to the hospital with a diagnosis of urinary tract infection (UTI), problems with urinary flow and is placed on antibiotics.

Suggested Courses/Content/Concepts

- Fundamental nursing courses at all levels of education
- Principles of asepsis
- Symptoms of infection
- Assessment
- Clinical reasoning
- Documentation
- Standards and scope of practice
- Decision making

Suggested Questions to Guide Critical Reflection/ Self-Reflection/Dialogue

1. What are your assumptions and expectations for the responsibilities and role performance standards of each member of the health care delivery team?

2. If you had been the LPN charge nurse in this situation, what, if anything, would you have done? Why?
3. What could have been causing the pain?
4. What other information would you need to make decisions related to this resident?
5. After the indwelling catheter was ordered, what would you have documented on the plan of care related to the catheter?
6. List all elements missing from the above documentation. Why would this be important information to document?
7. What information do you know at this point about assessment, infection, immunology, etc.?

CASE STUDY 13

An 87-year-old female is a resident in your facility. Her medical diagnoses include: UTI, atrial fibrillation, hypertension, and cerebrovascular accident (CVA) with right hemiparesis. The minimum data set (MDS) has the resident coded as having short- and long-term memory problems with severely impaired cognitive skills. She is totally dependent on staff for ADLs. The resident has an order for a Hoyer Lift when she is placed in a geri chair and back to bed with assist of two staff. Documentation in the nurses' progress notes include:

3/2/2012 10:15 a.m.: Summoned to resident's room by CNA who stated that while transferring the resident using the Hoyer lift, it tilted, and the resident slipped out. Resident is now complaining of pain in the right upper arm and right hip. Resident is also noted to have a cut above her left eye.

3/2/2012 10:28 a.m.: On-call physician notified and new orders received to X-ray right upper arm and right hip.

3/2/2012 10:30 a.m.: Went down to check on resident, knot and bruise noted on middle of forehead. Resident complaining of headache. Tylenol ×2 administered.

3/2/2012 1:30 p.m.: Summoned to resident's room by family member. Resident complained of pain on right side and head.

3/2/2012 1:40 p.m.: Beeped on-call physician concerning pain on side and head and asked if he could talk to a family member. Family member spoke with on-call physician concerning resident. New orders for Darvocet N 100 mg q. 4 hours ordered and PRN.

3/4/2012 8:15 a.m.: Resident moaning—states that she is in pain. Daughter at bedside. States resident had a fall on Thursday, but no X-rays done. Both eyes have purple color bruise around them. Resident complaining of pain in face and "head all over." Will notify doctor.

3/5/2012 11:50 a.m.: Resident noted vomiting again despite Phenergan this morning.

3/6/2012 12:00 a.m.: Resident vomited moderate amount this a.m. Daughter at bedside and requesting Phenergan 25 mg IM given.

3/6/2012 2:05 a.m.: Resident taken to hospital via ambulance. Admitted with a diagnosis of traumatic subarachnoid hemorrhage and subdural hemorrhage.

Although not documented in the nurses' notes, the family member tells the ED physician that her mother has been delirious, not sleeping well, and constantly tugging at her head since her fall.

Suggested Courses/Content/Concepts

- Fundamental nursing courses at all levels of education
- Assessment
- Clinical reasoning
- Documentation
- Standards and scope of practice
- Ethical/legal principles
- Decision making

Suggested Questions to Guide Critical Reflection/ Self-Reflection/Dialogue

1. What are your assumptions and expectations for the responsibilities and role performance standards of each member of the health care delivery team?
2. What ethical principles apply to this case study?
3. What legal principles apply to this case study?
4. Self-reflect to identify what you know at this point in time that would be needed to provide care for this person. Are there any patterns of knowing from which you identify additional knowledge is needed? If so, in what way do you desire obtaining that information?
5. If you had been the LPN charge nurse in this situation, what, if anything, would you have done? Why?
6. What information do you know at this point about symptoms of pain after trauma, infection, cognitive changes, etc.?
7. What other information would you need to make decisions related to this situation? Why?
8. List all missing elements from the above documentation. Why would this be important information to document?
9. If this resident died after arrival at the emergency department, would this influence your level of commitment to actions or decisions in any way? If so, why? If not, why?

CASE STUDY 14

Ms. Smith was admitted to XYZ LTC on 3/8/2012 with diagnoses of CVA, neurotic depression, hypertension, organic brain syndrome (OBS), dysphagia, and arteriosclerotic dementia. According to the MDS, her impairments included long- and short-term memory loss and severely impaired skills for daily decision making. Ms. Smith is designated to receive no resuscitation. On 3/23/2012 at 5:00 p.m., a CNA summons the charge nurse to Ms. Smith's room. Upon entering the room, the nurse notes that the resident is coughing excessively. She also notes that the resident is coughing up clear phlegm. The nurse leaves the room and returns with

10 cc of Robitussin expectorant mixed with nectar (resident has order for thickened liquids). The LTC facility has standing orders for meds such as cough medicines, Tylenol, etc. When the nurse tries to give Ms. Smith the medication, she spits most of it out. The nurse also notes that Ms. Smith's supper tray is on the bed side table and that the CNA has not attempted to feed her due to the excessive coughing. The nurse stays with the resident for about 5 minutes and then returns to administering 5:00 p.m. medications. The 5:30 p.m. notation in the nurses' notes made by the nurse is "Ms. Smith is responding somewhat better, coughing is decreased, alert." At 6:08 p.m., a CNA calls the RN supervisor to the room stating that Ms. Smith has no pulse, and her color is ashy. Ms. Smith is pronounced dead, and her family is notified. The nurse returns to the desk after passing medications to find out that the resident has died.

Suggested Courses/Content/Concepts

- Fundamental nursing courses at all levels of education
- Leadership/management
- Assessment
- Clinical reasoning
- Documentation
- Standards and scope of practice
- Ethical/legal principles
- Decision making

Suggested Questions to Guide Critical Reflection/ Self-Reflection/Dialogue

1. What are your assumptions and expectations for the responsibilities and role performance standards of each member of the health care delivery team?
2. What ethical principles apply to this case study?
3. What legal principles apply to this case study?
4. If you had been the charge nurse in this situation, what, if anything, would you have done? Why?
5. What information do you know at this point about respiratory status, swallowing, medications, etc.?
6. What other information would you need to make decisions related to this situation? Why?
7. List all missing elements from the above documentation. Why would this be important information to document?
8. Does the fact that the resident died influence your level of commitment to actions or decisions in any way? If so, why? If not, why?
9. Dialogue with a classmate related to each of your feelings at this point regarding the responsibilities and roles of nurses and concerns you have.
10. Dialogue with a classmate to discuss how each of you arrived at the answers to these questions. Did either of you use a decision making framework? If so, which one? Would there be another method to use that could potentially lead to consideration of more than one possible effect of actions (e.g., effect-based reasoning)?

CASE STUDY 15

Ms. Roberts is 86 years old and has recently been admitted to XYZ LTC. Her admission diagnoses are diabetes, glaucoma retinopathy, and dementia of the Alzheimer's type. Ms. Roberts lived with her husband until 6 months ago when he suddenly died of a myocardial infarction. After his death, Ms. Roberts needed help with all of her ADLs, and her niece arranged for home care assistance, 6 hours daily. About one month ago, she started getting up and wandering outside at night. Once, she wandered off at 4:00 a.m., resulting in the police returning her to her home. After this episode, she was afraid to be alone. She agreed to be admitted to a LTC because she could not afford to pay for 24-hour assistance in the home. During the first week in the LTC facility, Ms. Roberts was cooperative with the staff and sociable with the other residents. She was resistant to the morning schedule of getting up at 6:00 a.m. and eating breakfast in the dining room at 7:30 a.m., but she passively complied when the staff firmly directed her. Her niece visited her daily and accompanied her to social and recreational activities with other residents. Ms. Roberts has been in XYZ facility for 10 days and is becoming very resistant to staff efforts to get her dressed for breakfast. When she attends group activities, she is very disruptive and stands up and yells about being a hostage in a monastery. Ms. Roberts tells other residents that she was tricked into coming to this place and that the only reason she has to stay is because her niece has taken over her house and is living there with her family. She frequently paces up and down the corridors and says she has to find her niece to take her home because her husband is sick, and she needs to take care of him. When you walk up and down the hallway with Ms. Roberts, she says, "I don't know why they keep me locked up here, I can't do anything like I used to do at home. It's like a monastery where you have to get up in the middle of the night and they make you get cleaned up and eat breakfast when it's still dark out."

Suggested Courses/Content/Concepts

- Fundamental nursing courses at all levels of education
- Assessment
- Clinical reasoning
- Chronic care/caregiver burden/cognitive changes
- Communication
- Standards and scope of practice
- Ethical/legal principles (autonomy, health care proxy, etc.)
- Decision making

Suggested Questions to Guide Critical Reflection/ Self-Reflection/Dialogue

1. What are your assumptions and expectations for the responsibilities and role performance standards of each member of the health care delivery team?

2. What ethical principles apply to this case study?
3. What legal principles apply to this case study?
4. If you were Ms. Roberts' niece, describe some of your feelings.
5. If you had been the nurse, how would you respond to this situation? Why?
6. If you were the nurse with whom Ms. Roberts discusses the monastery perception, how would you respond? Why?
7. What information do you know at this point about cognitive changes, therapeutic communication techniques, client autonomy versus safety, etc.?
8. What other information would you need to make decisions related to this situation? Why?

CASE STUDY 16

In 2010, Stone was elected President of his state nursing association and served a 2-year term. Stone is speaking to a group of his colleagues and shares the following story:

> I learned more about myself as a leader during those two years than I had over my long nursing career. My most memorial, let's call it a leadership moment, during my tenure as President unfortunately was not a positive experience, but it was nevertheless a learning moment. The situation involved me residing over the annual House of Delegates for the nursing association. Once a year all the districts in the state send delegates to a meeting to discuss changes to bylaws and to make resolutions for the upcoming year's agenda. As you might surmise the first time presiding over the meeting was quite daunting and yes frightening to me as I like to be in control. I have, let's call it an irrational fear of being placed in a situation where I do not know the answer to questions or do not know what may happen next, or cannot even anticipate what might happen. The majority of followers in this particular situation recognized my legitimate power and trusted me as a leader. While I do not know if all the followers were self-aware about themselves as followers, they were willing to be led in my particular leadership moment. Although I did not do a formal assessment of their readiness to be led, I did believe that most were willing for me to be the leader. However, there were some that were not which became obvious to me when several delegates from one district began to question me about the rationale for a particular bylaws change. Although I knew the answer, it was not something that I was willing to share with all the delegates and I therefore tried to be diplomatic in my answer. Sharing the "real" reasons for the proposed change to the bylaws would have caused several leaders at one other district level to be embarrassed. The delegates that had asked the question, however, were having no part of my evasiveness. They were demanding that I tell them the reason(s) for the proposed change to the bylaws. It became apparent as they continued to talk loudly that the association's goals were not the same as the goals at the district level. The goals were actually in conflict. As the constituents continued to demand answers, I will have to admit to you all, I was quite disturbed and frustrated by what was happening.

Suggested Courses/Content/Concepts

- Development of skills in self-reflection
- Civility
- Professionalism
- Ethical principles
- Advocacy
- Leadership of nursing organizations

Suggested Questions to Guide Critical Reflection/ Self-Reflection/Dialogue

1. What are your assumptions and expectations for the responsibilities and role performance standards of each member of nursing organizations?
2. What ethical principles apply to this case study?
3. Analyze Stone's characteristics of effective leaders?
4. If you were Stone, describe some of your feelings.
5. If you had been Stone, how would you have responded in this situation? Why?
6. If you were a member of the constituent assembly during the attack on Stone's leadership, how would you have responded? Why?
7. Why is this case important to me as a future nurse?
8. What are my own assumptions and expectations for membership in professional organizations?
9. What other information would you need to make decisions related to this situation? Why?

CASE STUDY 17

Twenty-five years ago when John was 17, he and four friends attempted to rob a fast food restaurant. When the manager tried to defend the store and his customers, John and his friends started shooting. Ten people were either killed or injured. Several of the injured were females who were paralyzed and had to be maintained on a ventilator. Two of the women died 10 years after the incident, but one remains alive. Two of John's friends hung themselves in jail after they were arrested, and the other one died in prison 15 years after the incident. John was tried as an adult, as he had his 17th birthday the week before the shooting. John was sentenced to death by lethal injection. As his time draws near, his lawyer asks the governor to commute his client's sentence to time served. John says he does not want a pardon, but that after 25 years, he is no threat to society and is a changed person. He says he is no longer the 17-year-old kid that committed the crime. He argues that he deeply regrets what happened, but he has changed so much and experienced so much that he simply is "not the person who committed the crime." The survivors and the victims' families have objected to any change in John's sentence. They think that the death sentence should be carried out. The families of the paralyzed women who died 10 years after the attack argue that John should suffer death just like their loved ones did. They say John may look different and say he's sorry, but the jury's sentence should remain if people are to have faith in the judicial system. The victim, who is still alive and on a ventilator, believes that John's sentence, should be commuted. You are the nurse working in the prison, and the prison warden tells you that you will start the IV for the lethal drugs to be administered.

Suggested Courses/Content/Concepts

- Ethical issues/ANA Code of Ethics
- Legal issues
- Public policy
- Advocacy
- Family theory
- Grief/bereavement
- Value conflict and clarification

Suggested Questions to Guide Critical Reflection/ Self-Reflection/Dialogue

1. What are your assumptions and expectations for the responsibilities and role performance standards of each member depicted in the scenario?
2. What ethical principles apply to this case study?
3. What legal principles apply to this case study?
4. If you were the nurse, describe some of your feelings.
5. Reflect on possible feelings toward John.
6. Would the victim's request for John's sentence to be commuted influence your thinking in this situation? If so, describe with rationale.
7. If you were a family member of one of the victims on the ventilator, how would you respond in this situation? Why?
8. If you were this nurse, how would you respond? Why?
9. Why is this case important to me as a future nurse?
10. What other information would you need to make decisions related to this situation? Why?

CASE STUDY 18

Thirty years ago, Susan began her nursing career as an LPN. She worked in a four-bed ICU for 10 years before returning to school to obtain her associate degree in nursing (ADN). After passing boards and becoming registered as an RN, Susan was appointed supervisor of the ICU. She worked in this position for 5 years when she realized that she loved being a leader and manager, and if she were going to advance in her career, she needed to return to school. Over a 5-year span, Susan obtained a BSN and MSN. In a month, she will assume a new position as chief nursing officer (CNO) at XYZ hospital.

Suggested Courses/Content/Concepts

- Leadership
- Lifelong learning
- Public policy
- Transition to professional nursing

Suggested Questions to Guide Critical Reflection/ Self-Reflection/Dialogue

1. Is Susan's educational trajectory important? If so, why? If not, why?
2. What is the relationship of education, lifelong learning, past personal and professional experiences?
3. Is there any relationship among education, leader, and manager roles? If so, describe. If not, describe.
4. Is there any relationship between personal passion, commitment, and role performance? If so, describe. If not, describe.

Susan has been the CNO for 6 months now and is well liked by her subordinates. The other day, one of Susan's managers came to her and asked for every Thursday off so she could attend college to complete her BSN. Susan told her she would "make it happen." Two days ago, she received a call from a graduate student who is attending a MSN program in the area. Susan agreed to mentor the student in completion of requirements for a leadership course. At the last staff meeting, Susan told her employees that she would support anyone who wanted to attend a workshop for continuing education or take courses to advance their careers. In fact, she told her staff that she is working with a local 4-year college to bring an RN to MSN program on site. Several staff nurses are overheard in the cafeteria discussing how health care reform will impact the hospital. One of the nurses states, "Never fear, Susan will embrace the changes that are coming!"

Suggested Questions to Guide Critical Reflection/ Self-Reflection/Dialogue

1. If you were Susan, identify your personal assumptions and expectations about leadership/followership, formal education, and past experiences.
2. Do you believe that Susan's behaviors are based on a need for approval from her subordinates? If so, why? If not, why? What other values may be motivating her behaviors?
3. Susan's behaviors model which leadership style/theory? Identify which behaviors with rationale for your choices.
4. Other than CNO, what are other roles that a macrosystem leader/manager might assume?

During a weekly manager meeting, Susan is discussing the upcoming budget workshop in preparation for the new budget. Susan realizes that this year's budget preparation will most likely be very difficult as a number of microunits have operated in the *red*. Several of these units have new managers, and Susan wants to make sure that they are prepared for the workshop as she understands that the Chief Financial Officer (CFO) is focused on the bottom line and may not be open to listening to the fact that many units are experiencing high acuity levels, thus resulting in increased overtime. As Susan listens to several of the managers discuss how they will frame dialogue with the CFO, she knows that she does not have the *luxury* of thinking about one unit, she must broaden her thinking related to economics to a macro-perspective.

Suggested Questions to Guide Critical Reflection/ Self-Reflection/Dialogue

1. What are your assumptions about nursing's role in economic issues?
2. What educational or life experience preparation in health care economics is needed to function effectively as an advocate for nurses within the current organizational climate?
3. How might your current assumptions impact your future competencies as a leader/manager at either the microlevel or macrolevel?
4. Why is Susan concerned about her managers defending their budgets to the CFO?
5. Why is it important for a macrosystem leader to understand how health care is reimbursed?
6. What impact does reimbursement have on patient care delivery at the point of care?
7. What impact does reimbursement have on provider performance?
8. What impact does reimbursement have on patient outcomes?
9. How does reimbursement impact the financial resources for use at microlevels and macrolevels?

As soon as the management staff meeting is concluded, Susan must hurry to her next meeting. Since the passage of the *Patient Protection and Affordable Care Act*, Susan's hospital has been holding monthly administrative meetings to discuss the impact of this legislation on reimbursement to XYZ. Susan is very concerned, not only about the direct economical impact of this policy, but also realizes that the policy will force social, cultural, and ethical change in her community. Susan smiles as she enters the room as she is thinking about where she started in her career and where she is now. She would have never thought that as a patient side nurse, she would need to have political acumen. If someone had told her she would need to know the types of policies, the policymaking process, points of entry into the process, strategies for lobbying policymakers, etc., she would have laughed. Susan sits at the table with other macrosystem leaders confident that she will offer intelligent alternatives to solutions. This confidence comes from the fact that Susan critically self-reflects to understand her personal and professional values and how these drive decision making and ultimately actions.

Suggested Questions to Guide Critical Reflection/ Self-Reflection/Dialogue

1. Identify what level of confidence you have at this point in time and how commitment related to personal and professional values influence on your decision making and actions.

2. Identify what level of confidence you have at this point in time and commitment related to systems thinking.
3. Compare and contrast health care financing from a micro-perspective and macro-perspective.
4. Why would you, as a staff nurse, need to understand health care reimbursement from a macro-perspective?
5. What are you democratic values, and how do these impact your political point of view?
6. How might the *Patient Protection and Affordable Care Act* impact the local community from a social, cultural, ethical, and legal perspective?
7. What skills do you currently possess to help you be a politically savvy nurse?

As the meeting begins, the CFO stands up and says we must address Mr. X's issue. He states, "We simply cannot keep ignoring the issue." Susan knows about Mr. X as he is a 50-year-old undocumented migrate worker who was admitted to XYZ a month ago with end-stage renal disease. Mr. X needs a kidney transplant and was placed on the list ahead of a number of patients who are citizens of the United States. Mr. X's case has been the topic of formal and informal conversations for several weeks now. The CFO begins the discussion by stating, "This patient's current bill is over $300,000." He turns to Susan and asks her for a health status update. Susan acknowledges that a number of the nurses have loudly voiced concerns regarding Mr. X and his potential for receiving a kidney over someone who is a citizen. Susan states, "Mr. X's case is not the only hot button issue. My nurses are seeing more and more cases of disparity related to the needs of those who are mentally ill or older."

Suggested Questions to Guide Critical Reflection/ Self-Reflection/Dialogue

1. How does an organizations culture influence decision making and actions of the staff?
2. How would your assumptions, values, and beliefs impact professional decision making and actions regarding Mr. X?
3. How do the following statements relate to Mr. X specifically and to health care disparities from a broader perspective:
   a. We are human beings, caring for other human beings.
   b. We are all caregivers (Planetree, 2010. Retrieved from http:www. plantree.org/about.html).

Erin, Susan's assistant, asks her if she is familiar with a 2007 systematic review related to reducing racial and ethnic disparities in health care. Susan says she is not and asks Erin to share this information. Erin explains that the concept of cultural leverage is offered as an alternate to thinking and redesigning organizations. According to Fisher et al. (2007), cultural leverage is a "focused strategy for improving the health of racial and ethnic communities by using their cultural practices, products, philosophies, or environments as vehicles that facilitate behavior change of patients and practitioners" (p. 245S). Erin goes on to explain that cultural leverage can be used in conjunction with existing strategies as a proactive alternative for addressing cultural interventions that improve behaviors. *Source*: Fisher, T., Burner, D., Huang, E., Chin, M., & Cagney, K. (2007). Cultural leverage: Interventions using culture to narrow racial disparities in health care. *Medical Care Research and Review, 64* (5 Suppl.), 243S–282S.

Suggested Questions to Guide Critical Reflection/Self-Reflection/Dialogue

1. Erin's use of evidence demonstrates what professional value?
2. What are the ways that disparities impact health care from a socioeconomic perspective?
3. What are your assumptions related to access to health care?
4. How do your assumptions related to access to health care impact your decision making and actions?
5. As a future nurse, in what way could you use concepts related to cultural leverage in your practice? As a change agent, describe the change process you could use to implement the strategy.
6. How could alternative thinking impact decision making and actions?
7. Is there a relationship between access to health care and quality health care? If yes, why? If no, why not?

Susan is grabbing a quick lunch at her desk when her secretary reminds her of the community advisory board meeting at 2:30 p.m. As the meeting begins, the vice president of the group states that recent reports from various quality agencies might be the impetus for dialogue. A consumer on the community board states, "I don't see the connection between those reports and health care in our community or in our state for that matter." Everyone on the committee stares at Susan. Susan then says, "Let's talk more about the reports and why the reports do impact health care locally and state-wide."

Suggested Questions to Guide Critical Reflection/Self-Reflection/Dialogue

1. What are your thoughts about how Susan responded to the consumer? How would you have responded if you were Susan?
2. What are your assumptions about quality health care and policy creation/implementation?
3. What is the role of advocacy related to this topic?
4. Why is Susan a member of a community advisory board?
5. Why should Susan be concerned about interest groups in relation to XYZ hospital?
6. Using quality reports such as those from the Institute of Medicine (IOM) and the Agency for Healthcare Research and Quality, what strategies could XYZ use to implement recommendations from the reports? Reflect on this question from the perspectives of policy development, professional education, and collaboration with professional organizations.
7. How do the responsibilities of a staff nurse or a manager differ from Susan's in relationship to quality improvement? Describe the responsibilities and your reasons for specifying.

8. What is the relationship of quality care to patient outcomes?

The conversation quickly turns to a recent newspaper report where a patient is suing XYZ for a medication error. Members of the advisory board ask Susan, "What happened? Aren't your nurses competent?"

Suggested Questions to Guide Critical Reflection/ Self-Reflection/Dialogue

1. Imagine that you are Susan, how would you respond to these questions?
2. What legal or ethical principles might come into play here?
3. Reflect on the relationship of working conditions to patient outcomes and safety.
4. How do working conditions affect the rate and type of medical/nursing errors?

During a brief break, a reporter from the local newspaper approaches Susan and asks her for some comments on how she anticipates that the new regulations related to Medicare and Medicaid reimbursement will impact XYZ hospital.

Suggested Questions to Guide Critical Reflection/ Self-Reflection/Dialogue

1. What are your initial feelings in response to being asked for an interview?
2. Identify any assumptions or expectations that you have regarding your personal and professional values, political values, and your points of view about reimbursement for older, indigent, and disabled people.
3. Imagine that you are Susan, and identify how you would respond to these questions.
4. Are there any issues or concerns that Susan should be aware of before she responds to the reporter?

As the Community Advisory Board meeting is ending, a Dean at a local university asks Susan how her nurses are reacting to the recent increase in licensure fees. He goes on to state that when he mentioned this to a group of nursing students they "looked unconcerned." Additionally, he asks Susan to share her thoughts about a recent change in the State Nurse Practice Act that increased the ratio of students to clinical faculty in all settings of care.

Suggested Questions to Guide Critical Reflection/ Self-Reflection/Dialogue

1. What are your initial assumptions about licensure fees?
2. What are your expectations from licensed persons versus those who are unlicensed?
3. Describe how the Dean's questions to Susan could influence your practice of nursing upon your graduation, then the potential effect throughout a 40-year nursing career.

4. Why would the Dean expect the CNO of a local hospital to provide an opinion regarding these questions? Would the Dean have the same expectations for a staff nurse?
5. Do you have any assumptions/expectations regarding Susan's professional or political organization involvement? Would you have the same expectation for any staff nurse? Why or why not?

Susan is leaving the hospital for the day. It has been a long 12 hours and she would like nothing better than to go home and relax. However, there is a meeting of the state nursing association board this evening, and as the secretary of this organization, Susan is obligated to attend. The meeting tonight centers on the association's agenda for the upcoming legislative session. Susan's state association has been lobbying for increased state funding for nursing scholarships if the recipients will agree to serve at least 2 years as nurse educators in this state.

Suggested Questions to Guide Critical Reflection/ Self-Reflection/Dialogue

1. What are your initial assumptions or expectations about those who participate in nursing organizations?
2. What are your initial assumptions or expectations about nursing organizations' involvement in political activity?
3. Describe how your personal and professional values may be in conflict regarding various expectations for your time.
4. Describe your opinion regarding scholarship funding that has a requirement attached.
5. What values do you identify that Susan has that would relate to the issue of state-funded scholarships?
6. Should the government be involved in the nursing shortage? If so, how and why? If not, how and why not?
7. Describe characteristics of interest groups. Is the state nurses association an interest group? If so, how? If not, why not?
8. In what way do interest groups influence health policy? According to your personal, professional, and political values and points of view, what role should interest groups have in political processes?

The state nursing association meeting is ending. Several nursing students from a local college have attended the meeting to fulfill course requirements. One of the students asks Susan about health care reform legislation. Specifically, the student asks about possible impact on XYZ hospital from the regulation related to all citizens being required to purchase acceptable health care insurance coverage by 2014 or pay a penalty if they do not. Susan responds by asking the students to do the following:

Suggested Questions to Guide Critical Reflection/ Self-Reflection/Dialogue

1. Research possible effects from the regulation on citizens in the state and their local community.

2. Research possible effects from the regulation on the health care and insurance industries.
3. Research possible effects from the regulation on themselves as future nurses.
4. Ponder why the particular provision regarding required insurance purchase was of concern to the student rather than other provisions.
5. Discuss the role of nursing as a profession and nurses as individuals in the health care reform implementation and in policymaking processes.
6. Critically reflect about the point of entry for individual nurses into the political process.

CASE STUDY 19

Ms. Grassley was admitted to a LTC for short-term rehabilitation on April 15, 2011. During her one month stay at the facility, she received physical therapy for a fracture to her right hip. She progressed well and was scheduled for discharge on May 15, 2011. The social worker began discharge planning with the client and family on the day of admission. The family had agreed all along that Ms. Grassley would return home after her rehab. On May 14, arrangements were made for Ms. Grassley to be transported via ambulance to her daughter's home. On May 15 at 8:30 a.m., two ambulance drivers arrived at the facility to transport Ms. Grassley. It was documented that she left the facility via stretcher at 8:37 a.m. One hour later, the ambulance drivers arrived back at the facility with Ms. Grassley and stated to the unit charge nurse, "No one was at home. The neighbor told us that the daughter was out of town. What do you want us to do with Ms. Grassley?" The director of nursing (DON) and administrator were called to the unit. After a brief private meeting between the charge nurse, DON, and facility administrator, the ambulance drivers were told that Ms. Grassley could not be readmitted because she had been discharged, and they had no new orders to admit her back into the facility. The ambulance drivers did not know what to do. They decided to take her to another facility where she had been a former resident. When they arrived at that facility, they were told that she could not be admitted there. The ambulance drivers then decided to take Ms. Grassley to the emergency medical service (EMS) office. They parked the ambulance and decided to leave her in the back of the ambulance on the stretcher. Ms. Grassley was on the stretcher for 6 hours without food or water or anyone checking on her. After 6 hours, the chief EMS officer instructed the drivers to take Ms. Grassley to the local ED. When they arrived at the ED, Ms. Grassley was taken to a room, and she was asked by the triage nurse, "What is going on?" Ms. Grassley replied, "I feel horrible and like an idiot. My daughter was not at home and the ambulance drivers left me in the back of the ambulance all day. I have not had anything to eat or drink since leaving the nursing home at 8:30 this morning." Ms. Grassley was seen by the ED physician and admitted with diagnoses of dehydration and hypoglycemia.

Suggested Courses/Content/Concepts

- Foundational courses across all levels of education
- Ethical issues
- Legal issues
- Decision making
- Person-centered care
- Quality
- Safety
- Transitions of care across health care delivery systems
- Health care financing
- Regulation

Suggested Questions to Guide Critical Reflection/ Self-Reflection/Dialogue

1. What are your initial assumptions or expectations about this situation?
2. What are your initial assumptions or expectations about the health care delivery team responsibilities at transition across each of the settings?
3. Describe how your personal and professional values may be in conflict regarding expectations for care that was or was not provided in this case.
4. What values do you identify that would relate to the issues involved in this case?
5. What is the influence of government regulations for reimbursement on this case?
6. Describe choices made at each point. Did each decision maker consider all potential effects of the decision? If so, how? If not, why not?
7. To achieve a different outcome, what information was needed at what point in time?
8. How would government regulations related to long-term care impact the facilities in this situation?

CASE STUDY 20

At 4:30 a.m., a CNA notified the nursing staff that Mr. B had not slept much during the night due to multiple trips to the bathroom resulting in a total of four liquid stools. The staff nurse assessed Mr. B and documented his color as slightly pale, abdomen slightly distended, dried blood around his mouth, and his bed smeared with feces (color and consistency not described). Vital signs were B/P 100/60, 70, 25, 100.5 (orally). At 5:45 a.m. the CNA reported that Mr. B became unsteady while exiting the bathroom and was lowered to the floor to prevent him from falling. At 6:00 a.m., the staff nurse documented that Mr. B's skin was cold and clammy to touch and pale in color. Vital signs at this time were B/P 88/50, 85, 30 with O_2 saturation at 93% on room air. Oxygen per nasal cannula at 5 L per minute was initiated per standing orders, and the physician was called. At 6:25 a.m., Mr. B remained on the floor outside of his bathroom. Documentation included that he was combative, trying to remove his nasal cannula, and insisting on sitting up. Vital signs included B/P/ 80/50, 67, 28. Other observations include sallow skin color and coffee ground drool from both corners of his mouth. At 6:45 a.m., Mr. B is now unresponsive without blood pressure, pulse, or respirations. Cardiopulmonary resuscitation was initiated, but Mr. B was declared dead at 7:00 a.m.

Suggested Courses/Content/Concepts

- Foundational courses across all levels of education
- Pathophysiology
- Ethical issues
- Legal issues
- Decision making/prioritization
- Clinical reasoning
- Quality
- Safety
- Scope of practice

Suggested Questions to Guide Critical Reflection/ Self-Reflection/Dialogue

1. What are your initial assumptions or expectations about this situation?
2. What are your initial assumptions or expectations about the nurse's responsibilities?
3. What are your initial assumptions or expectations about the CNA's responsibilities?
4. Describe how your personal and professional values may be in conflict regarding expectations for care that was or was not provided in this case.
5. What values do you identify that would relate to the issues involved in this case?
6. Describe choices made at each point. Did each decision maker consider all potential effects of the decision? If so, how? If not, why not?
7. To achieve a different outcome, what information was needed at what point in time?
8. What were critical assessment findings that could have led to a different outcome?
9. Findings in this case suggest what ethical/legal issues?
10. How would you feel if you were Mr. B?
11. How would you feel if you were Mr. B's family?
12. Would your commitment to decisions or actions be influenced if this was based on an actual or contrived situation? Why?

CASE STUDY 21

A home health nurse has been assigned to assess and provide wound care for Ms. C twice a week. Upon arrival at the rural home, the nurse enters a dilapidated wooden structure with several missing front steps.

Ms. C called from the bedroom for the nurse to enter. The nurse observed several stacks of old newspapers, shredded papers, rat droppings, and general disarray in the bedroom. There was a strong odor of urine, and an unemptied bedside commode chair was in the corner of the room. Ms. C was alone with remains of a cinnamon roll near her pillow. The nurse begins her assessment. Vital signs include B/P 90/60, 88, 24, 101 (orally). Skin turgor at forehead returns in 6 seconds, and skin is dry to touch and flaking on all extremities. Hands and feet are cool to touch with capillary refill in 7 seconds. Pedal pulses are weak bilaterally and left foot has +2 pitting edema. A 3-inch gauze is wrapped loosely around Ms. C's left calf. Removal of the dressing reveals a stage 3, 2 × 5 cm stasis ulcer with black edges and yellow-green exudate that smells like soured apples. The nurse cleans the wound with sterile saline and applies a dry 4 × 4 to the area and rewraps with clean 3-inch gauze. The nurse documents her assessment findings and wound care and tells Ms. C that she will return in 2 days. The nurse returns 2 days later to find Ms. C in the same situation with the bedside commode overflowing. Vital signs include B/P 80/40, 110, 30, 102 (orally), and skin is cool and clammy. The nurse now asks Ms. C if anyone has been to see her since the prior nurse visit. Ms. C responds that her family has told her that she has become more than they can handle and keep their jobs. The family tells her they will check on her on the weekends. Ms. C changes the subject from her family by stating that she has become weaker and does not have energy to get to the kitchen, asking what would be involved to receive meals on wheels. Ms. C further states that she has not had a bowel movement (BM) since 3 days ago, and she is worried that she only voids small amounts of urine.

Suggested Courses/Content/Concepts

- Foundational courses across all levels of education
- Community
- Pathophysiology
- Ethical issues
- Legal issues (abuse and neglect)
- Decision making/prioritization
- Clinical reasoning
- Quality
- Safety
- Scope of practice
- Community resources
- Family theory

Suggested Questions to Guide Critical Reflection/ Self-Reflection/Dialogue

1. What are your initial assumptions or expectations about this situation?
2. What are your initial assumptions or expectations about the nurse's responsibilities?

3. What are your initial assumptions or expectations about Ms. C's family's responsibilities?
4. Describe how your personal and professional values may be in conflict regarding expectations for care that was or was not provided in this case.
5. What values do you identify that would relate to the issues involved in this case?
6. Describe assessment findings from the initial visit that are pertinent to this situation. In what way would these findings influence your decisions and actions if you were the nurse?
7. To achieve a different outcome, what information was needed at the first visit?
8. Did the nurse consider all potential effects of the initial assessment? If so, how? If not, why not?
9. Findings in this case suggest what ethical/legal issues?
10. How would you feel if you were Ms. C?
11. What community resources would apply to this situation?
12. Reflect on any prior experiences that may influence your thinking and actions in a positive or negative manner. Turn to a classmate and share this experience and how it has influenced your point of view.
13. After your critical reflection about this case, what level of commitment do you feel toward any responsibilities you may have for a family member or as a nurse?

CASE STUDY 22

Read the following article as background information: Jackson-Allen, P. L., & McGuire, L. (2011). Incorporating mental health checkups into adolescent primary care visits. *Pediatric Nursing, 37*(3), 137–140.

Barry is a 13-year-old who is beginning a new public junior high school in a mid-sized community. Several of his friends are attending other schools, but he has a friend from the past 2 years who is in several of his classes on the first day of the school year. Barry anticipates that he and the prior friend will sit together in the classes and finds the friend to discuss this. However, when Barry attempts to talk with the prior friend, he is told to "Go away, I don't have the time to talk with the likes of you." After this comment, the prior friend pushes Barry away, causing him to fall in the hallway in front of a group of adolescents who have gathered at the lockers. All of those in this group begin to laugh at Barry, stating, "What a loser!" Barry leaves the area as quickly as possible, unsure what all has just happened or why. He remains quiet for the rest of the school day. When he speaks with his mother that evening, he expresses anger at her stating, "I am not going back to that stupid school." His mother admonishes him for his outburst, replying, "You most certainly are going back!" Barry becomes sullen and remains so for the rest of the week, eating very little at meals, and becoming unkempt in appearance. One of his teachers referred him to the school nurse.

Suggested Courses/Content/Concepts

- Pediatric courses across all levels of education
- Growth and development courses
- Assessment courses
- Mental health courses
- Safety versus bullying
- Community resources
- Family theory

Suggested Questions to Guide Critical Reflection/ Self-Reflection/Dialogue

1. What are your initial assumptions or expectations about Barry's situation?
2. What are your initial assumptions or expectations about the school nurse's responsibilities?
3. What are your initial assumptions or expectations about Barry's family's responsibilities?
4. What values do you identify that would relate to the issues involved in this case?
5. Describe assessment findings from the initial visit with the school nurse that would be most pertinent in this situation. In what way would these findings influence your decisions and actions if you were the nurse?
6. What other information does the school nurse need to obtain at the first visit?
7. If you were the school nurse, how could you consider all potential effects of findings from the initial assessment? If desired, incorporate effect-based reasoning to guide your thinking processes.
8. Findings in this case suggest what ethical/legal issues?
9. How would you feel if you were Barry? Barry's mother? The school nurse? Barry's teacher?
10. What community resources would apply to this situation?
11. Reflect on any prior experiences that may influence your thinking and actions in a positive or negative manner. Turn to a classmate and share this experience and how it has influenced your point of view. (If in an online environment, share through e-mail with one classmate or through a discussion posting.)
12. After your critical reflection about this case, what level of commitment do you feel toward any responsibilities you may have for an adolescent such as Barry or his family?

CASE STUDY 23

Hana is a 9-year-old fourth grader who is best friends with Gretchen. They do everything together. They are both involved in taking gymnastics. Two weeks ago, Gretchen complained of fatigue and showed Hana several bruises that she had on her back. Gretchen was taken to the pediatrician and has been diagnosed with leukemia. Hana's mother decides to wait until Gretchen is feeling better to let Hana visit. However, Gretchen perceives that Hana is afraid that she will catch leukemia and will never come to visit her again. Gretchen's parents have had to decide if she will receive treatment locally or at a children's cancer center. If Gretchen has to travel to the cancer center, her parents will be unable to remain with her because Gretchen's father is unemployed and seeking temporary employment to cover anticipated health care costs and the needs of Gretchen's four younger siblings.

Suggested Courses/Content/Concepts

- Pediatric courses across all levels of education
- Growth and development courses
- Assessment courses
- Mental health courses/anticipatory grieving
- Community resources
- Family theory

Suggested Questions to Guide Critical Reflection/ Self-Reflection/Dialogue

1. What are your initial assumptions or expectations about Gretchen's situation?
2. What are your initial assumptions or expectations about the nurse's responsibilities when Gretchen is admitted for treatment?
3. What are your initial assumptions or expectations about Gretchen's family's responsibilities?
4. What values do you identify that would relate to the issues involved in this case?
5. How could you assess and plan for meeting Gretchen's developmental needs according to at least four different developmental theories?
6. Describe assessment findings from the admission that would be most pertinent in this situation. In what way would these findings influence your decisions and actions if you were the nurse?
7. What other information would the nurse need to obtain at admission?
8. If you were the nurse, how could you consider all potential effects of findings from the admission assessment? If desired, incorporate effect-based reasoning to guide your thinking processes.
9. How would you feel if you were Gretchen? Hana? Gretchen's parents? The nurse?
10. What community resources would apply to this situation?
11. Reflect on any prior experiences that may influence your thinking and actions in a positive or negative manner. Turn to a classmate and share this experience and how it has influenced your point of view. (If in an online environment, share through e-mail with one classmate or through a discussion posting.)
12. After your critical reflection about this case, what level of commitment do you feel toward any responsibilities you may have for a child such as Gretchen and her family?

CASE STUDY 24

Mr. Smith is a 55-year-old male of Hispanic background. He has managed his insulin-dependent diabetes mellitus by self-administering insulin each morning until he experienced a stroke 3 weeks ago that resulted in his right side being paralyzed and some expressive aphasia. He had previously had an above-the-knee amputation of his lower left leg from a traumatic injury that became gangrenous. He needs total assistance for his activities of daily living and has lost 10 pounds during his hospitalization due to reluctance to eat/difficulty swallowing. His wife visits every other day for 3 hours, describing how hard Mr. Smith worked and how much he was respected by his religious group. She states how difficult it must be for Mr. Smith not to be able to participate in his usual religious practices that had always been such strength for him. As a student, you have been assigned to provide care for Mr. Smith.

Suggested Courses/Content/Concepts

- Fundamental nursing courses across all levels of education
- Growth and development courses
- Assessment courses
- Mental health courses
- Spirituality
- Cultural influences on communication
- Community resources
- Family theory

Suggested Questions to Guide Critical Reflection/
Self-Reflection/Dialogue

1. What are your initial assumptions or expectations regarding Mr. Smith's situation?
2. What are your initial assumptions or expectations about your responsibilities for caring for Mr. Smith?
3. What are your initial assumptions or expectations about the Smith family's strengths and needs?
4. What values do you identify that would relate to the issues involved in this case?
5. Describe assessment findings that you anticipate to be most pertinent in this situation. In what way would these findings influence your decisions and actions as you assume care?
6. Findings in this case suggest what ethical issues?
7. How would you feel if you were Mr. Smith? Mrs. Smith?
8. What community resources would apply to this situation?
9. In what creative ways could you help to meet Mr. and Mrs. Smith's spiritual needs?
10. Reflect on any prior experiences that may influence your thinking and actions in a positive or negative manner.

11. After your critical reflection about this case, what level of commitment do you feel toward any responsibilities you may have for a client such as Mr. Smith or his family?

CASE STUDY 25

Mr. Jones is a 74-year-old African American who served in the Korean War and is now hospitalized at the local Veteran's Affairs Medical Center for prostate cancer that has metastasized to his pelvic bones and spine. He is alert, oriented, and talkative most of the time but is now unable to get out of bed without assistance using a Hoyer lift due to severe pain with movement. During his talkative periods, he recounts his military service, meeting his wife in Korea, and his remorse that he did not seek earlier assessment for decreased strength of his urine flow. He has recently developed skin breakdown at his sacral area. The staff nurse has just begun dressing change when a group of children from a nearby school enter the room without knocking on the door. Although the nurse quickly covers Mr. Jones, the children obviously are shocked by the appearance of Mr. Jones' sacral area. However, one child walks toward Mr. Jones, stating "We brought you some flowers and a flag for Veteran's Day. Thanks for your service to our country." The children then turn and leave the room. Mr. Jones begins to sob.

Suggested Courses/Content/Concepts

- Fundamental courses across all levels of education
- Geriatric or life span development courses
- Mental health courses
- Loss/grieving concepts
- Communication
- Reminiscence therapy

Suggested Questions to Guide Critical Reflection/ Self-Reflection/Dialogue

1. What are your initial assumptions or expectations about Mr. Jones' situation?
2. What are your initial assumptions or expectations about the staff nurse's responsibilities?
3. What values do you identify that would relate to the issues involved in this case?
4. Why do you believe that Mr. Jones begins to sob? Compare your response to one of your classmates.
5. Describe the thinking process that you would use if you were Mr. Jones' nurse to identify and prioritize his needs.
6. Dialogue with a classmate about how you would phrase your communication with Mr. Jones immediately after the group of children left his room.

7. How would you obtain information about Mr. Jones' psychosocial, cognitive/emotional, developmental, and spiritual needs?
8. In what way would these findings influence your decisions and actions if you were the nurse?
9. What other information does the nurse need to obtain from Mr. Jones?
10. How would you feel if you were Mr. Jones? The staff nurse?
11. What community resources would apply to this situation?
12. Reflect on any prior experiences that may influence your thinking and actions in a positive or negative manner. Turn to a classmate and share this experience and how it has influenced your point of view.
13. After your critical reflection about this case, what level of commitment do you feel toward any responsibilities you may have for a client such as Mr. Jones?

CASE STUDY 26

A clinical instructor is taking a group of intermediate-level nursing students to a local Veteran's Affairs hospital. She assigns two students to provide nursing care for Mr. B., a retired Navy medic who has been hospitalized for his chronic unstable diabetes. Mr. B. has had bilateral below-the-knee amputations due to vascular insufficiency secondary to his diabetes. As a result of a stroke about a year ago, his right side is paralyzed, and he drools saliva from both corners of his mouth. When the instructor enters Mr. B.'s room with the two students right behind her, she states to Mr. B., "Good morning Mr. B. I have two new students here. Are you ready to whip them into shape today?" Mr. B. smiles lopsidedly and nods yes. The instructor tells the students that Mr. B. desires assistance getting into his motorized wheel chair and likes to have a towel around his neck to use to wipe his chin using his left hand. The instructor further tells the students that Mr. B. will let them know what to do. The students look bewildered by this comment due to the difficulty Mr. B. has with verbal communication. At the end of the shift of care, the instructor invites Mr. B. to participate in the beginning period of the post-clinical conference with all students in the clinical group. She tells Mr. B., "You worked most of your life as a Navy medic and know all about providing health care. Would you please share some of your words of wisdom with these students?" Mr. B. attempts to speak, but due to difficulty, reaches with his left hand for the instructor's pen and paper. He painstakingly and slowly prints in large underlined letters **LET ME DO IT MYSELF!**

Suggested Courses/Content/Concepts

- Clinical courses across all levels of education
- Geriatric or life span development courses
- Mental health courses
- Effective coping concepts
- Theories of nursing
- Communication
- Reminiscence therapy

Suggested Questions to Guide Critical Reflection/ Self-Reflection/Dialogue

1. What are your initial assumptions about Mr. B? Why?
2. What are your expectations about the staff nurse's responsibilities based on various nursing theories?
3. Identify your feelings in response to what Mr. B. wrote. Share with a classmate.
4. Why do you think the instructor assigned students to care for Mr. B?
5. Why do you think the instructor said what she did initially to Mr. B?
6. What values do you identify that relate to Mr. B?
7. Why do you believe that Mr. B. wrote what he did in response to the nursing instructor? Compare your response to one of your classmates.
8. Describe the thinking process that you would use if you were the student caring for Mr. B.
9. Dialogue with a classmate about how you could best communicate and provide care for Mr. B.
10. What is the most important lesson that you have learned from Mr. B?

CASE STUDY 27

Mary is enrolled in an ADN program in a small junior college. During almost all of Mary's clinical assignments, she has known most of the clients she was assigned to care for because the hospital is located in a small community. Today, she is assigned to observe on the labor and delivery unit. During her second day on the unit, Mary attended the delivery of a premature infant. After delivering the tiny baby, the physician walked to a nearby room, placed the infant on a metal utility table, turned to the nurses and stated, please do not touch this infant, her mother is mentally and physically handicapped, was raped, and she does not want this baby. Because the infant is premature, it is unlikely she will survive in the best of situations; nevertheless, Mary is shocked and begins to ask the OB nurses what they are going to do. She states, "I am going to call my clinical instructor, this is murder!" It is obvious to Mary that the other nurses are also struggling with the situation and are just as shocked and upset as Mary.

Suggested Courses/Content/Concepts

- Clinical courses across all levels of education
- Ethical/legal issues
- Values conflict

Suggested Questions to Guide Critical Reflection/ Self-Reflection/Dialogue

1. In this situation, do you believe that the end justifies the means? Why or Why not?

2. Utilitarianism holds that an action is judged as good or bad in relation to the consequences or outcomes that are derived from it. If the physician was thinking in terms of utilitarianism, what could have been the arguments to support his actions?
3. Assume that the infant is rescued. Reflect on as many possible outcomes as you can imagine. Share these with a classmate or in a threaded online discussion.
4. Identify four arguments in support of and in opposition to the physician's decision.
5. Considering her position as a student in the hospital, what are Mary's options?
6. What thoughts would have gone through your mind if you were in the situation?

CASE STUDY 28

June is a 14-year-old junior high school cheerleader. She presents to the local health department family planning clinic requesting birth control pills. June is attractive, dressed appropriately, and appears very anxious. A primary care nurse practitioner begins June's physical examination and is disturbed when she finds numerous bruises over her back in various stages of healing and has obvious cigarettes burns to her buttocks. After June is dressed, the care provider caringly begins to question June about the findings. June begins to sob uncontrollably and blurts out that her mother's boyfriend hits her, and when he is very angry will burn her with his cigarettes. She reports that she has told no one, not even her mother about the abuse. As she continues to cry, she admits that he is also sexually abusive, and she just cannot tolerate the abuse any longer. She states, "I came here today to get some pills so I don't get pregnant by him." As a student nurse, you are aware that state law requires that the nurse report any suspicion of child abuse. However, both the nursing code of ethics and federal law require that the nurse maintain client confidentiality.

Suggested Courses/Content/Concepts

- Clinical courses across all levels of education
- Ethical/legal issues

Suggested Questions to Guide Critical Reflection/ Self-Reflection/Dialogue

1. What assumptions, expectations, or prior experiences would influence your thinking about this case?
2. What ethical principles are involved in this situation?
3. Does the nurse's legal obligation to report the incident of child abuse supersede the ethical obligation to maintain confidentiality—particularly considering the patient requested confidentiality? What if June were 18 years old?

4. What are the nurse practitioner's options related to June's situation?
5. What are the possible outcomes of the different options?
6. Does June's autonomy outweigh the nurse's responsibility to report the abusive situation?

CASE STUDY 29

The day has finally arrived—your first clinical day as a nursing student. You are assigned to a resident in a long term care facility who has a diagnosis of Alzheimer's dementia with a history of falls and wandering. You are assigned to help the resident ambulate with a special walker. While you are sitting with the resident in the dining room, one of your classmates asks if you want to go on break. You tell your patient that you will be back in 15 minutes. When you return, the resident is lying on the floor in a pool of blood, bleeding from the nose and ears with a large hematoma and laceration on his head. You are horrified and scream for help.

Suggested Courses/Content/Concepts

- Clinical courses across all levels of education
- Ethical/legal issues
- Clinical reasoning
- Quality and safety

Suggested Questions to Guide Critical Reflection/ Self-Reflection/Dialogue

1. What are your expectations regarding your first day of clinical experience?
2. What are your assumptions related to caring for residents in long-term care settings?
3. How would you begin thinking about and planning for your role in providing care for your first clinical patient?
4. What areas do you consider your strengths as you begin your clinical experiences?
5. What resources do you think you would prefer to use if you were uncertain about your responsibilities in a clinical setting?
6. Imagine that you are this student's nursing instructor. What would you do?

CASE STUDY 30

Twelve-year-old Jennifer is a patient on the pediatric unit with a diagnosis of terminal stage Ewing's sarcoma. She has three brothers ages seven, six, and three, who are presently being cared for by a grandmother. Jennifer's dad is self-employed as a long distance truck driver and is often away for weeks at a time. Her mother has never worked outside the home. Both parents never graduated from high school, and their primary activities outside of family responsibilities are church-related. They belong to a small rural church and state that they have faith that God will heal Jennifer. Before her illness, Jennifer was a healthy child. The family does not have health insurance. About a year ago, Jennifer began limping. The family attributed the limp to a playground injury. When she continued to complain of pain and the limp persisted, her mother took her to the local health department. Above-the-knee amputation followed diagnosis, but metastasis was evident, and chemotherapy has only been palliative. The physician has many times discussed Jennifer's poor prognosis with the parents, recommending hospice care. The parents say they want everything possible to be done for Jennifer. The entire family holds nightly prayer sessions at Jennifer's bedside, affirming that God is healing her. Two days ago, Jennifer asked one of the student nurses assigned to care for her if she was going to die. The astute student nurse asked Jennifer's mother what Jennifer had been previously told about her condition. The mother responded, "She knows God is trying us and we must have faith." The mother continues to supervise Jennifer's care relentlessly, at times irritating the staff with questions and demands. She keeps a notebook record of Jennifer's care, including medications, times of care, intake and output, and personal assessments. Although Jennifer used to love to talk with the nursing staff and especially with the student nurses, she now appears frightened and remains quiet, sleeping intermittently.

Suggested Courses/Content/Concepts

- Clinical courses across all levels of education
- Ethical/legal issues
- Pediatrics
- Family theory
- Spirituality
- Coping/anticipatory grief

Suggested Questions to Guide Critical Reflection/ Self-Reflection/Dialogue

1. What is your first personal reaction to this situation? Identify your values relative to the situation.
2. What do you perceive to be the values of those involved?
3. Identify value incongruencies that might lead to conflict. Give specific examples of how such conflict can potentially affect patient care.
4. Identify specific nursing interventions to manage the conflict in a professional manner, and give examples of how the Code of Ethics would guide such actions.
5. Critically self-reflect to identify your own strengths and limitations as you consider dealing with this situation.

CASE STUDY 31

Monica has been the nurse manager of a busy acute care unit for the past 9 years and is highly regarded by her subordinates and nursing administration. For the past several months, however, Monica has been feeling more frustrated and less satisfied with her work due to staffing and budget cuts and other decisions related to the pending health care reform legislation. Providing quality care to meet patient needs has always been the most rewarding part of her job. However, recently, Monica believes that she has been forced to overlook these needs and attend more to the needs of the organization. She discusses with another manager that she is considering quitting her job even though she has seniority, good benefits, and three children to support. She is also aware that her distress at work is affecting her family because she carries the frustration of her job home with her.

Suggested Courses/Content/Concepts

- Clinical courses across all levels of education
- Ethical/legal issues
- Leadership/management courses
- Public policy courses

Suggested Questions to Guide Critical Reflection/ Self-Reflection/Dialogue

1. Identify values evident in this situation. Which of these reflect your personal values?
2. What conflicts might arise from these values?
3. What do you think Monica should do?
4. If you were in Monica's position, what beliefs, ideals, or goals would guide you in making a decision to stay or leave? Identify potential consequences of each choice.

CASE STUDY 32

Anne Smith is an experienced nurse. She has worked in the same intensive care unit for the past 15 years. During one night shift, Anne assesses Mr. Gordon who has been a patient on the unit in the past. The patient's vital signs are within normal limits, and there is no significant change from past readings. However, Anne feels uneasy. Not only does Mr. Gordon complain of pain, but he looks sick to Anne who senses something is seriously wrong. Anne calls the hospitalist who instructs her to callback if there are any changes in the vital signs. As the shift progresses, Anne becomes convinced Mr. Gordon is getting sicker by the minute. However, there are still no changes in Mr. Gordon's vital signs. Anne calls the physician a second time. This time the physician yells at

Anne telling her to stop bothering the physician. After a couple of hours, Anne decides to call her supervisor, who checks Mr. Gordon and encourages Anne to "get a grip." Anne repeatedly checks on Mr. Gordon who remains awake throughout the night. The next morning, Anne reports her assessment to the oncoming charge nurse and asks the nurse to make sure someone evaluates Mr. Gordon's abdominal pain. The charge nurse responds. "Don't worry about him. If there is anything seriously wrong, he will let us know." When Anne returns after 2 days off, she learns that Mr. Gordon died the prior evening of a ruptured abdominal aortic aneurism. Anne spends that evening crying at the nurses' station, barely able to take care of her patients.

Suggested Courses/Content/Concepts

- Clinical courses across all levels of education
- Ethical/legal issues
- Clinical reasoning
- Intuitive thinking
- Quality and safety
- Interprofessional communication

Suggested Questions to Guide Critical Reflection/ Self-Reflection/Dialogue

1. What is the ethical dilemma in this case?
2. Were Anne's actions sufficient?
3. What were the institutional and professional constraints to action?
4. How could Anne have responded to the situation in a way that would result in a better outcome?
5. Would you label Anne's reaction as moral distress or moral reckoning? Why?
6. How could Anne prevent a similar situation in the future?

CASE STUDY 33

Inez is a 69-year-old African-American woman who lives in a substandard apartment in a housing project with a high crime rate. She draws a small Social Security check that does not cover living expenses. Her income is supplemented by food stamps, housing assistance, and by providing ironing twice a week for customers who pay approximately $50 a week. She uses public transportation when she has to buy groceries or go to the doctor. Inez is an alcoholic, and most of the $50 she earns goes to buying cheap wine. Inez has two daughters who try to visit her at least once a month. Neither of Inez's children can afford to contribute to her household expenses and state that even if they could afford to help, they would not because of Inez's drinking problem. Inez weighs 250 pounds. She has hypertension, with her blood pressure ranging from 200/90 to 250/110. She is on medication for her blood pressure, and the physician has ordered home health services to encourage a diet and simple exercise regime for her obesity and hypertension. Unfortunately, Inez has developed a small ulcerated area on her right ankle. The home health nurse visits Inez and instructs her in the care of her ulcer, advising her to keep her right foot elevated as much as possible. This is, of course, almost impossible as Inez stands long hours to do the ironing. The nurse spends considerable time explaining a 1,200-calorie diabetic diet with moderate sodium restriction to Inez and talks with her about the need to begin walking as soon as the ulcer heals. Inez tells the nurse, "I've lived sixty-nine years without walking and I do not believe I have anything to lose if I never walk. Anyway, it is not safe to walk in this neighborhood and who wants to walk after standing on their feet all day ironing?"

Suggested Courses/Content/Concepts

- Clinical courses across all levels of education
- Values clarification and conflict
- Ethical/legal issues
- Community courses
- Health promotion and motivation for behaviors
- Substance abuse
- Health care financing
- Family theory

Suggested Questions to Guide Critical Reflection/ Self-Reflection/Dialogue

1. What assumptions do you have regarding Inez's situation?
2. What are your thoughts about Inez's daughters' comments about not providing financial assistance due to her alcohol intake?
3. Consider Inez's decision to ignore recommendations regarding diet, exercise, and, perhaps, care of her ankle ulceration in relation to autonomy, beneficence, and nonmaleficence.
4. As the principle of beneficence requires actively doing good for Inez, who decides what is good?
5. Discuss implications of the value of social justice in relation to health care for Inez.
6. How would you approach Inez about her health issues?
7. Critically self-reflect about your level of commitment to provide quality and safe care for individuals such as Inez.

Appendix C: Examples of Learning Modules/Lesson Plan

LEARNING MODULE EXAMPLES FOR ONLINE COURSES

Example 1: Basic Concepts for Leading and Managing at the Microsystem Level

Concepts
Organizational theory
> Structure
> Process

Organizational design
Leadership theory
Leadership styles
Decision making and problem-solving methods
> Related to patient care
> Related to unit management
> Ethical decision making

Change process

Teaching Strategies/Methodologies
In-class seminars
Voice-over PowerPoints

Learning Activities
Pre-assessments and post-assessments
Required readings
Notes: *leadership moment model*
Links
Transformative learning activities

Introduction
As you complete the readings, suggested pre-, post-, and further study assignments, and the transformative learning activities for this module, you will be moving toward the outcome of providing person-centered professional care. This module sets the stage for thinking about your role as a leader by addressing how ethical nurse leaders evolve and how they creatively, legally, and ethically handle issues/problems in today's complex, evolving systems of health care at microlevel and macrolevels. The theoretical underpinnings include

leadership, organizations, change, and decision making. Consider the term *creative leadership* as you are reading. What does this mean to you? To me, it means a leader who is willing to take risks, one who does not embrace the status quo. Creative leaders influence followers to accomplish goals by helping followers to imagine solutions to problems by applying theory to practice situations.

In this first module, you will learn about organization at the macrolevel, specifically organizational design and structure within the context of nurse leadership. The readings and learning activities in this first module will help you develop important leadership skills for roles such as change agent, problem solver, and decision maker to become a creative nurse leader. It is imperative as a professional nurse that you can hone these skills by applying modern leadership theories and by functioning legally and ethically in not only patient-situated care (microlevels) but also in situations at the organizational level. Enjoy!

Pre-Assessment
Go to the website provided in the syllabus and create a free student account. Once the account is created, enter the site. At the top of the welcome page, you will see a drop down menu under the title of the book at the top of the page. Click on the down arrow next to the word "go" and then click on Chapter 1. Then click "go." On the menu on the left-hand side, click on "My Hospital Unit." Complete activity 1 for your own learning. You do not need to submit for grading.

Learner Outcomes
Upon successful completion of this module, the student will be able to:

1. Analyze the professional, historical, and social factors that affect health care delivery in an organization.
2. Examine the effects of organizational design, leadership theory and style, and basic management functions on health care delivery.
3. Relate decision-making models to patient, microenvironment management, and the structure of an organization.
4. Use change theory to inform the interdisciplinary relationships and decision-making and problem-solving methods that are applied to issues of diversity, consumer care, and microenvironment management.
5. Explore ethical issues applicable to the microenvironment that affect the delivery of health care in an organization.

Assigned Required Readings
Chapter 1—Leadership Text
Chapter 2—Leadership Text
Chapter 3—Leadership Text
Chapter 4—Leadership Text

Transformative Learning Activities—Putting Thoughts Into Action

1. Identify three lessons learned from the information in the readings and describe how the information can be used in your practice setting.

2. Design a problem statement for a research study focused on the transformational leadership theory. Write a PICO for a study regarding transactional leadership. Refer to information in your EBP text for help with this activity.
3. Identify a change that needs to take place in your work setting. Imagine you are the change agent, and using your text or through an Internet search, identify the most appropriate change theory to guide the change, and state why you selected this theory.
4. What is the relationship of ethical, legal, and political issues at the microsystem level?
5. Using the information about transactional and transformational leadership types, create a brief scenario that would illustrate both styles of leadership (two scenarios would need to be created).
6. Respond to this statement by Anita Finkleman: *It is not easy to describe effective leadership. There is certainly no magic formula that will guarantee effective leadership* (p. 13). (Answer must be supported with evidence and must be at least two to four paragraphs in length.)
   Source: Finkleman, A. (2012). *Leadership and management for nurses* (2nd ed.). Boston, MA: Pearson.
7. On page 17 in your leadership text, three components are asked within the question, Who is a nurse leader? Respond to the three components by incorporating evidence from the readings.
8. According to Maas and Specht (as cited in Finkleman, 2001), "Governance or self-regulation has long been recognized as a privilege given to professions that earn the public trust by demonstrating accountability for their specialized practices" (p. 318). After pondering on this statement, answer the following questions: (1) How does this relate to the concept of shared governance? (2) How is shared governance demonstrated on your work unit? (3) As a manager at the microsystem level, how would you ensure shared governance?
   Source: Finkleman, A. (2012). *Leadership and management for nurses* (2nd ed.). Boston, MA: Pearson.

For Further Study
Complete any of the student resources offered in your leadership text. Remember you must set up a free student account to access these resources.

Post-Assessment
Complete any of the student resources offered in your text. Remember you must have or you must set up a free student account to access these resources.

Example 2: The Ethical Nurse Leader

Introduction
Hamric and Delgado as cited in Hamric and Spross (2009) state "the moral position of nursing in the health care arena is distinct" (p. 315). What does this mean to you? Assuming that this is a true statement, what is the impact to your role as an advanced practice nurse? Ethics, doing what is "good," is critical to all of the domains of leadership. In today's highly complex, technologically

advanced health care environment, it is imperative that nurses adhere to the American Nurses Association Code of Ethics when providing person-centered care, when leading at system levels, when influencing the political and regulatory process, and when serving as a member of the profession.

Source: Hamric, A. B., Spross, J. A., & Hanson, C. M. (2009). *Advanced practice nursing: An integrative approach.* Philadelphia, PA: Saunders.

A qualitative analysis of 63 graduate students enrolled in a nurse practitioner program showed that the ANA Code of Ethics was an essential framework in helping graduate students understand human dignity as it related to the advanced role (Kalb & O'Conner-Von, as cited in Hamric, Spross, & Hanson, 2009). The researchers' primary thesis is that prior educational and clinical experiences should serve as a foundation for essential ethical education at the graduate level.

Source: Hamric, A. B., Spross, J. A., & Hanson, C. M. (2009). *Advanced practice nursing: An integrative approach.* Philadelphia, PA: Saunders.

The management of ethical dilemmas in the clinical setting, while complex, is something that most nurses have thought about and/or faced on an almost daily basis. Ethical decision making in the policy arena, however, is not an area where many nurses have experience. As changes brought about by recent health care reform legislation become a reality, doing what is good and right (deciding who will get what and when [rationing]) will present nurses with new ethical dilemmas. Understanding and using the ANA Code of Ethics, understanding ethical principles, and how to use frameworks for decision making will be invaluable to the graduate nurse as more complex roles are assumed.

The assumption is that all of you had a basic ethics course at the undergraduate level. The reading in your text covers all the major topics related to ethics including principles and theoretical thought and should be a review.

Learner Outcomes
After completing this module, the learner should be able to:

1. Describe professional ethics.
2. Identify major ethical dilemmas at the system level.
3. Analyze health policy from an ethical perspective.

Assigned Required Reading
Chapter 11

Weblinks

- ANA Center for Ethics and Human Rights, www.nursingworld.org/ethics
- Center for Bioethics and Human Dignity, http://www.cbhd.org/
- The Nurse Friendly, http://www.nursefriendly.com/nursing/directpatient care/ethics.htm
- Ethics Center of Continuing Education, http://www.learnwell.org/alleth ics.htm

- Ethical and *Bioethical Issues in Nursing* and Health Care—A PowerPoint presentation, http://www.google.com/search?q=bioethical+issues+in+nursing&ie=utf-8&oe=utf-8&aq=t&rls=org.mozilla:en-US:official&client=firefox-a
- The Hastings Center, www.thehastingscenter.org
- What Are Political Ethics, http://www.wisegeek.com/what-are-political-ethics.htm

Module Learning Activities

Select one of the following activities to complete.

1. Using the *Phases of Development of Core Competency for Ethical Decision Making* on pages 321–322 of your textbook, create a measurement tool that would allow the graduate nurse to evaluate individual ethical competency.
2. Imagine that a *Death With Dignity Bill* is being debated in the state legislature. Write a one-page letter to your senator asking him or her to support the bill. You must include evidence to support your points of view in the letter.
3. Imagine that a *Death With Dignity Bill* is being debated in the state legislature. Write a one-page letter to your senator asking him or her to vote no on the bill. You must include evidence to support your points of view in the letter.
4. Imagine that you are the chief nursing officer of a large metropolitan hospital. There are two patients who need a transplant. With equal risk factors and life situations (i.e., age, gender, race, past medical history, current medical condition, etc.), use one of the alternative ethical approaches discussed on pages 324–326 of your text and the sample ethical decision-making framework in Box 11-3 on page 328 of your text to decide who will get the heart. One patient is an American citizen, and one is an illegal immigrant.
5. Imagine that you are a lobbyist for the state nursing association. A very important bill related to expanding the scope of practice for nurse practitioners is being discussed in the Healthcare Committee. The chair person of the committee is a nurse and an active member of the state nursing association. During a social gathering, this nurse (the chair person) seeks you out and asks for a donation for her upcoming campaign for re-election. She says to you, "I will get your Bill out of committee and can guarantee that it will get a vote in the legislature if the state nursing association will give me $10,000." Reflect on the *Code of Lobbying Ethics* in your text. Is the request for funds legal and/or ethical? How would you respond to the senator's request?

Example 3: Regulatory and Quality Control

Introduction

Milton Friedman, an economist once stated, "regulation is a disease of government, it is not government." Reflect upon this quote: What does it mean to you personally and professionally? Share your comments in the dialogue room in the course management system.

Pre-Assessment
1. What role does the regulatory process play in policymaking?
2. What role does regulation play in the profession of nursing?
3. What do you, as a leader at the systems level, need to know about regulation to influence the process?

All of these questions are the focus of this module. As a professional whose practice is regulated, it is critical that you understand regulatory processes and the direct influence that individual nurses and the profession have on the process. As you read the information in the chapters, pay close attention to how quality and regulation interact. This is critical information for you as a nurse leader in the four leadership domains.

Learner Outcomes
After completing this module, the learner should be able to:

1. Articulate the interaction between regulatory controls and quality control within the health care delivery system.
2. Analyze regulation and legislation governing quality and safety.

Assigned Required Readings
Chapter 22
Chapter 9
PowerPoint presentation: Practical ethics

Weblinks
- JONA's *Healthcare* Law, Ethics, and *Regulation*, www.ovid.com/site/catalog/Journal/1238.jsp
- The Federal Register, www.archives.gov/federal-register
- Senate Appropriations Committee, http://appropriations.senate.gov
- The Joint Commission, http://www.jointcommission.org/
- National Council of State Boards of Nursing, https://www.ncsbn.org/
- Quality Indicators, http://www.cms.gov/
- Comparison site for consumers and providers of health care, http://www.hospitalcompare.hhs.gov/
- Institute of Medicine home page, http://www.iom.edu
  - *To Err Is Human: Building a Safer Health System (1999)*. http://www.iom.edu/report.asp?id=5575
  - *Crossing the Quality Chasm (2001)*. http://www.iom.edu/report.asp?id=5432
  - *Envisioning the National Health Care Quality (2001)*. http://www.iom.edu/report.asp?id=5441
  - *Guidance for the National Healthcare Disparities Report* http://www.iom.edu/report.asp?id=4353
  - *Unequal Treatment: Confronting Racial and Ethnic Disparities in Health Care (2002)*. http://www.iom.edu/report.asp?id=4475

- *Health Professions Education: A Bridge to Quality (2003)*. http://www.iom.edu/report.asp?id=5914
- *The Future of the Public's Health in the 21st Century (2003)*. http://www.iom.edu/CMS/3793/4720/4304.aspx
- *Keeping Patients Safe: Transforming the Work Environment for Nurses (2003)*. http://www.iom.edu/report.asp?id=16173
- *Leadership By Example: Coordinating Government Roles in Improving Health Care Quality (2003)*. http://www.iom.edu/report.asp?id=4309
- *Patient Safety: Achieving a New Standard for Care (2003)*. http://www.iom.edu/report.asp?id=16663
- *Priority Areas for National Action: Transforming Health Care Quality (2003)*. http://www.iom.edu/report.asp?id=4290
- *Health Literacy: A Prescription to End Confusion (2004)*. http://www.iom.edu/report.asp?id=19723

Module Learning Activities
Select one of the following activities to complete.

1. Interview the Director of Nursing/Chief Nurse in your institution. Ask him or her to respond to this statement: *Health care in America is one of the most highly regulated industries in our country*. Analyze the response in a one-page paper in terms of assumptions and points of view expressed by the person.
2. In one page, argue for the NDNQI project.
3. In one page, argue against the NDNQI project.
4. Answer this question in one page: How are regulation and quality control interrelated? Use evidence from your readings to support your points. How does your political ideology influence your thinking related to regulation and quality control?
5. In your own words, define health care quality. Create a scenario that would illustrate your definition.
6. Write an Opinion-Editorial related to the role of regulation in nursing practice.

LESSON PLAN FOR FACE-TO-FACE CLASSROOMS

Example 4: Lesson Plan for Basics of Communication

Concepts:
Communication
with patients;
Interprofessional
Communication

Duration:
Three 50-minute sessions
with 10-minute breaks
after each session

Location:
200-seat auditorium with
unmovable desks

Learner outcomes:
Session One 9:00–9:50 a.m.
At the end of this session,
learners will be able to:
1. Identify personal
assumptions/expecta-
tions regarding nurse–
client communication
2. Therapeutic communi-
cation skills
a. Theoretical
background
b. Interpersonal
relationships
c. Communication
processes
d. Therapeutic
communication
techniques
e. Barriers to
communication

Teaching/learning activities:

Pre-class reading
assignments: Chapter X
PowerPoint presentation
Videos:
Therapeutic communication
(20 minutes);
Barriers to communication
(20 minutes)

*Transformative learning
activities:*
Critical self-reflection,
Using "1 minute paper"
at beginning of class
meeting to identify
personal assumptions
and expectations
regarding nurse–client
communication processes
Critical self-reflection:
Consider which barriers or
therapeutic techniques
are most often used
in your current
communication practices.

Learner outcomes:
Session Two 10:00–10:50 a.m.
At the end of this session,
learners will be able to:
1. Identify key points/
questions from session
one
2. Accurately apply
content to situations
representative of
practice

Teaching/learning activities:

Review pre-class reading
and content from
session one;
In-class electronic
response system
to answer practice
questions
Learners will pair for
application activity.
See Appendix A,
*Interpersonal Process
Recording*

*Transformative learning
activities:*
Critical self-reflection:
Identify areas of needed
improvement from
2-minute in-class
interpersonal dialogue.
Dialogue:
Sharing points of view
about what techniques
were most effective in
application practice and
why.

Learner outcomes:
Session Three 11:00–11:50 a.m.
At the end of this session,
learners will be able to:
1. Identify key points/
questions from session
three
2. Use the TeamSTEPPs
framework for
interprofessional
communication.

Teaching/learning activities:
PowerPoint presentation
Weblink: www.ahrq.gov
Video clips of SBAR
Call-out, Check-Back,
I-PASS-the-BATON (see
Appendix A)

*Transformative learning
activities:*
Critical reflection and
dialogue:
Learners will apply each of
these techniques to the
situation in Case Study 31
(see Appendix B)

Learner outcomes:
Additional opportunity for enrichment activities for self-regulated learning

Teaching/learning activities:
Videotape a 5-minute role-play. One learner will assume the role of nurse, and the other will assume the role of a person seeking health care. The student portraying the nurse will use as many therapeutic communication strategies as appropriate. Both learners will view the videotape to identify nonverbal and paraverbal barriers or therapeutic strategies.

Transformative learning activities:
Critical self-reflection and dialogue:
Compare perceptions of what techniques were effective and what was perceived as a barrier.

Assessment/ evaluation of learning

Activities:
Interpersonal process recording (formative)
15 multiple choice exam items

Transformative learning activities:
Effective use of therapeutic communication in clinical settings
Effective use of TeamSTEPPS strategies in clinical settings
Commitment to continued development of effective communication

Index